Medical Problems in Women over 70
When Normative Treatment Plans do not Apply

Edited by

Margaret Rees MA DPhil FRCOG
Reader in Reproductive Medicine
John Radcliffe Hospital
Oxford, UK

and

Louis G Keith MD PhD
Professor Emeritus of Obstetrics and Gynecology
Northwestern University
Chicago, IL, USA

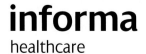

informa
healthcare

© 2007 Informa UK Ltd

First published in the United Kingdom in 2007 by Informa Healthcare, 4 Park Square, Milton Park, Abingdon, Oxon OX14 4RN. Informa Healthcare is a trading division of Informa UK Ltd. Registered Office: 37/41 Mortimer Street, London W1T 3JH. Registered in England and Wales number 1072954.

Tel: +44 (0)20 7017 6000
Fax: +44 (0)20 7017 6699
Email: info.medicine@tandf.co.uk
Website: www.informahealthcare.com

Although every effort has been made to ensure that all owners of copyright material have been acknowledged in this publication, we would be glad to acknowledge in subsequent reprints or editions any omissions brought to our attention.

Although every effort has been made to ensure that drug doses and other information are presented accurately in this publication, the ultimate responsibility rests with the prescribing physician. Neither the publishers nor the authors can be held responsible for errors or for any consequences arising from the use of information contained herein. For detailed prescribing information or instructions on the use of any product or procedure discussed herein, please consult the prescribing information or instructional material issued by the manufacturer.

A CIP record for this book is available from the British Library.
Library of Congress Cataloging-in-Publication Data

Data available on application

ISBN-10: 0 415 37352 2
ISBN-13: 978 0 415 37352 4

Distributed in North and South America by
Taylor & Francis
6000 Broken Sound Parkway, NW, (Suite 300)
Boca Raton, FL 33487, USA

Within Continental USA
Tel: 1 (800) 272 7737; Fax: 1 (800) 374 3401
Outside Continental USA
Tel: (561) 994 0555; Fax: (561) 361 6018
Email: orders@crcpress.com

Distributed in the rest of the world by
Thomson Publishing Services
Cheriton House
North Way
Andover, Hampshire SP10 5BE, UK
Tel: +44 (0)1264 332424
Email: tps.tandfsalesorder@thomson.com

Composition by Exeter Premedia Services Private Ltd, Chennai, India
Printed and bound in India by Replika Press Pvt Ltd

Contents

Contents

Contributors

Laura A Berman LCSW PhD
Berman Center and The Feinberg School of
  Medicine at Northwestern University
Chicago, IL
USA

Isabelle Bourdel–Marchasson MD PhD
CHU de Bordeaux
Geriatric Department, Xavier Arnozan Hospital
Pessac
France

Sarah Cullum BSc MRCPsych MPhil MSc PhD
Thornbury Hospital
Bristol
UK

Thomas R Dening MA MD FRCPsych
Older People's Mental Health Service
Fulbourn Hospital
Cambridge
UK

Sally Edmonds MD FRCP
Stoke Mandeville Hospital
Aylesbury
UK

Roger P Goldberg MD
Feinberg School of Medicine
Northwestern University
Evanston, IL
USA

Themos Grigoriades MRCOG
St Albans City Hospital
St Albans
UK

Andrew Hextall MD MRCOG
St Albans City Hospital
St Albans
UK

Alyson L Huntley PhD
Peninsula Medical School
Universities of Exeter and Plymouth
Exeter
UK

Sean Kehoe FRCOG
John Radcliffe Hospital
Oxford
UK

R Sari Kovats
Public and Environmental Health Research Unit
  (PEHRU)
London School of Hygiene and Tropical Medicine
London
UK

Franck Lamouliate MD
CHU de Bordeaux
Geriatric Department, Xavier Arnozan Hospital
Pessac
France

Guy W Lloyd MD FRCP
East Sussex Hospitals NHS Trust
Eastbourne District General Hospital
Eastbourne
UK

Jo Morrison MA BM BCh MRCOG
John Radcliffe Hospital
Oxford
UK

James David Price
John Radcliffe Hospital
Oxford
UK

Margaret Rees MA DPhil FRCOG
John Radcliffe Hospital
Oxford
UK

Rossana Salerno-Kennedy MD
Department of Food and Nutritional Sciences
and Department of Medicine
University College Cork
Cork
Ireland

Liv Wergeland Sørbye RN CAND PHILOL
Diakonhjemmet University College
Oslo
Norway

Leila Toiviainen
School of Philosophy
University of Tasmania
Hobart
Australia

Susan Tucker RMN RGN BA MSc
Personal Social Services Research Unit
School of Medicine
University of Manchester
Manchester
UK

Stephanie Wai
Northwestern University
Chicago, IL
USA

Kathleen E Walsh DO MS
Monroe Clinic and University of Wisconsin
  School of Medicine
Madison, WI
USA

Susan Welsh MRCPsych MPhil
Older People's Mental Health Service
Fulbourn Hospital
Cambridge
UK

Paul Wilkinson FRCP
Public and Environmental Health Research Unit
  (PEHRU)
London School of Hygiene and Tropical Medicine
London
UK

Hilary A Wynne MA MD FRCP
Department of Care of the Elderly Services
Royal Victoria Infirmary
Newcastle-upon-Tyne
UK

Preface

According to recently published data from the US government, over the next 25 years the elderly population is projected to grow in both relative and absolute terms. This circumstance has important implications for health care providers because, to date, most of the research upon which modern medicine is based has been performed on individuals who were at best young to middle age and healthy. It is only recently that women have been included in general medical trials and even more recently that so-called 'older' women were given the opportunity to participate in any such evaluations. Thus, the actual data pertaining to provision of health care to women over age 70 is relatively modest, and many probationers are unaware of it. This book was conceived during one of our meetings in Oxford when we recognized the existence of this literature gap and that the provision of health care to women might be improved if members of the health care professions had access to a book that was both gender specific, evidence based and related to women over age 70.

The book's approach is holistic covering demographics, climate change, common medical conditions, gynecological problems and delivery of health care. The authors are international in scope to provide a wide focus.

Rereading all the page proofs was not a chore; rather it was a treat, because it reaffirmed the value of our original decision to produce this volume. We have, with the help of the authors of the various chapters, brought together a great deal of useful information about the medical conditions that are prominent in women over the age of 70 and the best approaches to treat them. In this regard, the book will be useful because it is a comprehensive overview of the subject, probably the first of its kind.

The readers will be presented with evidence, the best that is available on the topics that represent the main chapter titles. The reader will also be enlightened where evidence is poor or lacking and where research is desperately needed.

All in all, we believe that this book fulfills our plan and expectation, that is, to gather the available evidence about treating a variety of conditions in women over 70 into one useful compendium. We hope that readers will agree.

Margaret Rees, Oxford
Louis G Keith, Chicago

Section I

Epidemiology and scope of problem

Population changes and new social structures

1

Leila Toiviainen

INTRODUCTION

The proportion of older women is increasing in all developed as well as in many developing Asian countries. Statistically, women outnumber men because they live longer. Increasing life expectancy and decreasing fertility rates worldwide define, as it were, the basis of an aging population. In 2002, 440 million people were older than 65 years; this was about 7% of the world population (Figure 1.1).[1]

POPULATION GROWTH OF SPECIFIC AGE GROUPS: 2002–2050

This figure is projected to increase rapidly, and it is estimated that the elderly will constitute nearly 17% of the global population by 2050. The percentage of elderly people varies between countries, ranging from a high of 22% in Monaco to a low of 1.7% in Mayotte, an island in the Mozambique Channel. In general, the percentage of elderly persons is higher in the developed

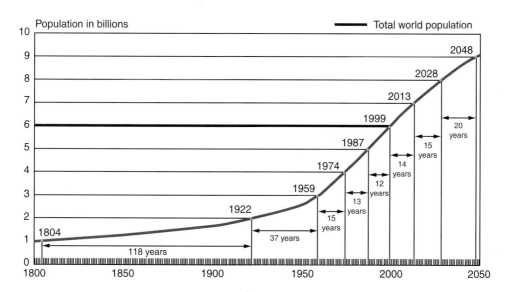

Figure 1.1 Annual additions and the annual growth rate of the global population. The growth of global population has peaked. Source: United Nations, World Population Prospects: The 1994 Revision; US/Census Bureau. International Programs Center, International Data Base and unpublished tables.

world and very low in Africa and the Near East. In the UK, the total population is projected to increase by 7.2 million by 2031. Life expectancy at birth will continue to rise from 81 in 2004 to 85 years in 2031 in women (Figure 1.2).[2]

Women over 70 to date have not attracted the attention of researchers as subjects of interest. As Hughes and Mtezuka aptly note, 'If coverage in academic literature is a valid measure of importance, then older women must be singularly unimportant'.[3] Both feminists and social workers have failed to consider problems such as gender inequities that result in lack of retirement income, independence, and choices for a meaningful old age for women. This is particularly disappointing as many prominent feminists are themselves by now in their 70s. As the key to successful aging is continuing to find meaning in life, social workers should be at the forefront of those who are more

aware of how financial as well as emotional poverty limits the options of any older person.

Policymakers, economists, and the public need to recognize the financial pressures of an aging population. Feminist economists, in particular, are drawing attention to the problems facing women over 70 and this is essential to the provision of healthcare in the 21st century.

PROFILE OF WOMEN OVER 70

Women over 70 do not represent a homogeneous group with the same needs and interests in the same way that they, as a group, differ from younger women. Growing older entails both positive and negative life changes that women deal with as individuals. Perhaps, most significantly compared to the last generation, women in their 70s today no longer see themselves as 'old' in the sense that

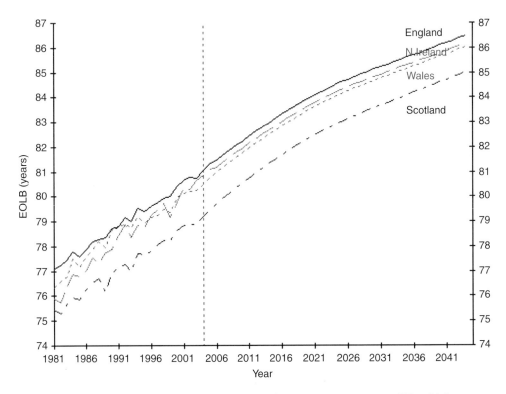

Figure 1.2   Period expectation of life at birth, 1981–2044 (females). EOLB, expectation of life at birth.

their advancing age signifies the closing off of life choices. Indeed, the lives of many older women are characterized by increasing flexibility, independence, information, and involvement.[4]

That having been said, the availability of a wider range of choices presents many women with new challenges which can lead to tensions in interpersonal relationships. More women today, including those in their 70s, choose to divorce in order to assert their individuality, and to free themselves from the subjugation of decades of marriage, or divest themselves of the care of others at the expense of personal growth. Following divorce, women often choose to live alone in order to exercise a broader range of choices that were not available in conventional marriages; others choose to live with a partner without marriage. Entering into these new forms of families and relationships is also available to women newly confronted with widowhood. At the same time, the traditional forms of family life remain strong; older women become involved in the lives of their children and grandchildren and provide them with practical and psychological support.

As well as being more independent, the transformation of everyday life for the woman over 70 has been described in terms of 'inclusivity, community participation, and reduced moral and financial dependence'.[5] Many older women have recently retired after working and possess good disposable incomes and benefit from the knowledge and information that comes with professional achievement. In part, the increasing longevity of such women is largely the result of better education and understanding of personal health issues, as well as the capacity and opportunity to prevent the onset of illnesses and frailties associated with aging. Without doubt, more women over 70 in good health are living independently at home. Even those in poor health may live at home while receiving home care services due to the lack of suitable nursing home accommodation.

The improved financial status of some older women means that they are no longer invisible passive recipients of social services but are recognized as consumers of services such as car ownership, Internet use, and extensive travel plans. Access to all these activities further enhances their independence, adds to the interests and hobbies that they can engage in, and improves their mental and physical health.

Even in rich nations, it is possible for women in their 70s to suffer from poverty because they have never been employed outside the home and may have lost financially as a result of divorce; or the society in which they live has no social security provisions for the elderly. Gender inequalities come into sharp focus because of past life histories of broken work patterns; these, in turn, determine the kind of future a woman in her 70s will have.

One feminist scholar, Carolyn G Heilbrun,[6] argues that her life in many respects began after 60 because only then could she become the person she really wanted to be. The anticipated closeness of death brought her already full life to a particular 'intensity, that constant awareness of newness and brightness' that only used to happen 'with the parting of friends and lovers in the days before direct communication over distances was possible'. However, anticipating physical frailties and unexpected health problems as well as social losses is essential to avoid loneliness.

THE LIVES OF WOMEN OVER 70

Women live longer than men. In 2004 women in the UK could expect to live to 81 years compared with 76 for men.[2] The UK charity Age Concern estimated that 72% of those aged 85 and over in 2003 were women, and that by the age of 90 the ratio of women to men is three to one.[4] In the United States, 'women make up 58% of the population age 65 and older, and 70% of the population of aged 85 and older. Older women are less likely than older men to be currently married and are more likely to be alone'.[7] In 1997, life expectancy at birth in the US was 79 years for women and 74 years for men.[7] In Australia, life expectancy for women at birth according to 1994–5 statistics was 80.1 years and for men 75.2 years. According to the same statistics, at age 65 women can expect to live another 19.6 years and men another 15.8 years. Of Australian women over 85, 72% are widowed in comparison with 42.7% of men.[8]

A similar ratio that favors women over men in the older age groups is also true of Asia. In the overall Asian population among those aged 75 and above, there are only 70 men to every 100 women. Japan has the oldest population in Asia, with 17% aged 65 and above.[9] In Asia, older single women are not common; most are either married or widowed. In South Korea, 52% of all women aged 65–69 are widows; the percentage of widowers in the same age group is only 8%. These numbers are expected to go down as the life expectancy of both men and women rises; it is projected that South Korean widows in the 65–69 age group by 2050 will be down to 17%. As long as these societies maintain their present traditions, however, there will always be more widows than widowers.[9]

Home care

Many women over 70 still live in their own homes, albeit receiving home care. In a recent US survey, 13 women interviewed about their experiences were aged between 82 and 96. The authors note, however, that everyday experiences have not been analyzed in research literature. They also found that home care mainly consists in providing treatment to already existing conditions such as leg ulcers while there was no focus on the prevention of falls.[10] In other words, women of this age group were perceived as passive recipients of a narrow range of services. They are not being asked about their needs or their interests, either because researchers assume that they are so few, or they are regarded as a collection of diseases

of aging (dementia and cardiac disorders) rather than as individuals with specific requirements.

Short-term, piecemeal solutions for care of the elderly are preferred by economists and policy-makers of many developed and developing nations. Thus, service providers are left to focus on 'the importance of undertaking (and assisting with) primary "tasks" such as feeding and toileting' at the expense of the recipients' emotional and psychological needs, which are generally ignored because of lack of time and resources (see Chapter 15). In reality, interaction between the older person and the carer is an important opportunity for each to voice concerns about serious issues which might prevent many future physical and mental health problems. Lack of coordinated, client-centered care is also illustrated in an interview survey of 55 users of care services in seven English local authorities or municipalities. Seventy-one percent of the women interviewed lived at home and received some form of care, whereas the corresponding figure for men was 29%; also, 83% of the total number of women received nursing care in contrast to the figure for men of 17%.[11] The findings of the interviewers supported earlier results showing that older people do not want to complain lest there be repercussions or because they feel that they ought to be 'grateful for what they get'.[12] The researchers found this disconcerting, as in some instances, such as when a carer simply does not turn up or exhibits overtly antagonist behaviour, a formal complaint would have been appropriate.[12] The overall conclusion of both research groups was that services to older people in their own homes was fragmented. The shortage of domiciliary services in rural areas and shortages of services in respite care or services for the elderly mentally ill have also been identified as areas of concern, at least in the UK.[13]

Shortages of appropriately qualified and committed care staff will remain acute as long a caring for older people in the community and in institutions is associated with low pay and status. It is hard for the carers to value their clients if they do not feel valued by the community for whom they provide these services. Having recognized that, researchers have consistently found that what both the care recipients and care givers value is the opportunity for personal contacts between individuals. Although not of a monetary nature, this benefit is invaluable.

Cultural differences

The ways in which women perceive their own health status differ between cultures. Although it is assumed in the West that Asian women are stoical about growing older and frailer, according to South Korean statistics, 63% of women and 46% of older men in that country regarded their health as poor or very poor.[14] This is in contrast to British research that demonstrates that although older women have more health problems than men, they are less likely to report them.[3] Older men who are more mobile and have less chronic illnesses are twice as likely to complain that less serious illnesses prevent them from undertaking activities of daily living regarded as feminine, such as washing clothes, preparing meals, and doing small sewing jobs. The authors postulate that women, because of their experiences of childbirth and discomforts associated with menstruation, are expected to endure illness and to cope with pain without complaining about it.[3]

Maintaining independence

Men and women over 70 can remain independent and involved in their communities if they are assisted in their endeavors to keep in touch with the people around them. In order to enhance the lives of older people, the state government of Tasmania in Australia has formulated eight key principles for positive aging. The last three of these are:

- Older people have a right to have access to information that enables them to make informed choices and to be included in making decisions about their lives.
- Partnerships between individuals, communities, including businesses, and governments are required in the planning and delivery of services for older people.
- Intergenerational community participation and opportunities enhance aging in a positive manner.

The government assists older people to participate in their communities by providing computer-training classes specifically geared to older people through the department of education. As a result of community consultation with older individuals, the use of technologies at the banks in particular was identified as an area that needed special attention.[15]

According to Heilbrun, governments should not only enable school children to access the Internet but also assist older people to access Internet and email. She would like to see personal computers in every retirement home and argues for the benefits of older people being able to keep in touch with their families and friends in a more immediate, instant fashion, as well as to avail themselves of educational opportunities that are provided easily and at little cost by the Internet.[6]

In Tasmania, a state with a population of half a million people, 6.4% or 2861 of the students enrolled in Adult Education courses in 2005 were women over 70 according to state government statistics.[16] Computing, business, and professional studies were the second most popular courses, with 378 students being women over 70; only art and craft courses were more popular, with 413 students. The third most popular classes were health and well-being, with 283 students being women over 70.

Starting from computer courses offered for beginners in the over-55 age group, women over 70 enrolled in a total of 59 different computer courses offered by the Tasmanian Adult Education courses. Amongst their choices were courses entitled Financial Essentials for Women, iPods – What are they?, Photo Editing for over 55's, Successful Retirement – How to Prepare Financially, as well as courses on starting and managing share portfolios and on how to deal with computer viruses.[16]

Apart from traditional adult education courses, informal education for older people in Australia is offered by the University of Third Age. The purpose of Third Age Learning is, as emphasized by one of its teachers, 'to help people, and particularly older people, to remain active, independent and useful, by providing them with all sorts of choices for mental, physical and social activities'.[17] The author argues that the beneficiaries of this continuing education are not only the older individuals undertaking the activities but also those around them: 'Happy active people not only stay healthy, they put back some of the energy into that community'.[17]

Wealth and poverty of women over 70

For women over 70 to engage in adult education classes and continue other interests that enhance social networking, they need adequate personal income in order to exercise independence. They also need government assistance, such as adult education services and transport at reduced rates as well as doorstopper buses and car pooling.

Data from the Luxembourg Income Study shows that 'poverty is especially a problem amongst women 75 or older who are living alone'.[18] The social security provisions in the Nordic countries ensure that this is less of a problem, whereas poverty amongst women in the same age group in the US and in the UK is more prevalent, as similar provisions for older women are lacking or non-existent.[19,20] According to British statistics, the median disposable incomes of women living within pensioner couples is 34% of that of their partners. According to the same survey, women are amongst the same cohort of the underprivileged as ethnic minorities and disabled people, in being at a particular risk of being 'underpensioned'.[21]

Potential solutions are that women stay longer in the paid workforce in order to accumulate superannuation and other benefits including sick leave entitlements. The charity Age Concern in the UK advises the government to overturn its previous decision on mandatory retirement age. Even if the life expectancy of women has risen, many Asian countries still have retirement ages of 55 years and lower for women; such limits were set during the 1950s when the life expectancy of women was only 41 years.[22] In South Korea, life expectancy of women has risen from 66.1 in 1970 to 80 in 2004; the corresponding figures for South Korean men are 59.0 in 1970 and 72.8 in 2004.[23]

To address the obvious discrepancy between increasing life expectancy and early retirement age, Singapore has extended the retirement age from 55 to 62 and will perhaps extend it beyond this in the near future.[24] It must be remembered, however, that in many more traditional, rural Asian societies women have not been in the workforce for as many years as they have been in Singapore, Taiwan, and Korea as well as in Japan. Traditionally, they have been expected to take care of domestic chores and childcare and so have not been able to make any provisions for independent old age. This poses difficult challenges to policymakers in the less-developed countries of Asia.[25]

Legal provisions in the case of divorce should take account of the amount of unpaid work performed as homemakers and mothers. In Australia, women now have access to their husband's superannuation as a joint asset to be equally distributed in property settlements.[26] Nations that do not have social security systems ideally should develop them, but this is an increasingly difficult proposition at a time when the proportion of older people is increasing in relation to the number of working younger adults.

Early retirement can bring many benefits to the retiring individuals and the communities to which they retire. If women live healthy, useful lives into their 80s, then for them retiring early means that they can still have two decades of enjoying new interests and challenges. A compromise between early retirement and working until one's 70s would of course be working part-time to ensure a better balance between work and leisure and to ensure a steady income to fund the pursuit of education and hobbies. Sweden has been a world leader in making this compromise financially viable by providing half of the person's actual work income as a pension, so that the income of an older person working half-time remains that of the person continuing full-time work.[27]

Intergenerational relationships

Because of their longevity, women over 70 tend to remain a parent of adult children (who may reach retirement during their life time) for longer than they were parents bringing up a minor or grandparents.[28] Such relationships between two adults in one family are different from those in the past in that sons and daughters can now share more life experiences with their mother but on an adult basis.[29] At the same time, the relationship may also be a source of friction if the sons and daughters expect the mother to provide financial assistance and free childminding services when the mother wants to be free of these roles.

In the popular media, terms such as 'generation boom' and 'the sandwich generation' are used to describe the ways in which families live today. As people live longer, children are more likely to meet their great-grandparents. Even though families are smaller in size, they are larger across generations, because of second and even third marriages of members of the 'sandwich generation'. Such individuals married young for the first time and then remarried and started a second family in their late 30s or early 40s. An example of such a woman is Pru Goward, the Australian Federal Sex Discrimination Commissioner. She has two daughters in their 30s and one aged 17. She has been 'sandwiched' in between the needs of her career, of her youngest daughter, and the needs of her parents in their late 70s; she maintains that often the needs of her youngest child have to come second to those of her parents who are in need of more care. Despite all this, she considers herself lucky because her father 'remarried a woman who is 10 years younger than him and a wonderful carer' and her mother moved to live nearer to her brother, thus relieving some of the pressure on her.[30]

Much research documents that many older adults are satisfied in their traditional roles as parents and grandparents. In the French Transition from Working Life to Retirement survey, for example, 65% of male and 71% of female respondents aged 75 reported that they both provided help to and received help from one or more children.[31] The women who were either divorced or widowed received the most help: 64% of 70–75-year-old unmarried women reported receiving help from a child, compared with 43% of married women.[32] Traditional ways of intergenerational transfers are also reflected in the pension system of many countries, including Australia. Thus the arrangements could be considered as follows: 'a compact between successive generations: generation B supports generation A in the expectation that it will be supported by generation C'.[33] Unfortunately, these assumptions can no longer be maintained at a time when generation A is expanding, generation B is shrinking, and the future of generation C in terms of education and employment as well as its size remains uncertain. That each generation should look after itself and not expect anything from the other seems the obvious answer, yet intergenerational transfers not only involving money but also time and caring remain desirable.

Another point of view is put forward by Heilbrun, who argues that there is too much emphasis on the wisdom transmitted by older individuals to the young. In reality, transmission can go both ways. Experiences of the young can provide those older people who are prepared to listen 'the feel of life, its beat as it sounds each day'.[6] In her view, young want older people to be 'there [for them]. We reassure them that life continues, and if we listen, we assure them that it matters to us that it continues'.[6]

In a similar manner, Californian women over 70 questioned by Vaillant about what they have learnt from children, replied that the young people provided them with a freshness of outlook that renewed their own youth.[34] For a meaningful interaction, both young and old individuals should be able to live in ways in which each generation can enrich the other. The uses of modern technology are but one means by which these communications can be enhanced; simply speaking to each other and listening to each other respectfully still ensures that we value each other. The same can be said for email.

FEMINISM AND WOMEN OVER 70

The portrayal of women in feminist literature demonstrates and conflicts between generations of women the invisibility of women over 70. For example, in a page-long discussion under the heading 'aging' in a recent feminist encyclopedia, the half devoted to the menopause portrays it as if it was the end of a woman's worthwhile life; indeed, women in their 40s and 50s are classified as older in this entry.[35] The same volume describes the celebrations of women's suffrage in South Australia in 1994. Although someone protested against 'A conference for all women at $135 a day?', the author praises the 'dominance of such economic issues as women in big business, superannuation' and the delegates being asked to turn off their mobile phones. Amazingly, no mention is made of older women who have not had access to paid work in their lifetime, even less to superannuation or mobile phones.[36] Although the comments quoted are a decade old, much current literature supports the argument that feminist researchers have not considered issues that are important to women over 70; women in their 40s and 50s are still considered older by them. The Older Women's Network, an international organization, lists under its Australian links 'Feminist Lesbians Over Forty'.[37] In contrast the British 'Older Feminists Network' does not set any age limits to their members but allows self-definition. Although their brief is to support not only women's issues but also 'peace movements, anti-racism and the environment', their first link is titled 'Midlife and Menopause: changing bodies, changing lives'.[38] The information provided is illustrated by an embroidered cloth uterus; readers can only draw the conclusion that even old feminist ladies over 40 and 50 do crafts.

In contrast to the feminists, the Australian Rural Women's Network tells the stories of women on the land and offers practical services such as the Drought Hotline. Posted on the site is the story of Bessie Jennings, who at 75 'works as a part-time relationship counsellor, part-time University of Third Age (U3A) tutor, and a self-published performing bush poet'.[39] It could be postulated that country people who live closer to nature regard aging as a natural part of the life cycle. As well, it could be expected that people living on the land must find more creative, flexible solutions to problems not encountered by their city counterparts.

THE FUTURE OF WOMEN OVER 70

In this chapter describing how women over 70 live in various countries, several key factors that make lives meaningful have been identified across cultures and geographical locations. Among these are the following. First, aging should be regarded as a positive, lifelong process; the transition from one phase of life to another should be smooth rather than abrupt. Secondly, those things that provided meaning when the person was younger are likely to be the same things that continue to provide meaning in old age. This is not to demand that the person continue along the same tracks, but rather suggest that new challenges and interests can be picked up on the way.

The perspective on aging as an ongoing creative physical and cognitive process is supported by prospective American studies of white Harvard college males born in 1920, and of a female comparison group of 90 women born between 1908 and 1914, initially studied by Lewis Terman of Stanford University and continued by his present-day successors.[34] Based on the thesis that successful aging is a continuation of a lifelong development beginning in childhood, the researchers have identified several positive and protective factors, such as the capacity to plan and to hope and to be with people, that enhance the quality of life of individuals of all ages, including the final years of life.[40] Continuing this theme, Swedish studies of cognitive capacities of older adults show that 70 year olds today have the same level of mental fitness as 65 year olds 30 years ago.[41,42]

Aging should be a positive experience, not only for those women who have been properly educated and have financial support to enjoy it. Regardless of whether they remain in reasonable health, women should have access to the healthcare of their choice. Women over 70 need proper access to educational and healthcare facilities by means of better public transport and security while going about their business of living as individuals of worth.[43] The future of women over 70 should be one of self-growth, self-discovery, and self-fulfillment. They will then be sources of strength, wealth, and the continuity of values for those around them.

REFERENCES

1. US Census Bureau. Global population at a glance: 2002 and beyond. Washington, DC: US Census Bureau, 2004. Available at: http://www.census.gov/ipc. Accessed 18.1.2006.
2. Office for National Statistics and Government Actuaries Department, UK. http://www.gad.gov.uk. Accessed 18.1.2006.
3. Hughes B, Mtezuka M. Social work and older women: where have older women gone? In: Langan M, Day L, eds. Women, Oppression and Social Work. London: Routledge; 1992: 220–41.
4. Metz D, Underwood M. Older Richer Fitter. London: Age Concern; 2005.
5. Gilbert T, Powell JL. Family, caring and ageing in UK. Scand J Caring Sciences 2005; 19: 53–7.
6. Heilbrun CG. The Last Gift of Time: Life Beyond Sixty. New York: Ballantine Books; 1997.
7. Older Americans 2000: Key Indicators of Well-Being: Federal Interagency Forum on Aging-Related Statistics. http://www. agingstats. gov/chartbook2000/highlights/html. Accessed 18.1.2006.
8. Department of Health and Human Services. Older People in Tasmania: A Profile. Hobart: Department of Health and Human Services; 1999: 6–7.
9. Jaijagcomel W. Asia's aging population. In: The Future of the Population in Asia. Honolulu, Hawaii: East-West Centre; 2002: 83–95.

10. Porter EJ, Ganong LH. Older widows' speculations and expectancies concerning professional home-care providers. Nursing Ethics 2005; 12: 507–21.

11. Ware T, Matosevic T, Hardy B, et al. Commissioning care services for older people. Ageing and Society 2003; 23: 411–28.

12. Hardy B, Young R, Wistow G. Dimensions of choice in the assessment and care management process: the views of older people, carers and care managers. Health and Social Care in the Community 1999; 7: 483–91.

13. Department of Health, UK. Three Year Programme for NHS Reform and Expansion. Department of Health; 2002: 31–45.

14. Chung K, Aejeo C, YoungHee O, et al. Living Profiles and Welfare Service Needs of Older Persons in Korea. Seoul: Korea Institute for Health and Social Affairs; 1998: 20–43.

15. Department of Health and Human Services, Tasmanian Plan for Positive Ageing 2000–2005. Hobart: Department of Health and Human Services; 1999.

16. Moore E. Women Over 70 Years – Participation in Adult Education. Adult Education Tasmania; 2005: 1–7.

17. MacKean R. All you need is a door: access to Third Age Learning in Tasmania. Austr J Adult Learning 2002; 42: 353–63.

18. Smeeding TM, Sandstrom S. Poverty and income maintenance in old age: a cross-national view of low-income older women. Feminist Economics 2005; 11: 163–74.

19. Bjorklund A, Freeman R. Generating equality and eliminating poverty – the Swedish way. In: Freeman R, Topel R, Swedenborg B, eds. The Welfare State in Transition: Reforming the Swedish Model. Chicago: University of Chicago Press; 1997: 17–35.

20. Harrington Meyer M, Wolf DA, Himes CL. Linking benefits to marital status: race and social security in the US. Feminist Economics 2005; 11: 145–62.

21. Herklots H, ed. The Age Agenda 2005. London: Age Concern Reports; 2005.

22. Caldwell JC. Asian fertility decline in perspective. Innovation 2004; 5: 46–7.

23. Chung K, AeJeo C, YoungHee O, Duk S. 2001 Survey of Care-Giving Status and Welfare Needs of Older Persons in Korea. Seoul: Korean Institute for Health and Social Affairs, 2001: 45–60.

24. Goh VHH. Aging in Asia: a cultural, socio-economical and historical perspective. The Aging Male 2005; 8: 90–6.

25. Straughan P. The power of work in the family. Innovation 2004; 5: 48–9.

26. Weston R, Smyth B. Financial living standards after divorce. Family Matters 2000; 55: 11–15.

27. Swedish Institute. Social Insurance in Sweden (one of the Fact Sheets on Sweden): 1995. Stockholm, Sweden.

28. Grundy E, Murphy M, Shelton N. Looking beyond the household: intergenerational perspectives on living kin and contacts with kin in Great Britain. Population Trends 1997: 19–27.

29. Grundy E, Shelton N. Contact between adult children and their parents in Great Britain 1986–1999. Environment and Planning 2001; 33: 685–97.

30. Heirich K. Tug of love. Family Circle 2005; September: 87–9.

31. Delbes C, Gaymu J. The shock of widowhood on the eve of old age: male and female experiences. Population 2002; 57: 885–914.

32. Grundy E. Reciprocity in relationships: socio-economic and health influences on intergenerational exchanges between Third Age parents and their adult children in Great Britain. Br J Sociolo 2005; 56: 231–55.

33. Hancock K. The economics of retirement provision in Australia. Economic Papers 1981; 20: 1–23.

34. Vaillant G. Aging Well: Surprise Guideposts to a Happier Life from the Landmark Harvard Study of Adult Development. New York: Little, Brown and Company; 2002.

35. Caine B. Ageing. In: Caine B, Gatens M, Grahame E, et al., eds. Australian Feminism:

A Companion. Melbourne: Oxford University Press; 1998: 378–9.

36. Bulbeck C. Class, ethnicity and generations. In: Caine B, Gatens M, Grahame E, et al., eds. Australian Feminism: A Companion. Melbourne: Oxford University Press; 1998: 32.

37. The Older Women's Network: http://www. own.org.au/links.php#au. Accessed 16.12.05.

38. Older Feminists Network: http://www.ofn. org.uk/. Accessed 16.12.05.

39. Rural Women's Network: http://www.agric. nsw.gov.au/rwn/. Accessed 16.12.05.

40. Vaillant G. Aging Well: Surprising Guideposts to a Happier Life from the Landmark Harvard Study of Adult Development. Boston: Little, Brown and Company, 2002; 305–6.

41. Svanborg A. The Gothenburg longitudinal study of 70-year-olds: clinical reference values in the elderly. In: Bergener M, Ermini M, Stahelin HB, eds. Thresholds in Aging. London: Academic Press; 1985: 231–9.

42. McClearn GE, Johansson B, Berg S, et al. Substantial genetic influence on cognitive abilities in twins 80 or more years old. Science 1997; 276: 1560–3.

43. Age Concern. The Age Agenda 2005: Public Policy and Older People. London: Age Concern; 2005: 50.

Health effects in the elderly from heat and cold

2

R Sari Kovats and Paul Wilkinson

INTRODUCTION

Climate affects health in both time and space. Seasonal patterns in mortality were described as soon as routine data on deaths became available in the 19th century. Since at least the early decades of the 20th century, when infectious disease mortality was greatly reduced, populations in temperate regions have patterns of deaths that are higher in winter than in the summer.[1,2] Occasionally, during the summer months, episodes of very high temperatures will cause peaks in mortality. In the past, this mortality often went undetected and unreported. Following a major heat wave event that occurred in Western Europe in 2003 however, steps have been taken to protect elderly people from heat as well as cold.

This chapter reviews the current state of knowledge about health risks in the elderly in relation to both extremes of temperature. We also discuss the main determinants of risk – which are different for heat and cold – as well as the ongoing development of specific intervention measures.

PHYSIOLOGICAL EFFECTS OF AGING ON THERMOREGULATION

Most healthy individuals are able to regulate their body temperature within a wide temperature range. An individual gains body heat from food and muscular activity and loses it through convection, conduction, radiation, and sweating to maintain a constant body temperature or heat balance. When body temperature drops even a few degrees below its normal range, blood vessels constrict, decreasing peripheral blood flow to reduce heat loss from the skin surface. Shivering generates heat by increasing the body's metabolic rate.

When environmental temperatures increase, on the other hand, an individual needs to lose heat by evaporation of sweat, convection (warming of air or water around the body), respiration (inhaled air is usually cooler and dryer than exhaled air), long-wave radiation, or by conduction (contact with solids; e.g. floor). When air temperature approaches that of the skin, heat loss by convection approaches zero, and heat gain may even be possible under these circumstances; the main (and sometimes only) route for heat loss becomes sweat production and evaporation. When humidity increases with air temperature, even this will be compromised. High temperatures can cause certain well-described clinical syndromes such as heat stroke, heat exhaustion, heat syncope, and heat cramps.[3] Heat stroke is the only syndrome that is clearly attributable to ambient temperature, and it has a substantial case-mortality ratio. Severe heat stroke occurs when the core body temperature reaches 40.6°C. Multiple organ dysfunction ensues, and death may occur very rapidly (within hours).

Age and illness are important comorbid conditions that accentuate the likelihood of heat stress, as age correlates highly with increasing illness, disability, medication use, and reduced fitness. A range of clinical risk factors bear on the likelihood of clinical heat illness,[4] including dehydration due to reduced food and liquid uptake, intestinal problems (such as diarrhea and vomiting), and the use of diuretics or excess alcohol intake. Specific medications can affect thermoregulation by a variety of mechanisms. For example anticholinergic drugs such as atropine, antihistamines, tricyclic antidepressants, and phenothiazines cause decreased sweating and do not allow the body to cool. Drugs that cause vasoconstriction also create an obstacle for the body to lose heat. These include sympathomimetic agents such as epinephrine, cocaine, and amphetamine. Fitness tends to decrease with age, owing to a reduced physical activity level in the elderly. Therefore, high environmental temperatures put greater strain on the cardiovascular system, and any activity performed becomes more stressful. Cardiovascular reserve is especially relevant to thermoregulation, as it determines the capacity to move heat from the body core to the skin for dissipation.[5,6] Under such circumstances, impaired fitness, leading to reduced activity, can exacerbate heat stress in an individual.

Gender may play a role in the physiology of heat stress. Adult women generally have higher core body temperatures and skin temperature[7] and would appear to be at higher risk, from the epidemiological studies of heatwaves. In theory, menopause may produce an adverse effect on thermoregulation during heat exposure over and above any effect on cardiovascular fitness, but little research exists to support or refute this possibility.

The perception of ambient temperature is impaired in the elderly for heat as well as cold. A comparison of the responses of elderly men and young adults to changes in temperature[8] found that, whereas both age groups preferred the same room temperature (22–23°C), the older volunteers manipulated the temperature controls much less precisely than did the younger age group. Thus, the threshold for a behavioral response to perceived discomfort due to cold is higher in elderly persons.

Knowledge related to the pathophysiological mechanisms for mortality in relation to heat and cold is incomplete. Few deaths that are attributed to heat and cold are actually certified as being due to hyperthermia/heatstroke or hypothermia, respectively. Although exposure to higher temperatures causes hemoconcentration,[9] heatwaves have little or no effect on the risk of myocardial infarction or emergency admissions for cardiovascular problems.[10] Dehydration and impaired kidney function also play an important role in heat stress-related admissions, as admission for renal disease increases at higher temperatures[10] and diabetes is also a risk factor for heat-related mortality.[11,12]

Evidence suggesting that cold has adverse effects on the circulation and hemostasis that may predispose to thrombotic events is more robust.[13–16] Cold alone is probably not a sufficient cause of death unless there is concomitant atheromatous narrowing of the coronary and cerebral circulations, which is common in the elderly. On the other hand, cold may lead to constriction of the peripheral vasculature, with reduction of plasma volume, hemoconcentration, and consequent increased risk of thrombosis. In someone already at risk of a myocardial infarction or stroke, the additional effect of cold may be sufficient to precipitate a clinical event.

EFFECTS OF HIGH TEMPERATURES AND HEAT WAVES

Heat waves, short episodes of extremely high temperature, cause short-term increases in mortality in the elderly. This is illustrated in Figure 2.1, which shows the peak in mortality associated

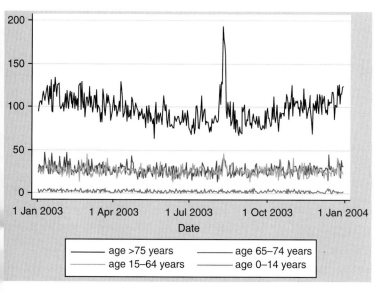

Figure 2.1 Daily deaths per day in Greater London during 2003, by age group. Mortality data from the Office for National Statistics.

with a heat wave in the first 2 weeks of August 2003 in Greater London. This heat wave, with temperatures exceeding 32°C in the South of England for a 10-day period, caused an estimated 2091 deaths in England and Wales, of which 1781 (85%) were of people aged over 75 years. The excess mortality associated with heat waves can be considerable, as experienced in continental Europe during the same summer. More than 14 800 deaths were attributed to the 2003 heat wave in France[17] as temperatures exceeded 40°C in some places, and night-time temperatures were also very high. It was the hottest summer in Western Europe since 1500.[18]

There is an increasing risk of heat-related mortality as age increases. The effect of the heat wave in Europe on mortality was found to be greater in women than in men, even after adjusting for differences in longevity.[12,19] For example, in Italy, the odds ratio for dying on a hot day in women compared with men (all ages over 35) was 1.45 (95% CI 1.27, 1.42).[12] The heat wave in Chicago in 1995 was atypical because it affected men more than women in all age groups. It was

suggested that this was due to cultural differences, particularly the lack of social support networks in poor urban elderly men in the US.[20] In general, it has not been possible to disaggregate the physiological from the social and environmental determinants that make elderly women more at risk from extreme hot weather.

There are contrasting patterns between impacts on mortality and hospital admissions during heat waves by age group and cause or diagnosis. Excess mortality is typically greatest for cardiovascular and respiratory diseases in the elderly. Hospital admissions during heat waves increase for adults as well as for the elderly, and for the classical heat-related illnesses (heat stroke, heat exhaustion) and related conditions (dehydration), neurological conditions, renal disease, and neurological illness. However, when compared with mortality, the relatively low increase in admissions for the elderly indicates that persons dying in heat waves do so quickly, before they can be admitted to hospital, or persons are dying before they come to the attention of others, either because they live alone or because of failures in care.[10]

Variations in risk

Evidence from the US indicates that air conditioning is an effective intervention to prevent heat stroke and heat-related illness,[21] both in private houses and in nursing homes.[22] Benefits seem to be associated with inbuilt air conditioning, rather than free-standing units.[23] Air conditioning is energy intensive, however, and is not recommended when alternatives are available, such as natural ventilation. Further, although air conditioning reduces mortality during weather extremes, it also takes away the natural stimuli that normally induce acclimatization to cold or heat and are beneficial in preventing temperature-related illnesses.

Additional important determinants of risk for heat wave mortality relate to housing and social support networks. These factors are much less well studied, as information at the individual level is not readily available. Studies in the US indicate some effect of deprivation, because only low income groups are without functioning air conditioning.[24–26] In Paris and in Italian cities, low-income groups were more affected by the 2003 heat wave.[27]

The elderly in hospitals and institutions, such as residential care homes, are vulnerable to heat-related illness and death in Europe (Table 2.1).[28] An almost twofold increase in mortality rate was reported in geriatric hospital inpatients (but not other inpatients) during the 1976 heat wave in the UK.[29] In Europe, such institutions are unlikely to be air conditioned. In France, death rates in retirement homes doubled during the heat wave in 2003.[17] A larger than expected excess was also reported in northern Italian nursing homes.[30] Assessment of the 2003 heat wave on mortality in the South East of England, by place of death, found that excess mortality due to the heat wave occurred in both nursing and residential homes, but not in hospices.[31]

Whereas it is generally acknowledged that people in nursing homes are frail and have a higher risk of death than the general population,

Table 2.1 Summary of environmental and social determinants of heat- and cold-related mortality for the UK population

Heat	Cold
• Elderly	• Living in houses with low thermal efficiency, particularly older houses
• Living in residential care and nursing homes	
• Chronic diseases, particularly cardiovascular diseases and diabetes	• Rural populations
	• Inappropriate clothing and protection from cold outdoors
• Urban populations	• Women more at risk than men
• Women more at risk than men	

it is only recently that it has been made clear that those in charge of such facilities must take steps to protect their residents from temperature extremes. In the past, this guidance, more likely than not, was related to extremes of cold, but it now extends to heat illness that can also easily be prevented.[32] It is also possible that some institutionalized or hospitalized individuals are more at risk from heat exposures than they might be in their own homes.[33]

EFFECTS OF COLD AND EXCESS WINTER MORTALITY

As is the case with heat, the risk of cold death rises steeply with age and is highest (but not confined to) people over the age of 70 years. The problem of excess winter mortality has perhaps been better addressed in the UK than heat-related issues, as there exist long-standing health promotion campaigns to protect the elderly from cold, both indoors and out.

Death rates during the winter months are appreciably higher than in other months of the year. The absolute number of winter excess deaths in the UK varies somewhat from year to year, but is generally in the range 30 000 to 50 000. Comparison of mortality in winter and non-winter months does not properly reflect the true magnitude of seasonal fluctuations, which become apparent from examination of daily mortality rates. Even on the basis of a monthly running mean, the peak of winter deaths is more than 40% greater than that occurring during the summer nadir. The largest part of this excess is attributable to cold, with other fractions due to winter respiratory infections – especially influenza and respiratory syncytial virus (RSV) – and other seasonal factors that may include variations in behavior and micronutrient intake.

The cold excess is apparent only in statistical terms, in that the number of deaths overall, and of cardiorespiratory disease in particular, is higher on cold days than it is on warmer days. At its simplest, the relationship between temperature and mortality can be characterized by a plot of the daily rate of death against daily temperature, as shown in Figure 2.2 for London. There is a band of temperatures, around 18–27°C, at which daily mortality rate is at its lowest. Whereas the heat-attributable deaths are apparent as an increase in the daily mortality rate when the maximum

daily temperature is around 28°C, the cold-related deaths are represented by the increase in mortality below the cold threshold, which occurs at around 18°C maximum daily temperature. The increase in mortality below this threshold tends to be greater the colder it is. Such association with cold can be more formally quantified using (autoregressive) time-series methods, with adjustment for seasonally varying risk factors (influenza, air pollution, public holidays, and season itself). As a broad guide, these analyses suggest that cardiovascular mortality rises by about 2% for each °C decline in maximum daily temperature below the cold threshold of 18°C.

The increase in mortality after a cold day tends to occur with a time lag. Whereas some increase in mortality is usually apparent on the day of cold, it tends to rise for several days afterwards, reaching a peak around 4–5 days later. Deaths from cardiovascular disease (myocardial infarction, strokes) peak at around 3 or 4 days, and deaths from respiratory disease may be maximal more than 1 week after cold exposure. This suggests different pathophysiological mechanisms for different causes of death. In contrast, the effect of heat (temperatures above the threshold value) is only apparent for up to 3 days, and is relatively short-lived.

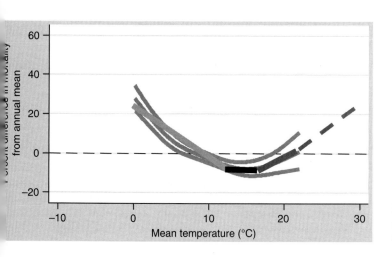

Figure 2.2 Relationship between daily mortality and daily mean temperature, London.

Variations in risk

One of the important observations in relation to cold-related mortality and morbidity is that vulnerability varies substantially between populations. The UK, for example, appears to have a larger seasonal fluctuation in mortality than many other countries of continental Europe and Scandinavia,[34] despite the fact that it has relatively mild winters because of the buffering effect of the surrounding seas and the impact of the warm air blown by the Gulf Stream. Other countries with high rates of 'excess' winter mortality in Europe are Portugal and Spain,[35] but their geography and living and social conditions are not similar to those in the UK.

Keatinge and colleagues are among those who emphasize the role of personal behaviors as the chief determinants of risk. They have argued that much of the excess winter mortality from arterial thrombosis is related to cold exposure from 'brief excursions outdoors rather than to low indoor temperature',[2,36] largely based on the results of the Eurowinter study, which compared relevant behaviors in a number of regions of Europe with varying cold-related mortality. These results suggested that for a day with a standard outside temperature of 7°C, the level of home heating tended to be warmer and personal clothing better adapted to cold in areas with lower winter temperatures (Figure 2.3). Moreover, temperature protection appeared more effective in countries with lower risk of cold-related mortality. Although there are complexities to this argument, the evidence nonetheless points to the

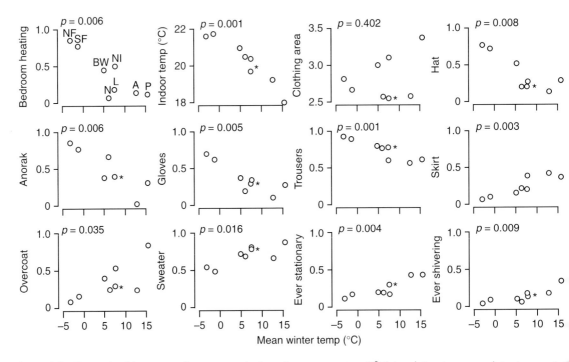

Figure 2.3 Personal cold exposure factors at standard outdoor temperature (7°C) in relation to mean winter temperature of region. Points from left to right: north Finland (NF), south Finland (SF), Baden-Württemberg (BW), Netherlands (N), London (L), north Italy (NI), Athens (A), Palermo (P). London given asterisk to distinguish from north Italy. Mean winter temperature in latter only 0.1°C higher than in London. (Reproduced from[2], with permission from Elsevier.)

fact that personal behaviors are an important risk determinant.

Research has also recently focused on the effect of housing quality;[37] analyses of cold-related deaths in England showed that the magnitude of the winter excess was greater in people living in dwellings that appear to be poorly heated.[37] The percentage rise in deaths in winter is greater in dwellings with low energy efficiency ratings/high costs of heating (Figure 2.4), and in dwellings predicted to have low indoor temperatures during periods of cold. There was also a gradient of risk with age of the property, the risk being greatest in dwellings built before 1850 and lowest in the more energy-efficient dwellings built after 1980. Absence of central heating and dissatisfaction with the heating system also showed some association with increased risk of excess winter death.

Surprisingly, however, there is little evidence that cold-related mortality varies with socioeconomic status. This is despite the fact that deprivation is a strong predictor of death rates overall and of cardiorespiratory mortality in particular. The lack of a socioeconomic gradient has been a consistent finding of UK studies, and has been reported in studies from elsewhere.[38–40] The explanation for this reality may be complex, but it is worthwhile to note that in England there is also very little socioeconomic gradient in winter indoor temperatures. This appears to be in part related to the fact that people from higher socioeconomic status tend to live in older, poorly heated dwellings.

There is some evidence that women are at slightly greater risk of winter- and cold-related death than men.[41] This may in part be expected from the fact that winter deaths rise steeply with age, and women tend to live longer. But the evidence suggests that women may be at increased risk independently of age effect, although the reason remains unclear.

INTERVENTIONS FOR HEAT AND COLD: KEY THEMES

Interventions for extremes of heat and cold have been developed in recent years. Unsurprisingly, there has been a rapid implementation of heat wave measures following the 2003 event in most countries in Western Europe. Interventions in relation to cold have often focused on addressing fuel poverty and home heating, which is part of the wider discussion on equity and poverty in the elderly. So far, there has been relatively little consideration of addressing heat and cold extremes into the integrated management of care of the elderly.

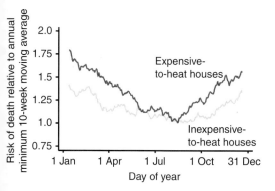

Figure 2.4 Seasonal variation in deaths from cardiovascular disease by standardized cost of home heating. England, 1986–1996. (Reproduced with permission from Wilkinson P, Landon M, Armstrong B, Stevenson S, McKee M. Cold comfort: the social and environmental determinants of excess winter death in England, 1986–1996. York: Joseph Rowntree Foundation; 2001.)

Housing quality

Housing quality is a key determinant of indoor temperatures. The evidence about the link between housing quality and cold-related death suggests that interventions aimed at improving the energy efficiency of the housing stock have the greatest potential for health benefits. In part motivated by health considerations, in 2000 the UK Government launched a Home Energy Efficiency Scheme in England (now known as Warm Front). This grant-funded program for tackling domestic fuel poverty provided (and continues to provide) packages of insulation – loft and/or cavity wall insulation, draught proofing, etc. – and heating measures (installation or upgrading of a central heating system, gas wall heaters, electric storage heaters, etc.), and is targeted at households on low incomes which may be in fuel poverty. A national evaluation of the health impact of this scheme found that the energy efficiency improvements of the scheme are associated with:

- increased winter indoor temperatures (by an average of around 2°C), the increase being greater in night-time bedroom temperatures than for daytime living room temperatures[42]
- reduction in 'normalized' relative humidity, condensation, and visible mold growth[43]
- some evidence for improvement in mental well-being
- indirect evidence of reduction in vulnerability to winter- and cold-related mortality from cardiovascular disease.

Among grant recipients, there was substantial improvement in satisfaction with the heating system, and fewer reports of difficulty paying (heating) bills and with draughts and damp in the home. Many householders reported improved well-being and, in several cases, the easing of symptoms of chronic illness. Warm Front improvements were also reported by some householders to improve family relations, expand the domestic space used during cold months, increase privacy within the home, and, finally, improve social interaction and comfort within the home.[44] Paradoxically, however, there was little evidence that Warm Front improvements altered ventilation or fuel consumption, even though theoretical considerations suggest that there should be significant savings.

Although there are risks of adverse effects on indoor air quality, they appear low and, over all the changes are broadly very positive – improving the indoor environment, contributing to psycho social well-being, and reducing the risks of cardiovascular events.

Health forecasting

A recent development in public healthcare has been 'health forecasting'. In the UK, the Met Office has established a dedicated health forecasting team which is aimed at developing systems for predicting and responding to forecast of temperature-related (mainly cold-related) risks. A pilot system focused on the management of chronic obstructive pulmonary disease (COPD) in primary care as well as emergency admission to hospital. Although clear evidence about the impact of such schemes has not yet been obtained a recent formative evaluation showed its potential. The (highly variable) risk of hospital admission from COPD was largely predictable from meteorological, infectious disease, and other data, and forecast of such risk appear to have the potential to be used for guiding clinical management. Where this had been tried, staff and patients have been generally positive to the scheme to improve quality of care through locally developed forecast-responsive care plans, with reported advantages including

- greater focus on prevention
- improved contact between high-risk patients and primary care staff
- more integrated, protocol-based care
- empowerment of patients to manage their own condition.

Although these benefits may be as much related to the increased focus on COPD as to the forecast themselves, the forecasts appear to be the essential catalyst. The evidence is sufficiently encouraging for wider testing, but formal assessment cost-effectiveness will be needed once more experience of how best to use health forecasting has been obtained.

Heat/health warning systems

An effective heat/health warning system (HHWS) requires the involvement of medical and social care institutions that have sufficient resources, capacity, knowledge, and political will to undertake the specific response measures.[45] An HHWS is implemented at the local level, and therefore provision and interventions deployed vary widely once a heat wave warning is triggered. Table 2.2 describes some of the interventions implemented during heat waves to prevent mortality. Advice focuses on the hazards of a heat wave, how to recognize the symptoms of heat exhaustion and heat stroke, and how to treat the effects of too much heat.

A range of strategies are used to encourage at-risk individuals to visit cool areas, based on

Table 2.2 Public health measures in European heat/health warning systems

Measure, strategy	Comments
Media announcements (radio, television)	Provide general advice on heat stress avoidance to general public. Elderly are mentioned as a vulnerable group
Bulletin or webpage	May be restricted access, to relevant professionals or accessed by anybody
Leaflets	General advice, and advice for nursing home managers. Often distributed at beginning of the summer via health centers, and places where vulnerable people may be
Telephone help-line	Either a dedicated telephone service is opened (e.g. Heatline in Portugal) or people are encouraged to phone a pre-existing general health advice line (e.g. NHS Direct in the UK)
Opening of special 'cooling centers'	Some evidence that cooling centers not used by high-risk individuals
Alert to hospital emergency rooms, ambulance services	Used to improve operational efficiency (e.g. if need to deploy extra staff). Needs to be based on local information and carefully evaluated
Home outreach visits to vulnerable persons	Requires some pre-existing register of 'vulnerable' individuals
Evacuation of vulnerable persons from their homes to cooling centers	Using a registry of vulnerable people, who are visited at home, and evacuated, if necessary
Electricity companies cease disconnection for non-payment	Most important where population relies heavily on air conditioning (as in the US)
Water companies cease disconnection for non-payment	
Fan distribution	Fans are effective when they circulate cooler air, but not above temperatures around 35–37°C

Source: based on reference 45.

the assumption that remaining indoors may be harmful. Local areas that are cooler can be used, such as public swimming pools, beaches, public parks, or large space-cooled buildings such as shopping centers. Anecdotal evidence from the US indicates that dedicated cooling centers were not well attended, and that the people who did attend were not those most at risk.[46]

For effective outreach, high-risk individuals need to be identified and outreach services initiated early. Heat waves are short-lived events, and any action must be triggered rapidly (within hours or days) in order to be effective. The outreach may be undertaken by professionals (health workers) or by volunteers, including friends or relatives. The Philadelphia HHWS was able to exploit a pre-existing community-based Buddy system that enables neighbours to check on vulnerable individuals.[47,48] Systems in Europe have used pre-existing registers of vulnerable people, or have asked persons to register themselves or their relatives voluntarily.[49]

Health promotion

A communication and public education strategy is an essential part of protection against climate extremes, and should be incorporated into any warning or forecasting system. Public health messages should be disseminated to all age and risk groups to increase awareness of symptoms of heat-related illness.[46] Given that perception of ambient temperature is generally poorer in the elderly, a person may not feel that that they are stressed, when in fact they are.[8] The most susceptible individuals are socially isolated, elderly, and those with an illness or disability that causes impairment of thermoregulation, or cognitive/behavioral problems. An understanding of human behavior and physiology during extreme weather events is therefore needed before the most appropriate messages can be developed and targeted.

There have been several campaigns at getting people to be warmer in winter. Searches of the published literature found no studies of the effectiveness of heat- or cold-awareness campaigns. Passive warnings for poor air quality, for example, are not thought to be particularly effective. A qualitative study in the UK found that, in general, elderly people were very interested in weather forecast information and used it to make decisions about daily activities.[50] However, the medium of the message was very important, as warnings delivered on television news programmes were not well understood as the information was delivered too quickly. Consideration must be given to the elderly with impaired vision or hearing.

COMMENTS

The burden of mortality and morbidity due to temperature extremes is considerable, and the majority of this burden falls on the elderly. Only recently has this burden been recognized as preventable. Effective measures are still being developed and evaluated for heat wave mortality. Acute responses linked to warning systems only address late-stage issues for primary prevention or early detection of clinical heat stress. Heat stroke deaths in individuals are easily preventable.[32] Many long-term interventions are necessary, such as training and education of staff and carers, improvements to domestic housing and healthcare infrastructure, and the care of the elderly at home. In France, the government has recommended that institutions for the elderly have at least one air-conditioned room.

Although heat deaths have received more attention in recent years, possibly because of the major heat wave in Europe in 2003 as well as the possibility of an increase in the frequency of such events under climate change, the large burden of temperature-related mortality and morbidity in mid-latitude Europe is in fact attributable to cold. The burden due to cold is particularly high in the UK, where milder winters mean that the population is poorly adapted to cold in comparison to countries with colder winters. Prevention measures will only be useful once the majority of houses have improved and are less expensive to heat.

REFERENCES

1. Sakamoto-Momiyama M. Seasonality in Human Mortality. Tokyo: University of Tokyo press; 1977.

2. Eurowinter Group. Cold exposure and winter mortality from ischaemic heart disease, cerebrovascular disease, respiratory disease, and all causes in warm and cold regions of Europe. Lancet 1997; 349: 1341–5.

3. Kilbourne EM. Heat waves and hot environments. In: Noji E, ed. The Public Health Consequences of Disasters. New York: Oxford University Press; 1997: 245–69.

4. Kilbourne EM. Illness due to thermal extremes. In: Last JM, Wallace RB, eds. Public Health and Preventative Medicine, 13th edn. Norwalk, Connecticut: Appleton & Lang; 1992: 491–501.

5. Havenith G, Inoue Y, Luttikholt V, Kenney WL. Age predicts cardiovascular, but not thermoregulatory, responses to humid heat stress. Eur J Appl Physiol Occup Physiol 1995; 70: 88–96.

6. Havenith G, Coenen JM, Kistemaker L, Kenney WL. Relevance of individual characteristics for human heat stress response is dependent on exercise intensity and climate type. Eur J Appl Physiol Occup Physiol 1998; 77: 231–41.

7. Havenith G. Temperature, heat balance, and climatic stress. In: Kirch W, Menne B, Bertollini R, eds. Extreme Weather Events and Public Health Responses. Berlin: Springer-Verlag; 2005: 70–80.

8. Collins KJ, Exton-Smith AN, Dore C. Urban hypothermia: preferred temperature and thermal perception in old age. Br Med J (Clin Res Ed) 1981; 282(6259): 175–7.

9. Keatinge WR, Coleshaw SR, Easton JC, et al. Increased platelet and red cell counts, blood viscosity, and plasma cholesterol levels during heat stress, and mortality from coronary and cerebral thrombosis. Am J Med 1986; 81: 795–800.

10. Kovats RS, Hajat S, Wilkinson P. Contrasting patterns of mortality and hospital admissions during heat waves in London, UK. Occup Environ Med 2004; 61(11): 893–8.

11. Schwartz J. Who is sensitive to extremes of temperature? A case-only analysis. Epidemiology 2005; 16(1): 67–72.

12. Stafoggia M, Forastiere F, Agostini D, et al. Vulnerability to heat-related mortality: a multicity population based case-crossover analysis. Epidemiology 2006; 17(3): 315–23.

13. Woodhouse PR, Khaw KT, Plummer M. Seasonal variation of blood pressure and its relationship to ambient temperature in an elderly population. J Hypertens 1993; 11(11): 1267–74.

14. Stout RW, Crawford VL, McDermott MJ, Rocks MJ, Morris TC. Seasonal changes in haemostatic factors in young and elderly subjects. Age Ageing 2006; 25(3): 256–8.

15. Godwin J, Taylor RS, Pearce VR, Read KL. Seasonal cold, excursional behaviour, clothing protection and physical activity in young and old subjects. Int J Circumpolar Health 2000; 59(3–4): 195–203.

16. Smolander J. Effect of cold exposure on older humans. Int J Sports Med 2002; 23(2): 86–92.

17. Hemon D, Jougla E. Estimates of excess mortality and epidemiological characteristics. Rapport d'etape 1/3. Paris: INSERM (Institute National de la Sante et de la recherche medicale); 2003.

18. Luterbacher J, Dietrich D, Xoplaki E, Grosjean M, Wanner H. European seasonal and annual temperature variability, trends and extremes since 1500. Science 2004; 303 (5663): 1499–503.

19. Michelozzi P, de Donato F, Bisanti L, et al. The impact of the summer 2003 heat waves on mortality in four Italian cities. Euro Surveill 2005; 10(7): 161–5.

20. Klinenberg E. Heat Wave: A Social Autopsy of Disaster in Chicago. Chicago: University of Chicago Press; 2002.

21. O'Neill M. Air conditioning and heat-related health effects. Appl Environ Sci Public Health 2003; 1(1): 9–12.

22. Marmor M. Heat wave mortality in nursing homes. Environ Res 1978; 17: 102–15.

23. Rogot E, Sorlie PD, Backlund E. Air-conditioning and mortality in hot weather. Am J Epidemiol 1992; 136: 106–16.

24. Smoyer KE. A comparative analysis of heat waves and associated mortality in St Louis, Missouri – 1980 and 1995. Int J Biometeorol 1998; 42: 44–50.

25. Smoyer KE. Putting risk in its place: methodological considerations for investigating extreme event health risks. Soc Sci Med 1998; 47: 1809–24.

26. Semenza JC, Rubin CH, Falter KH, et al. Heat-related deaths during the July 1995 heat wave in Chicago. N Engl J Med 1996; 335(2): 84–90.

27. Michelozzi P, de Donato F, Accetta G, et al. Impact of heat waves on mortality – Rome, Italy, June–August 2003. JAMA 2004; 291(21): 2537–8.

28. Faunt JD, Wilkinson TJ, Aplin P, et al. The effete in the heat: heat-related hospital presentations during a ten day heat wave. Aust NZ J Med 1995; 25: 117–20.

29. Lye M, Kamal A. Effects of a heatwave on mortality-rates in elderly inpatients. Lancet 1977; 1: 529–31.

30. Rozzini R, Zanetti E, Trabucchi M. Elevated temperature and nursing home mortality during 2003 European heat wave. J Am Med Dir Assoc 2004; 5(2): 138–9.

31. Kovats RS, Johnson H, Griffith C. Mortality in southern England during the 2003 heatwave by place of death. Health Stat Q 2006; Spring(29): 6–8.

32. Thomas ND, Soliman H. Preventable tragedies – heat disaster and the elderly. J Gerontol Socia Work 2002; 38(4): 53–66.

33. Ferron C, Trewick D, Le Conte P, et al. [Hea stroke in hospital patients during the summe 2003 heat wave: a nosocomial disease]. Press Med 2006; 35(2): 196–9. [in French]

34. McKee CM. Deaths in winter: can Britain lear from Europe? Eur J Epidemiol 1989; 5(2) 178–82.

35. Healy JD. Excess winter mortality in Europe: cross country analysis identifying key risk fac tors. J Epidemiol Community Health 2003 57(784): 789.

36. Neild PJ, Syndercombe-Court D, Keatinge WR et al. Cold-induced increases in erythrocyt count, plasma cholesterol and plasma fibrinoge of elderly people without a comparable rise i protein C or factor X. Clin Sci 1994; 86: 43–8

37. Wilkinson P, Armstrong B. Housing and exces winter death from cardiovascular disease i England, 1986–1996. London: London Schoc of Hygiene and Tropical Medicine; 2001 Report to Joseph Rowntree Foundation.

38. Aylin P, Morris S, Wakefield J, et a Temperature, housing, deprivation and the relationship to excess winter mortality in Grea Britain, 1986–1996. Int J Epidemiol 200 30(5): 1100–8.

39. Lawlor DA, Dews H, Harvey D. Investigatio of the association between excess winter mor tality and socio-economic deprivation. J Publi Health Med 2000; 22(2): 176–81.

40. Shah S, Peacock J. Deprivation and excess wint mortality. J Epidemiol Community Healt 1999; 53: 499–502.

41. Wilkinson P, Pattenden S, Armstrong B, et a Vulnerability to winter mortality in the elder in Great Britain: population based study. BM 2004; 329(7467): 647–51.

42. Oreszczyn T, Hong SH, Ridley I, Wilkinson Determinants of winter indoor temperatures low income households in England. Energ and Buildings 2006; 38: 245–52.

43. Oreszczyn T, Sung H, Ridley I, Wilkinson Mould and winter indoor relative humidity

low income households in England. J Indoor Built Environ 2006; 15(2): 125–35.

44. Gilbertson J, Stephens MJ, Stiell B, Thorogood N. Grant recipient's views of the Warm Front scheme. Soc Sci Med 2006; 63(4): 946–56.

45. Kovats RS, Ebi KL. Heatwaves and public health in Europe. Eur J Publ Health 2006; 16(6): 592–9.

46. Bernard SM, McGeehin MA. Municipal heat wave response plans. Am J Publ Hlth 2004; 94(9): 1520–1.

47. Ebi KL, Teisberg TJ, Kalkstein LS, Robinson L, Weiher RF. Heat Watch/Warning Systems save lives: estimated costs and benefits for Philadelphia 1995–1998. Bull Am Meteorol Soc 2004; 85(8): 1067–8.

48. Kalkstein LS, Jamason PF, Greene JS, Libby J, Robinson L. The Philadelphia hot weather-health watch warning system: development and application, summer 1995. Bull Am Meteorol Soc 1996; 77: 1519–28.

49. Michelon T, Magne P, Simon-Delaville F. Lessons of the 2003 heat wave in France and action taken to limit the effects of future heat waves. In: Kirch W, Menne B, Bertollini R, eds. Extreme Weather Events and Public Health Responses. Berlin: Springer-Verlag; 2005: 131–40.

50. Morgan K, Haslam R, Havenith G, Brace C, Tucker I. Forecasting the nation's health. Report to Help the Aged on a Pilot study to capture views and attitudes of older people in relation to the health aspects of cold weather early warning. Loughborough: Department of Human Sciences, Loughborough University; 2004.

Section II

Conditions affecting elderly women

Balance, falls, and osteoporotic fractures

3

Sally Edmonds

INTRODUCTION

Any discussion of the effects of aging must recognize the importance of two interrelated statistics:

- during the 20th century, a total of 30 years was added to the life expectancy of each individual born
- between 1990 and 2020, the global population of individuals aged over 75 is expected to increase by almost 140%.[1]

In contrast to the first number, which makes everyone happy, the second is fraught with numerous concerns for individual patients, their families, and society as a whole. As readers of this book have already discerned, women generally have a greater life expectancy than men. Given these circumstances, the numbers of older women at risk of falling and sustaining an osteoporotic fracture continues to rise at a significant rate, so much so that in terms of overall cost to the community, osteoporotic fractures have become an enormous public health burden. Not only is the high incidence of falls amongst older people of concern (young children and athletes have an even higher incidence of falls), but also this high incidence is accompanied by an extraordinary high susceptibility to injury. The propensity for fall-related injury in older people results primarily from the additional high prevalence of comorbid disease, especially osteoporosis.

The cost of osteoporotic fractures, particularly of the hip, both to the individual and to society, is high. In the UK the National Health Service's annual expenditure on the acute and after care of osteoporosis-related fracture is close to £1.7 billion. More important, approximately one-half of all older adults hospitalized for hip fracture never regain their former level of function, and up to one-third die within 1 year. In England, mortality rates following fractured femoral neck declined between the 1960s and the early 1980s, but stabilized thereafter[2] (Figure 3.1). Of patients over the age of 65 who are admitted to hospital with a hip fracture, about 80% are women. The estimated lifetime risk of hip fracture is about 14% in postmenopausal women, a figure that is more than

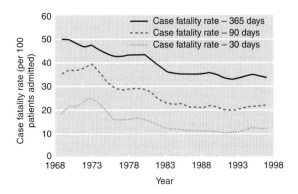

Figure 3.1 Age- and sex-adjusted trends in case fatality rates for fractured neck of femur after hospital admission, 1968-98. (Adapted from Roberts and Goldacre,[2] with permission: http://bmj.bmjjournals.com/cgi/content/full/327/7418/771.)

double that of men (6%).[3] Stated another way, the risk of hip fracture increases 10-fold with every 20 years of age.

One of the risk factors for sustaining a fracture is low bone density, and older postmenopausal women are more likely than older men to have low bone density. Bone density, however, is not the only risk factor, and it may be that risk of falling is more important, as more than 90% of hip fractures result from falls onto the greater trochanter.[4] Whereas bone density is measured routinely to assess fracture risk, little attention is paid to the assessment of fall risk, which may depend on balance, vision, hearing, and other senses as well as medications causing hypotension or sedation and environmental hazards in the home. Indeed, fall prevention strategies may be as, or more, important in the prevention of osteoporotic fractures than the use of bone-strengthening drugs such as the bisphosphonates.

BALANCE AND THE RISK OF FALLING

Falls, age, and disease

Whereas some osteoporotic fractures, principally vertebral fractures, are not the result of trauma, the vast majority of such fractures are sustained as the result of a fall. One-third of the population aged 65 and over fall each year, and this rate rises to 50% in the over-85 age group.[5–7] Older women living in the community experience significantly more falls than do older men;[6] even allowing for physical and social factors, women are 1.5 times more likely to fall than men.[8] Women start to fall more frequently by approximately 50 years of age. By the age of 70 years, some 20% of women fall at least once a year; by the age of 80 years, this figure has risen to 48%.[9] In addition, women who live alone are at greater risk of falling and sustaining an injury.[5] Given this reality, it does not require a great sense of logic to realize that prevention of falls is more likely than not to reduce the incidence of fractures in elderly women.

Maintaining balance is a complex task that is affected by aging and disease. This complexity is substantiated by the more than 400 potential risk factors for falling.[10] Whereas both men and women have an increased risk of falling as they age, women living in the community are more likely to fall than men, which may be due to a combination of reduced strength[11] and delayed execution of protective stepping responses.[12] Other important risk factors for fall include untreated visual impairments (including glaucoma and cataract), sedative use, and cognitive impairment,[13] all of which increase with age, and may not receive attention until the patient is referred for open access densitometry.[14] These considerations make a strong argument that a fall risk assessment should be part of the routine work-up when assessing osteoporotic fracture risk.

The presence of osteoporosis may bring with it a greater risk of falling than is experienced by those with normal bone mass.[15] One study looked at women between the ages of 64 and 75, matched for age and current activity level, and compared those with and without osteoporosis. A triad of fall risk factors (quadriceps strength, balance, and functional mobility) were compared between the two groups. Quadriceps strength and composite balance score were significantly worse in the osteoporotic group, suggesting that these women were at greater risk of falling.

Perhaps as important as identifying individual risk factors for falling is appreciating that multiple risk factors interact; several studies have shown that the risk of falling increases dramatically as the number of risk factors increases.[16,17] In one such study, multivariate analysis was used to simplify risk factors so that maximum predictive accuracy could be obtained by using only three factors (hip weakness, unstable balance, and taking four or more medications) in an algorithm format.[16]

Using this model, the predicted 1-year risk of falling ranged from 12% for people with no risk factors, to 100% in those with all three. Table 3.1 summarizes the risk factors for falling. As well as being more likely to fall, women are also more likely to sustain serious injury if they do fall. Serious injury is also more likely in those with cognitive impairment and two or more chronic conditions, such as arthritis and diabetes mellitus.[17]

Consequences of falls

In addition to the physical injury that may result from a fall, falls per se and the fear of falling may have important psychological consequences. In a quality of life survey of nearly 200 Australian women aged 75 and over, 80% suggested that they would rather be dead than suffer a 'bad' hip fracture; i.e. one that resulted in their permanent admission to a nursing home.[18] Admission to a nursing home was perceived as being synonymous with loss of independence and disastrous in terms of quality of life. This is not to say, however, that 80% of older women who experience a 'bad' fracture would prefer death to treatment. This study was conducted in a community where health and quality of life of older people equated with their ability to live and function independently, a circumstance which clearly does not translate to all communities, especially where the extended transgenerational family is the norm. It does, however, affirm the need for rehabilitation programs that not only focus on enhancing patients' mobility and functional abilities but also optimize their ability to once more live independently and participate in social and other aspects of community life.

FALL PREVENTION

Falls and their consequences can be the cause of catastrophic physical and psychological effects. Under these circumstances, fall risk assessments and fall prevention strategies are not only essential for the prevention of osteoporotic fractures but also for the prevention of the loss of quality of life which so often accompanies these injuries. The predictive validity of published fall risk assessment screens has been examined in recent reviews.[19,20] However, it may be that many of the tools used in such assessments either lack sensitivity or specificity and thereby classify too few or too many people as fallers.[19] Whereas further validation of screening tools for relevant populations is needed, good evidence exists to show that falls can be prevented in older people in a variety of populations and clinical settings. These include community-dwelling populations; care home residents; older people presenting to the emergency department having had a recent fall; hospital inpatients and those being discharged home from hospital. Collected data from 40 randomized controlled trials, involving nearly 14 000 patients, followed up for up to 10 years, suggest that interventions designed to reduce the incidence of falls in older people living in the community, in institutions, or in hospital care, can reduce the risk of falling by up to 20–50%.[21] Such interventions include programs to improve gait, balance, and muscle strength; tai chi exercises; tackling environmental hazards; and withdrawal of specific psychotropic medicines.

Table 3.1 Risk factors for falling

Advancing age
Female gender
Living alone
Impaired gait and mobility
Reduced muscle strength
Impaired stepping responses
Impaired visual acuity
Impaired cognition
Medical conditions, e.g. stroke, arthritis
Sedative use
Polypharmacy

The type, duration, and intensity of exercise that is optimal for fall prevention remains unclear, although the evidence is strongest for balance training.[22] In women of 80 years and older living in the community, individually designed exercise programs in the home that incorporate strength and balance training reduce both falls as well as associated injuries.[23] Moreover, for those women who continued to exercise, the benefits were evident even after a 2-year period. It is likely, however, that interventions targeting multiple risk factors are most effective. Collected data from five randomized controlled trials (involving nearly 3000 patients followed up for at least 1 year) suggest that interventions based on an assessment by a healthcare professional trained to identify intrinsic and environmental risk factors can reduce the risk of falling by about 20%.[24]

Fall prevention is being given higher priority at the national level. For example, in the UK, the National Service Framework (NSF) for older people was published in 2001.[25] Standard 6 of this document relates specifically to falls, and its aim is to 'reduce the number of falls which result in serious injury and ensure effective treatment and rehabilitation for those who have fallen'. A number of key interventions are recommended, including fall prevention at primary level and health promotion to include identification of those at risk. It also recommends the establishment of integrated falls services to improve care and treatment of those who have fallen, with emphasis on prevention of serious injury, and reduction of further falls. Table 3.2 is a list of fall prevention strategies.

EPIDEMIOLOGY OF OSTEOPOROTIC FRACTURES

Fractures are the clinically relevant endpoint of osteoporosis. Vertebral fractures may occur after minimal or no trauma, and may be asymptomatic, although new crush fractures may be associated

Table 3.2 Fall prevention strategies

Establishment of falls service
Identification of those at risk
Specific interventions:
    Exercise – strength and balance training
    Tackling environmental hazards
    Withdrawal of psychotropic drugs
    Cardiovascular assessment when appropriate

with severe back pain (Figure 3.2). More commonly, and particularly in older women, vertebral fractures lead to loss of height, kyphosis, and functional impairment. In addition, vertebral fractures are associated with increased mortality risk;[26] persons with previous vertebral fractures are at increased risk of new vertebral and non-vertebral fractures, including hip fracture.[27] The incidence of both vertebral and non-vertebral fracture – especially hip fracture – strongly increases with age in both women and men. Wrist fracture, for example, reaches a peak between 50 and 70 years.

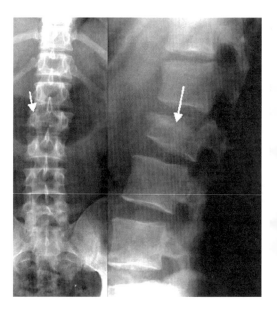

Figure 3.2 A vertebral crush fracture (arrowed). (From Rees M, Purdie DW. Management of the Menopause, 4th edn. Handbook of the British Menopause Society. London: BMS Publications; 2006).

RISK FACTORS FOR FRACTURE

Although falling is clearly one of the major risk factors for sustaining an osteoporotic fracture, it is not the only one (Table 3.3). Simply put, some falls result in fracture, whereas others do not. Whether a particular fall results in a fracture may be due to intrinsic differences in the fall phenomenon itself [28] or differences in bone strength, otherwise known as 'skeletal fragility'.

The combination of age and bone mineral density (BMD) are the two strongest independent risk factors for future fractures, both vertebral and non-vertebral, and in both men and women.[29] The incidence of hip fracture increases both with decreasing BMD and with increasing age, and these two factors independently add to fracture risk in women and men equally. In the US, one study showed that the four most significant risk factors for sustaining a hip fracture were personal history of previous fracture, family history of hip fracture, low body weight, and current smoking.[30]

In the UK, a more recent study confirmed that a personal history of previous fracture and a fall in the last 12 months were predictive of future non-vertebral, hip, and wrist fracture, and that increasing age was also predictive of non-vertebral and hip fracture, but not wrist fracture.[31] In addition, low body weight is also predictive of hip fracture, and has been shown to be a good surrogate marker for BMD in both women and men when used in a fracture risk prediction model.[32]

Bone strength

Bone strength is dependent on a number of factors, not the least of which is bone density. Whole bone strength is determined by the amount of bone (i.e. size or mass), the spatial distribution of the bone mass (i.e. shape or architecture), and the intrinsic properties of the materials that constitute the bone.[33] Bone mineral density measurements obtained by dual energy X-ray absorptiometry

Table 3.3 Risk factors for osteoporotic fracture

Risk factor	Example
Genetic	• Family history of fracture (particularly a first-degree relative with hip fracture)
Constitutional	• Low body mass index
	• Early menopause (<45 years of age)
Environmental	• Cigarette smoking
	• Alcohol abuse
	• Low calcium intake
	• Sedentary lifestyle
Drugs	• Corticosteroids >5 mg prednisolone or equivalent daily
Diseases	• Rheumatoid arthritis
	• Neuromuscular disease
	• Chronic liver disease
	• Malabsorption syndromes
	• Hyperparathyroidism
	• Hyperthyroidism
	• Hypogonadism

From: Rees M, Purdie DW, eds. The 2006 British Menopause Society Handbook. London: Royal Society of Medicine Press; 2006.

(DEXA) reflect some of the components of bone strength, including bone mass, degree of mineralization, and, to some extent, bone size. However, BMD measurements do not reflect other components of bone strength, including the three-dimensional distribution of bone mass, trabecular and cortical microarchitecture, and the intrinsic properties of the bone matrix. In many societies in which sitting near ground level (or squatting) is common in both sexes and almost all ages, hip fracture is rare, even when most women over the age of 65 years have osteoporosis. This apparent paradox may be due to the beneficial loading effects on the upper femur of regular standing up from a squatting position. One study has suggested that, as women age, their hip fragility increases because there is underloading of the femoral neck, which leads to loss of elastic stability in the bone.[34] Ordinary walking does not load the femoral neck sufficiently to prevent this loss of stability, and this may be another reason why older women have reduced bone strength and are therefore more susceptible to hip fracture. Nearly all community-based epidemiological studies have shown that lack of physical activity is a risk factor for osteoporotic fracture, and prolonged immobilization at any age is detrimental to bone health. However, in postmenopausal women, the balance between bone formation and resorption is already disturbed, and immobilization further upsets that balance and can considerably accelerate bone loss. As much as 40% of total skeletal mass may be lost within 6 months of immobilization and give rise to fracture.[35] Thus, an elderly woman may lose the same amount of bone in a week of immobilization as in 1 year of the natural history of 'uncomplicated' osteoporosis.

Fractures occur when the loads applied to bone exceed its strength. Therefore, strategies to reduce fractures should consider interventions aimed at reducing the loads applied to bone (fall prevention), as well as to maintaining or increasing bone strength.

IDENTIFYING THOSE AT RISK OF FRACTURE

Although BMD is a strong predictor of future fractures, population-based BMD screening is not sensitive enough to have a substantial influence on the population burden of fractures. Successful fracture prevention is therefore dependent on identifying those people at risk of osteoporotic fracture, either before they have suffered a fracture (primary prevention) or after their first fracture (secondary prevention). Theoretically, all post-menopausal women are at risk of developing osteoporosis and suffering an osteoporotic fracture, but only a relatively small subgroup of women are truly at high risk. The aim of case-finding is to identify those women. Van der Klift et al used a variety of risk factors to estimate an individual's fracture risk.[36] These included fracture after the age of 50 years; prevalent vertebral fracture; low body weight (<60 kg); severe immobility; and corticosteroid use (≥7.5 mg prednisolone equivalent daily). In practice, a number of risk factors need to be taken into consideration for deciding when to measure a woman's BMD. Premature menopause (<45 years), whether natural or surgical, is likely to increase a woman's risk of osteoporosis. Such women should be scanned, especially if the individual patient is undecided about taking hormone replacement therapy (HRT). Associated risk factors such as previous fragility fracture, maternal family history of hip fracture, smoking, and low body mass index will lower the threshold for scanning an individual woman. Of concern, it is not unusual to come across women over the age of 80 years who had a premature menopause but in whom HRT was never considered. Thus, it is essential to take a full medical history.

A number of the conditions that require long-term steroid treatment are more common in older women, e.g. polymyalgia rheumatica. Most clinicians start bone protective therapy at the same time as steroids are prescribed, and it is arguable, certainly in women over 65, that there is any need to scan such patients at all as their known risk of osteoporosis and fracture is so high. Whereas it remains controversial whether lower doses of oral steroids, inhaled or intermittent doses of steroids, may cause less significant bone loss, studies have demonstrated increased fracture risks on doses even as low as 2.5 mg of prednisolone daily.[37] The underlying condition for which steroid treatment is being administered also often contributes to loss of bone mass and increased fracture risk. A significant reduction in BMD at both the lumbar spine and femoral neck was noted[38] in patients with long-standing rheumatoid arthritis – a condition more common in women – who had not been treated with glucocorticoids.

Men tend to have stronger bones than women simply because their bones are bigger. Men attain greater bone mass than women, but also lose it steadily as they age. The higher a person's peak bone mass, the less likely they are to develop severe osteoporosis in older age. Strategies for preventing osteoporosis and osteoporotic fractures should also aim to maximize peak bone mass. The latter is outside the topic of this chapter, but preventing bone loss may be broadly divided into pharmacological and non-pharmacological approaches.

THE PREVENTION OF OSTEOPOROSIS AND OSTEOPOROTIC FRACTURES

Non-pharmacological approaches

Exercise

As previously discussed, exercise has a role in preventing falls, as well as helping to maintain or even increase bone density.[39] Physical activity is not only an important determinant of peak bone mass but also helps to maintain bone mass in later life. Exercise regimens can be very helpful in the management of established osteoporosis. Such regimens may not only improve an individual's sense of well-being and confidence but may also help chronic pain. Some people are reluctant to advise more active exercise for older people with osteoporosis for fear of further fracture, but, on the other hand, complete inactivity is clearly detrimental to bone health. Some sort of 'happy medium' therefore needs to be found, and exercises that are carefully structured according to the disability of the individual patient would seem to be a reasonable compromise. As far as the type of exercise is concerned, weight-bearing is most effective for improving bone strength, but the threshold of exercise, its type, degree, and periodicity that are optimal for bone mass are not known. In general, older people should be encouraged to take as much weight-bearing exercise as they are able to, supervised where necessary. In most cases this will include walking, but other forms of exercise such as cycling, swimming, and dancing, according to the individual's preference, may all provide similar benefit.

Smoking cessation

Smoking increases the overall lifetime risk of a woman developing a vertebral or hip fracture by 13% and 31%, respectively.[40] Smokers are generally thinner than their non-smoking counterparts, which may in part account for the risk. Adipose tissue is an important source of estrogen in the postmenopausal woman, and a decrease in body fat may explain this difference. Smoking may also increase the catabolism of estradiol, and, in addition, appears to reduce the beneficial effects of postmenopausal HRT on bone.[41] Clearly, the many reasons why smoking should be discouraged are well known, and bone health is one of them.

Diet and alcohol

All older people should be encouraged to eat a healthy, well-balanced diet and to moderate their alcohol intake. Excessive alcohol may not only be detrimental to bone health but may also greatly increase the risk of falling. The recommended intake for calcium for postmenopausal women is 1000–1500 mg/day and for vitamin D is 800 IU/day. A lot of older people have insufficient dietary calcium and many, particularly those living in institutions, are also lacking in vitamin D due to lack of exposure to sunlight. In addition, a decline in renal function in the elderly may lead to secondary hyperparathyroidism and disturbances in vitamin D metabolism. It may be impossible for older people to get enough calcium and vitamin D from their diet and, in some, supplementation should be considered.

Hip protectors

Hip protectors are plastic shields or foam pads which can be worn around the hips and are held in place by pockets within specially designed underwear (Figure 3.3). The aim of wearing hip protectors is to divert the impact of a fall away from the greater trochanter in order to prevent a fracture. A number of randomized controlled trials involving high-risk individuals in nursing homes or residential care show a significant reduction in the incidence of hip fracture in individuals wearing such protectors. However, a recent review of the evidence for the efficacy of hip protectors suggests that they are ineffective for preventing hip fracture in people living at home, and that their effectiveness in an institutional setting is uncertain.[42] Hip protectors are very bulky and many people do not like wearing them. Compliance is the major limitation to the efficacy of hip protectors, and many of the trials included in the systematic review[42] had compliance rates less than 40% by the end of the studies. The main reasons

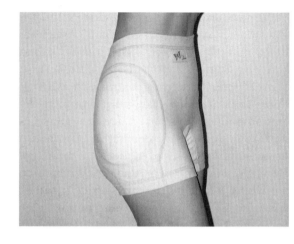

Figure 3.3 Hip protectors. (From Rees M, Purdie DW. Management of the Menopause, 4th edn. Handbook of the British Menopause Society. London: BMS Publications; 2006).

for poor compliance include not being comfortable (too tight/poor fit); the extra effort required to wear the device; urinary incontinence; and physical difficulties/illnesses. In spite of these limitations, hip protectors may be useful clinically as a hip fracture prevention strategy among those at high risk of falls who are willing and able to wear them.

Pharmacological approaches

Calcium and vitamin D

Calcium and vitamin D supplements reduce the number of non-vertebral fractures, including hip fractures, in the elderly, especially those who are institutionalized.[43] They may also reduce falls.[44] However, recent trials have shown that supplementation with calcium and vitamin D in non-institutionalized patients does not reduce fracture risk.[45] Furthermore, the Women's Health Initiative study of over 36 000 postmenopausal women randomly assigned to receive either 1000 mg of elemental calcium with 400 IU of vitamin D_3 daily or placebo calcium and vitamin D supplementation.

resulted in a small but significant increase in hip bone density, but did not significantly reduce the incidence of hip fracture.[46] In addition, the risk of renal calculi was increased. Given that fracture is the clinically significant endpoint of osteoporosis, there would seem little point in supplementing otherwise healthy postmenopausal women with calcium and vitamin D. On the other hand, it makes clinical sense to supplement the diets of elderly, mobile, institutionalized women with calcium and high-dose vitamin D in order to reduce their risk of hip fracture. This combination is widely available in both prescription and over-the-counter products around the world.

Hormone replacement therapy

Hormone replacement therapy is effective in preventing bone loss during and after the menopause and also in reducing the incidence of clinical vertebral and non-vertebral fractures. Protection against bone loss has also been reported in older postmenopausal women.[47] For many years, HRT was used as the first-line therapy for the prevention of postmenopausal osteoporosis, with its most beneficial effects seen when it was started early in the postmenopausal period. Newer drugs, such as bisphophonates, with a more robust evidence base, have largely superseded the use of HRT for this indication, and, in addition, recent large studies of HRT have forced the re-evaluation of its risk/benefit ratio, particularly with respect to breast cancer[48] and cardiovascular disease.[49] The Million Women Study[48] was a prospective cohort study of approximately 1 million women undergoing mammography. The incidence of breast cancer was rather higher in women using HRT than had been previously reported, but the study findings may have been confounded by factors relating to subject selection, surveillance bias, and incorrect treatment classification. Overall, HRT has probably had an unfairly negative press, and it remains a viable therapeutic option for some

women with osteoporosis, particularly those in their early menopausal years. Indeed, several articles have criticized the methodology of the Million Women Study, and thus many clinicians no longer hold the initial pronouncements as valid.[50,51] Older women with osteoporosis may also benefit from HRT, especially those with continuing menopausal symptoms, but clearly the risk/benefit ratio needs to be even more carefully considered in women over 60 years. For most women, the magnitude of the increase or decrease in absolute risk of diseases such as breast cancer and cardiovascular disease is small.[52]

Bisphosphonates and strontium ranelate

A number of therapeutic options, other than HRT, are presently available for the prevention of osteoporotic fracture in older women.[53] Of these, the bisphosphonates are the most commonly used and evidence shows that they reduce an individual's risk of fracture. When given daily for up to 5 years, the bisphosphonates reduce the risk of fracture in postmenopausal women with osteoporosis, and, in addition, the two worldwide approved bisphosphonates, alendronate and risedronate, reduce the risk of non-vertebral fractures, including those of the hip, as demonstrated by specifically designed randomized clinical trials.[54,55] Compliance has been a significant problem with the oral bisphosphonates, however, which, at the best of times, are absorbed poorly from the gut. They therefore have to be taken on an empty stomach, usually first thing in the morning, with a large glass of water. Dyspepsia is common, and in order to minimize this phenomenon, the individual must not lie down again after taking the drug. This can be a problem for many older people, and a significant number simply cannot tolerate oral bisphosphonates. This issue has been addressed somewhat by the fact that there are now bisphosphonates that can be taken weekly (alendronate and risedronate), and, more recently, a monthly bisphosphonate has come onto the market (ibandronate). In addition, bisphosphonates are available which can be administered intra-venously (pamidronate and zoledronate) and address both the problems of absorption and gastro-intestinal side effects. The drawbacks are that the patient has to come to hospital for the drug to be administered (although this is only once a year in the case of zoledronate), and the drugs tend to be costly.

A number of factors need to be taken into consideration when choosing between treatments. It is difficult to make direct comparisons between the various treatments, as no head-to-head studies with fracture as the primary endpoint have been conducted. However, one important considera-tion is whether a particular treatment has been shown to reduce fracture risk at both vertebral and non-vertebral sites, particularly the hip. Given that a fracture at any one site is an independent risk factor for further fractures at any other site, the ideal treatment should have proven efficacy against fracture at all commonly affected sites, particularly the spine and hip. Currently, only alendronate, risedronate, and strontium ranelate are approved for the prevention of vertebral and hip fractures. Whereas the bisphosphonates are antiresorptive, strontium is an anabolic agent, and appears to increase bone formation while, at the same time, decreasing bone resorption. Strontium has been shown to effectively reduce the incidence of both vertebral and non-vertebral fractures.[56,57] In the former study (the Spinal Osteoporosis Therapeutic Intervention trial), involving over 1600 post-menopausal women with osteoporosis, daily oral strontium ranelate in a dose of 2 g/day taken as a powder mixed with water was shown to reduce the risk of vertebral fractures by 49% at 1 year and 41% at 3 years. In the larger TROPOS (Treatment of Peripheral Osteoporosis) trial, strontium was shown, over 3 years, to reduce the relative risk for all non-vertebral fractures by 16%, and for the major fragility fractures (hip, wrist, pelvis and

sacrum, ribs and sternum, clavicle and humerus) by 19%. In a high-risk subgroup of women ≥74 years of age and femoral neck BMD T-score of ≤−3.0, the relative risk reduction for hip frac-ture was 36%. It would seem, therefore, that strontium may be a valuable therapeutic option in postmenopausal women, particularly in those who are intolerant of the bisphosphonates.

Raloxifene

The selective estrogen receptor modulators (SERMs), of which raloxifene is the only one used in routine clinical practice, exert selective agonist or antagonist effects in different estrogen target tis-sues. Clinical trials demonstrate that raloxifene can reduce the risk of vertebral fracture but have not yet unequivocally demonstrated an effect on non-vertebral fracture.[58] However, a continuation of the Multiple Outcomes of Raloxifene Evaluation (MORE) study has shown, in a post hoc analysis, a decreased risk of non-vertebral fracture in those with baseline prevalent vertebral fractures.[59] It is recommended, therefore, that raloxifene should be used mainly in postmenopausal women with milder osteoporosis as a preventive measure or for treatment in those with predominantly vertebral osteoporosis. It may also be useful as an alternative treatment in some women who are intolerant of bisphosphonates. There are drawbacks to ralox-ifene, however, the main one being that it may make menopausal symptoms worse, in particular hot flushes, and in some women may even initiate them.

Parathyroid hormone

No discussion regarding the pharmacological man-agement of osteoporosis and prevention of osteo-porotic fractures would be complete without the mention of parathyroid hormone (PTH). PTH, or teriparatide, significantly reduces the risk of vertebral and non-vertebral fractures.[60] This same study investigated the effect of PTH in post-menopausal women with osteoporosis, defined as having two or more moderate vertebral fractures or two or more mild vertebral fractures with T-score (spine or hip) <-1.0, or one mild fracture with T-score (spine or hip) <-1.0. In comparison with other treatments, PTH is costly, however, and at present is recommended primarily for the treatment of severe, treatment-resistant osteoporosis.

SUMMARY

The majority of osteoporotic fractures are sustained as the result of a fall, and elderly women are the group at greatest risk of falling. Fall prevention strategies should therefore play an important role in the prevention of osteoporotic fractures. Disorders of balance and gait are important risk factors for falling and are potentially remediable with exercise programs. Fracture risk is also dependent on bone strength, which itself is dependent not only on bone density but also on the amount of bone present as well as the microarchitecture of the bone. Of these, only bone density is readily measurable, usually with DEXA scanning. Population screening is generally not viable, and screening is therefore targeted towards 'at-risk' individuals. Individuals who have already sustained an osteoporotic fracture are at high risk of sustaining another. Secondary prevention of osteoporotic fracture aims to identify such individuals and treat them appropriately in order to prevent them suffering a further fracture. Treatment may be with a variety of pharmacological agents, of which the bisphosphonates are the most widely used. Hormone replacement therapy still has a role in the prevention of osteoporotic fracture in postmenopausal women for whom the risk/benefit ratio is favorable. Newer treatments, notably teriparatide, are reserved for postmenopausal women with severe osteoporosis.

REFERENCES

1. Murray CJL, Lopez AD, eds. The Global Burden of Disease, Vol. 1. Geneva: World Health Organization; 1996.
2. Roberts SE, Goldacre MJ. Time trends and demography of mortality after fractured neck of femur in an English population, 1968–98: database study. BMJ 2003; 327: 771–4.
3. van Staa TP, Dennison EM, Leufkens HG, Cooper C. Epidemiology of fractures in England and Wales. Bone 2001; 29: 517–22.
4. Youm T, Koval KR, Kummer FK, et al. Do all hip fractures result from a fall? Am J Orthop 1999; 28: 190–4.
5. Campbell AJ, Reinken J, Allan BC, Martinez GS. Falls in old age: a study of frequency and related clinical factors. Age Ageing 1981; 10: 262–70.
6. Prudham D, Evans JG. Factors associated with falls in the elderly: a community study. Age Ageing 1981; 10: 141–6.
7. Blake A, Morgan K, Bendall M, et al. Falls by elderly people at home – prevalence and associated factors. Age Ageing 1988; 17: 365–72.
8. Campbell AJ, Spears GF, Borrie MJ. Examination by logistic regression modelling of the variables which increase the relative risk of elderly women falling compared to elderly men. J Clin Epidemiol 1990; 43: 1415–20.
9. Winner SJ, Morgan CA, Evans JG. Perimenopausal risk of falling and incidence of distal forearm fracture. BMJ 1989; 298: 1486–8.
10. Oliver D, Hopper A, Seed P. Do hospital fall prevention programs work? A systematic review. J Am Geriatr Soc 2000; 48: 1679–89.
11. Lord SR, Sambrook PN, Gilbert C, et al. Postural stability, falls and fractures in the elderly: results from the Dubbo Osteoporosis Epidemiology Study. Med J Aust 1994; 160: 684–91.

12. Lord SR, Fitzpatrick RC. Choice stepping reaction time: a composite measure of falls risk in older people. J Gerontol 2001; 56: M627–32.

13. Tinetti ME, Speechley M, Ginter SF. Risk factors for falls among elderly persons living in the community. N Engl J Med 1988; 319: 1701–7.

14. Patel S, Tweed K, Chinappen U. Fall-related risk factors and osteoporosis in older women referred to an open access bone densitometry service. Age Ageing 2005; 34: 67–71.

15. Lui-Ambrose T, Eng JJ, Khan KM, et al. Older women with osteoporosis have increased postural sway and weaker quadriceps strength than counterparts with normal bone mass: overlooked determinants of fracture risk? J Gerontol A Biol Sci Med Sci 2003; 58: M862–6.

16. Robbins AS, Rubenstein LZ, Josephson KR, et al. Predictors of falls among elderly people. Results of two population-based studies. Arch Intern Med 1989; 149: 1628–33.

17. Tinetti ME, Doucette JT, Claus EB, Marottoli R. Risk factors for serious injury during falls by older persons in the community. J Am Geriatr Soc 1995; 43: 1214–21.

18. Salkeld G, Cameron ID, Cumming RG, et al. Quality of life related to fear of falling and hip fracture in older women: a time trade off study. BMJ 2000; 320: 341–5.

19. Oliver F, Daly FC, Martin FC, et al. Risk factors and risk assessment tools for falls in hospital in-patients: a systematic review. Age Ageing 2004; 33: 122–30.

20. NICE. Clinical practice guideline for the assessment and prevention of falls in older people. Nat Inst Clin Excell 2004. www.nice.org.uk/pdf/CG021publicinfoenglish.pdf

21. Drugs and Therapeutics Bulletin. Lifestyle advice for fracture prevention. Drugs Therapeut Bull 2002; 40: 83–6.

22. Panel on Falls Prevention. Guideline for the prevention of falls in older persons. J Am Geriatr Soc 2001; 49: 664–72.

23. Campbell AJ, Robertson MC, Gardner MM, et al. Falls prevention over 2 years: a randomised controlled trial in women 80 years and older. Age Ageing 1999; 28: 513–18.

24. Gillespie LD, Gillespie WJ, Cumming R, et al. Interventions for preventing falls in the elderly (Cochrane Review). In: The Cochrane Library 2000; Issue 3. Oxford: Update Software.

25. DOH. National Service Framework for older people. London: Department of Health; 2001.

26. Ensrud KE, Thompson DE, Cauley JA, et al. Prevalent vertebral deformities predict mortality and hospitalization in older women with low bone mass. Fracture Intervention Trial Research Group. J Am Geriatr Soc 2000; 48: 241–9.

27. Burger H, van Daele PL, Algra D, et al. Vertebral deformities as predictors of non-vertebral fractures. BMJ 1994; 309: 991–2.

28. Nevitt MC, Cummings SR. Type of fall and risk of hip and wrist fractures: the study of osteoporotic fractures. J Am Geriatr Soc 1993; 41: 1226–34.

29. de Laet CE, van Hout BA, Burger H, et al. Bone density and risk of hip fracture in men and women: cross sectional analysis. BMJ 1997; 315: 221–5.

30. Eddy DM, Johnston CC, Cummings SR, et al. Osteoporosis: cost-effectiveness analysis and review of the evidence for prevention, diagnosis and treatment. Osteoporosis Int 1997; Suppl 2: 1–72.

31. Porthouse J, Birks YF, Torgerson DJ, et al. Risk factors for fracture in a UK population: a prospective cohort study. Q J Med 2004; 97: 569–74.

32. Burger H, de Laet CDE, Weel A, et al. Added value of bone mineral density in hip fracture risk scores. Bone 1999; 25: 369–74.

33. Bouxsein M. Biomechanics of age-related fractures. In: Marcus R, Feldman D, Kelsey J, eds. Osteoporosis, 2nd edn. San Diego: Academic Press; 2001: 509–34.

34. Mayhew PM, Thomas CD, Clement JG, et al. Relation between age, femoral neck cortical stability, and hip fracture risk. Lancet 2005; 366: 129–35.

35. Epstein S, Inzerillo AM, Caminis J, Zaidi M. Disorders associated with acute rapid and

severe bone loss. J Bone Miner Res 2003; 18: 2083–94.

36. van der Klift M, de Laet CDE, Pols HAP. Assessment of fracture risk: Who should be treated for osteoporosis? Best Pract Res Clin Rheumatol 2005; 19: 937–50.

37. Van Staa TP, Leufkens HG, Cooper C. Use of inhaled corticosteroids and risk of fractures. J Bone Miner Res 2001; 16: 581–8.

38. Kroger H, Honkanen R, Saarikoski S, Alhava E. Decreased axial bone mineral density in peri-menopausal women with rheumatoid arthritis – a population based study. Ann Rheum Dis 1994; 53: 18–23.

39. Banciu M, Marza F, Ben Hadid R, et al. Recent findings on the role of physical exercise in osteoporosis. Osteoporosis Int 2005; 16: 187.

40. Ward KD, Klesges RC. A meta-analysis of the effects of cigarette smoking on bone mineral density. Calcif Tissue Int 2001; 68: 259–70.

41. Kiel DP, Barn JA, Anderson JJ, et al. Smoking eliminates the protective effect of oral estrogens on the risk for hip fracture among women. Ann Intern Med 1992; 116: 716–21.

42. Parker MJ, Gillespie WJ, Gillespie LD. Effectiveness of hip protectors for preventing hip fractures in elderly people: systematic review. BMJ 2006; 332: 571–3.

43. Chapuy MC, Arlot ME, Duboeuf F, et al. Vitamin D3 and calcium to prevent hip fractures in elderly women. N Engl J Med 1992; 327: 1637–42.

44. Boonen S, Bischoff-Ferrari HA, Cooper C, et al. Addressing the musculoskeletal components of fracture risk with calcium and vitamin D: a review of the evidence. Calcif Tissue Int 2006; 78: 257–70.

45. Porthouse J, Cockayne S, King C, et al. Randomised controlled trial of calcium and supplementation with cholecalciferol (vitamin D3) for prevention of fractures in primary care. BMJ 2005; 330: 1003–6.

46. Jackson RD, LaCroix AZ, Gass M, et al. Calcium plus vitamin D supplementation and the risk of fractures. N Engl J Med 2006; 354: 669–83.

47. Quigley ME, Martin PL, Burnier AM, Brooks P. Estrogen therapy arrests bone loss in elderly women. Am J Obstet Gynecol 1987; 156: 1516–23.

48. Million Women Study Collaborators. Breast cancer and hormone replacement therapy in the Million Women Study. Lancet 2003; 362: 419–27.

49. Rossouw JE, Anderson GL, Prentice RL, et al. Risks and benefits of estrogen plus progestin in healthy postmenopausal women: principal results from the Women's Health Initiative random-ized controlled trial. JAMA 2002; 288: 321–33.

50. Whitehead M, Farmer R. The million women study: a critique. Endocrine 2004; 24: 187–93.

51. Garton M. Breast cancer and hormone-replacement therapy: the Million Women Study. Lancet 2003; 362: 1328–31.

52. Pitkin J, Rees MC, Gray S, et al; British Menopause Society Council. Managing the menopause: British Menopause Society Council consensus statement on hormone replacement therapy. J Br Menopause Soc 2005; 11: 152–6.

53. Compston JE. Pharmacological interventions for post-menopausal osteoporosis: an evidence-based approach. Rheumatology (Oxford) 2000; 39: 1309–12.

54. Black DM, Thompson DE, Bauer DC, et al. Fracture risk reduction with alendronate in women with osteoporosis: the Fracture Intervention Trial. J Clin Endocrinol Metab 2000; 85: 4118–24.

55. Sorensen OH, Crawford GM, Mulder H, et al. Long-term efficacy of risedronate: a 5–year placebo-controlled clinical experience. Bone 2003; 32: 120–6.

56. Meunier PJ, Roux C, Seeman E, et al. The effects of strontium ranelate on the risk of ver-tebral fracture in women with postmenopausal osteoporosis. N Engl J Med 2004; 350: 459–68.

57. Reginster JY, Seeman E, Vernejoul MC, et al. Strontium ranelate reduces the risk of non-vertebral fractures in postmenopausal women with osteoporosis: TROPOS study. J Clin Endocrinol Metab 2005; 90: 2816–22.

58. Cranney A, Tugwell P, Zytaruk N, et al. Meta-analyses of therapies for postmenopausal osteoporosis. IV. Meta-analysis of raloxifene for

the prevention and treatment of postmenopausal osteoporosis. Endocrine Rev 2002; 23: 524–8.

59. Siris ES, Harris ST, Eastell R, et al. Skeletal effects of raloxifene after 8 years: results from the continuing outcomes relevant to Evista (CORE) study. J Bone Miner Res 2005; 20: 1514–24.

60. Neer RM, Arnaud CD, Zanchetta JR, et al. Effect of parathyroid hormone (1–34) on fractures and bone mineral density in postmenopausal women with osteoporosis. N Engl J Med 2001; 344: 1434–41.

Heart disease and stroke

4

Guy W Lloyd

INTRODUCTION

Heart disease and stroke ultimately kill more women than men. The gender difference lies in the disparate ages at which these conditions develop.[1] For men, heart disease, is a disease of middle age, with a steep rise in incidence begining in the sixth decade. Women, on the other hand, traditionally developed heart disease at older ages, the reasons for which remain obscure. This older age of presentation for women leads to a considerable distortion in the understanding of the disease process as well as its assessment and treatment, resulting in a poor representation of women in clinical trials of cardiac treatment and an underutilization of treatment strategies to improve the quality and increase the length of their lives. This chapter discusses specific issues relating to older women with coronary heart disease and cerebrovascular disease, assessment strategies, and responses to treatment.

EPIDEMIOLOGY OF HEART DISEASE AND STROKE

The vast majority (82%) of the total burden of cardiovascular disease in women occurs over the age of 75 years in comparison to 61% in men.[1] This difference largely results from the differences in coronary heart disease mortality and only to a lesser extent from stroke, where the gender advantage is less noticeable. As heart disease in women is a disease of the later years, the problems

of diagnosis and treatment are compounded by all the problems of physical and psychological comorbidity that go along with increasing age.

A steep decline in the age-standardized mortality for coronary disease amongst both men and women in Western Europe and the US has taken place over the past 35 years.[1,2] Although this phenomenon represents a major success of existing cardiac preventive policies, it has also shifted the burden of disease to an older age group. Some factors are less important in later years. For example, the clear gradient of coronary heart disease prevalence and socioeconomic status that is so striking in younger women (and men) is largely lost as the prevalence rises steeply in later life. Similarly, the presence of diabetes before the age of 75 neutralizes any female gender advantage.[1] In most contemporary cohorts, women with documented coronary disease are older and have significantly more comorbidities such as diabetes and hypertension than men; men, on the other hand, are more likely to be smokers. These measurable differences, as well as others that are harder to quantify such as social class and psychological factors, make the direct comparison of treatments for men and women difficult and prone to hidden bias.

CARDIAC RISK FACTORS

Women share the same cardiac risk factors as men, although the proportionate increase in directly attributable risk conferred by each factor varies. The factor that consistently confers the maximum additional risk is diabetes. Indeed, it is fair to say that the presence of either type I or II diabetes abolishes any female gender advantage.[3] As with men, various lipid and lipoprotein levels predict coronary disease, although the relative importance of each may vary. In men, total and low-density lipoprotein (LDL) cholesterol show a significantly stronger relationship with cardiovascular disease than they do in women, whereas in women a greater risk is associated with raised triglycerides. Characteristically, an elevated level increases risk by 30%.[4] On the other hand, the protective effect of an elevated high-density lipoprotein (HDL) cholesterol is observed in both sexes. Smoking more than trebles the lifetime risk of vascular disease, more so than in men. To make matters worse, smoking is not declining, especially in younger women.[5] Body fat distribution is as important in women as it is in men. Women appear to store fat in two ways: fat stored around the hips does not predict coronary disease, whereas that stored around the abdomen, and particularly intra-abdominal fat, confers a significant excess risk. This is likely to be related to a coexistent clustering of risk factors such as high circulating insulin, resistance to insulin, hypertension, and hypertriglyceridemia. This 'insulin resistant phenotype' per se confers an additional risk in women. Trials of lifestyle intervention in the form of a low-fat diet, such as the Women's Health Initiative, have shown no significant benefit for dietary modification on long-term cardiovascular risk.[6]

Social dominance and related factors are strong predictors of heart disease, particularly in younger women.[1] This combination may provide a theoretical link with sex hormones following the monkey model in which a recessive social status predicts both lower circulating estrogen levels and premature atherosclerosis.[7]

ASSESSING SYMPTOMS

Women present with a different symptom complex from coronary disease than do men, particularly in terms of acute coronary syndromes such as myocardial infarction (MI) and unstable angina.[8] A key difference appears to be the presence of a prodromal syndrome of fatigue, malaise, and breathlessness seen in women but not in men. Furthermore, women are 21% less likely to present with chest pain. This may be one reason why women are less frequently put forward for reperfusion procedures and why the time to diagnosis and treatment is characteristically longer.

Amongst women with stable angina the difference in symptoms between men and women is more controversial and the literature is divided on this point.[9] In the Euroheart study, women presenting with a suspected diagnosis of chest pain were less likely to undergo an exercise electrocardiogram (ECG) (odds ratio 0.81; 95% CI 0.69–0.95) and considerably less likely to be referred for coronary angiography (odds ratio 0.59; 95% CI 0.48–0.72).[10] Also, fewer women than men had significant coronary disease (defined as stenosis of ≥50% affecting one or more epicardial vessels) on angiography: 63% vs 87%.[10] However over 1 year in this study, just as many women as men suffered adverse coronary events and/or coronary death, suggesting an equal disease prevalence. But the investigational strategy resulted in only 21% of women being identified by angiography as having significant disease compared with 41% in men. This suggests that a significant proportion of women with early-stage or symptomatic disease might have been misdiagnosed by conventional modalities of assessment.

Investigating chest pain

One weakness of current strategies to detect coronary disease in women is that the cornerstone for the diagnosis of coronary disease remains the exercise test. However, most contemporary estimates put the sensitivity of the exercise ECG at no more that 60% for women.[11] The reasons for the poor performance of exercise testing are multiple. ECG ischemia only develops towards the end of the ischemic cascade (Figure 4.1), which begins early with inducible perfusion abnormalities, followed by wall motion abnormalities, and only finally by ECG abnormalities (see Figure 4.1). Therefore, in the ischemic patient, ST segment change is the last rather than an early sign. The investigation is highly dependent on pretest probability and performs poorly in those at low risk. As the probability of heart disease increases with age, fewer women are able to perform a satisfactory maximal exercise test, and the proportion of non-diagnostic investigations gets higher with age.[10] Furthermore. other factors may affect the performance of the exercise test; in particular, estrogen may affect the repolarization portion of the ECG in a similar way to digoxin, potentially resulting in a higher false-positive rate.[12]

The use of other imaging techniques, particularly myocardial perfusion imaging and stress echocardiography, significantly improves the detection of coronary disease and can help to reduce the need for coronary angiography,[13] but both modalities represent a significant change in the general approach to the investigation of coronary disease (Table 4.1). Both offer a superior sensitivity and specificity (with the possible exception of non-gated nuclear studies),[11] although both have their limitations. With myocardial perfusion imaging, the presence of breast and diaphragmatic attenuation can lead to erroneously positive scans, whereas stress echo is limited by window quality in some women. Both techniques remain influenced by pretest probability and therefore can result in false-positive and false-negative tests. The role of newer imaging techniques remains to be formally evaluated. Computed tomography (CT) scanning for coronary calcium[14] and non-invasive coronary angiography is also an increasingly important and available technique, and myocardial perfusion cardiac magnetic resonance imaging (MRI) offers many technical advantages over conventional nuclear techniques. Cardiac CT offers the potential of detecting early-stage disease, something poorly served by today's imaging technologies (Figure 4.2). It remains to be determined, however, whether this technology has significantly more to offer than current strategies.

BIOLOGICAL EFFECTS OF SEX HORMONES

The effects of endogenous estrogens remain the most favored explanation for the female gender advantage on three counts.

Table 4.1 The sensitivities of various non-invasive assessments for reversible myocardial ischemia

Technique	Sensitivity	Specificity
Stress ECG ($n = 3721$)	61%	70%
Stress echo ($n = 296$)	86%	79%
Nuclear (TI-201) ($n = 842$)	78%	64%
Nuclear (gated tech) ($n = 100$)	84%	94%

Reproduced from Kwok et al.[11]

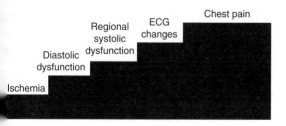

Figure 4.1 The ischemic cascade. A figurative representation of the development of myocardial ischemia with increasing myocardial oxygen demand during exercise or dynamic stress testing.

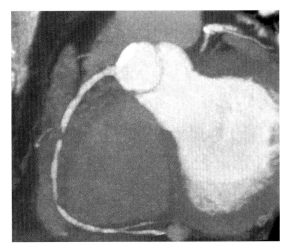

Figure 4.2 Computed tomography (CT) scan showing a functionally significant stenosis of the mid right coronary artery demonstrated by non-invasive CT coronary angiography using a standard 64-slice multislice CT scanner. (Courtesy of Dr Eric McWilliams.)

- The incidence of heart disease rises at around the time of menopause[15]
- estrogen and progestogens have a wealth of biological activities which ought to modulate cardiac risk
- replacement of the sex hormones at the menopause is associated with a lower subsequent heart attack risk.[16]

Although the acceptability and plausibility of this argument has been significantly undermined by more recent and robust findings from clinical trials, sex hormones nevertheless remain potent mediators of vascular function.

Lipids

Estrogen, regardless of whether oral, conjugated, or systemic, reduces LDL cholesterol and increases HDL cholesterol. The reduction in LDL cholesterol is of the order of 15%, whereas the increase in HDL cholesterol is between 4 and 5%.[17] Although these effects on cholesterol metabolism are clearly beneficial, unopposed oral estrogen also significantly raises triglyceride levels. Triglyceride level seem to predict a higher percentage increase in risk for women than it does for men.[4] Whereas the precise effects of the raised triglycerides remain obscure, it is likely that this increase brings about a reduction in the LDL particle size towards the more atherogenic small dense LDL phenotype. The particular effects on HDL and triglyceride can be significantly modified by the choice of progestogen.[18] The 19-carboxy steroids, typified by norethisterone acetate, have an androgenic effect on the lipid profile, reducing both HDL and triglycerides, whereas the 21-carboxy steroids, such a medroxyprogesterone, have less of an effect on lipids but seem to attenuate estrogen–derived vascular protection in experimental models of atherosclerosis. In contrast, parenteral estrogen, administered transdermally or subcutaneously, results in a much less obvious lipid modulation, because the liver does not receive the same supra-maximal doses as in oral treatment.[18]

Thrombosis

The effect of sex hormones on thrombosis is confusing. Sex hormones affect all levels of the coagulation and fibrinolytic cascade as well as, potentially, platelet function. A number of problems limit the usefulness of basic science in predicting in-vivo effects, however. The range of modulation encompasses both adverse reductions such as decreasing antithrombin III, as well as beneficial changes such as raising plasminogen activator inhibitor. These are but examples of the many and varied changes brought about by estrogen, and here again the choice of delivery route and progestin will effect any modulations.[19,20] It is therefore imperative to study the clinical data rather than focusing on individual segments of the coagulation cascade. In this instance, the message appears fairly clear from both observational cohorts and randomized trials. Overall, the risk of venous thromboembolism (and possible arterial embolism) is magnified by a factor of between 2 and 3 by taking oral estrogen.[21]

Other factors

There is a general acceptance of the proposition that damage to the vascular endothelium resulting in impaired nitric oxide release in response to various stimuli is one of the important pathogenic mechanisms in the development of atherosclerosis. Estrogen is well recognized as one agent (along with statins and some angiotensin-converting enzyme inhibitors) that can reverse this process, restoring endothelial function towards normal.[22] However, the importance of such a change in long-term vascular protection remains uncertain.

The other increasingly accepted pathogenic mechanism is that of local and systemic inflammation, as typified by a high level of C-reactive protein (CRP).[23] Whether CRP itself is pathological, or whether it represents a general increase in the systemic inflammatory response and hence increased cardiac risk, is unknown. Sex hormones elevate circulating CRP and this change may go some way to explaining the adverse event rates observed in some of the randomized trials.[24,25]

WHY DO WOMEN DEVELOP HEART DISEASE AND STROKE LATER IN LIFE?

The estrogen/menopause hypothesis

An enormous amount of time and resources have gone into exploring the observation that women are more likely to suffer from vascular disease after rather than before the menopause, and that women who take postmenopausal estrogen replacement are less likely to develop heart disease.

The flaw in most of the epidemiological evidence regarding the effect of menopause on the risk of heart disease is that it fails to take into account the exponential increase in the risk of heart disease, which occurs with time in both men and women, only later in women. Simply stated, around the age of 55 years, the maximum difference between men and women is observed, because men are already on the steep part of the exponential curve whereas women remain at a very low level. Once women also hit the steep portion, the difference between men and women rapidly declines, and this begins after the menopause. Furthermore, because increasing risk of heart disease is non-linear, in contrast to other comparators such as age, between the ages of 55 and 70 years small differences in age may account for quite large increases in cardiac risk. When incidence data are subjected to logarithmic transformation, thus rendering the exponential curve linear, no change in the rate of rise of heart disease is observed at or around the time of menopause. This 'steady state', as it were, can be directly compared to breast cancer, where the rate of rise declines as estrogen levels dwindle, thus providing the model of a hormone-sensitive disease[26] (Figure 4.3). Despite these facts, there are considerable data comparing aged-matched women before and after the menopause, demonstrating that postmenopausal women are more likely to have heart disease.[27] Dangers exist in these analyses, however, because the time of menopause has so many genetic and environmental components. Some causes of early menopause, such as smoking, which clearly would confound any association with coronary disease, are relatively easy to control for; others, such as social class, are infinitely more subtle.

Alternative hypotheses

As we live in the age of 'plan B', there has been considerable interest in the role of heavy metals in modulating cardiac risk. It is well accepted that women have relatively lower iron stores than men, as indicated by lower hemoglobin and

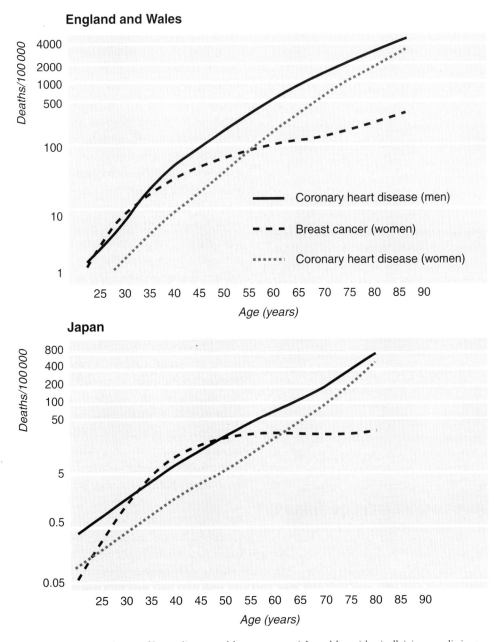

Figure 4.3 The rise in incidence of heart disease and breast cancer (plotted logarithmically) in two distinct population from the UK and Japan. (Reproduced with permission from Lawlor et al.[26])

ferritin values. Some evidence from the trans-fusion population where a relative iron deficiency is iatrogenically induced suggests that these patients have an appreciably lower cardiac risk. Furthermore, patients with higher oral iron intake appear to be at increased risk.[28,2] However, this finding has not been consistent in other similar investigations.[30]

Data from the Framingham Study suggest that women exhibiting type A behavior patterns are twice as likely as those with type B behaviors to develop heart disease, emphasizing the importance of psychological factors in mediating long-term risk.[31] One proposed explanation of the differential heart disease rates may relate to the traditionally different gender roles. A narrowing of the gender gap would be expected as gender roles become increasingly blurred, but this has yet to be observed. Finally, it may be that women, on average, demonstrate less risky behavior in particular with respect to diet and smoking habits, and this again may in part explain the differences.

HORMONE REPLACEMENT THERAPY AND THE RISK OF HEART DISEASE

The overwhelming body of observational evidence suggests that women who use postmenopausal hormone replacement therapy (HRT) have a lower risk of cardiovascular disease than those that do not. This remains true whether unopposed estrogen or estrogen and progestogen is used.[32,33] This, backed up by the biological plausibility of the cardioprotective effect of estrogen described above, presents a powerful rationale to use estrogen as a cardioprotective agent.

However, to date, randomized trials have not borne out this protective effect. There are now a number of well-conducted primary and secondary randomized trials of postmenopausal HRT and none have demonstrated an overall benefit. If anything a small adverse effect on heart disease and stroke has been observed[34–40] (Table 4.2). Studies have not been confined to a single form of HRT, and both opposed and unopposed estrogen have been examined. A tantalizing observation of the HERS study, also noted in patients with stroke in the WEST study, was a significant 'early risk' of events perhaps mediated through increased risk of thrombosis.[36,37,39] The question that remains unanswered is could the use of HRT at the menopause, long before any major atheroma is present and when the risk of events is very low, bring about a slow reduction in risk over many years through lipid risk factor modulation. This 'early risk/late benefit' model has some proponents from the randomized and observational Women's Health Initiative studies as well as the Nurse's Health Study.[41–44]

In women over 70 the main issue will be the secondary prevention of cardiovascular disease. The results of the randomized trials mean that

Table 4.2 The principal randomized trial results on the endpoints of stroke or myocardial infarction (MI)

Study acronym	HRT type	Target prevention population	Number	MI (% change in risk)	Stroke (% change in risk)
WHI[34]	CEE/MPA	Primary	16608	29%	41%
WHI (E)[35]	CEE	Primary	10739	−11%	39%
HERS[36]	CEE/MPA	Secondary	2763	−1%	NS
HERS II[37]	CEE/MPA	Secondary	2763	0%	NS
ESPRIT[38]	Estradiol valerate	Secondary	1017	0%	36%
WEST[39]	17-β estradiol, oral	Secondary	664	10%	0%
PHASE[40]	17-β estradiol, oral	Secondary	255	29%	NS

NS, not studied; CEE, conjugated equine estrogens; MPA, medroxyprogesterone acetate.

HRT can no longer be recommended at this age. Some women in their 70s may still have severe menopausal symptoms, however, and in such instances the benefits of HRT have to be balanced against the increased risk of cardiovascular disease.

Other hormonally active agents

Few long-term data with tibolone are available. Some studies have suggested an antianginal effect.[45,46] A prospective study evaluating carotid intimal medial thickness demonstrated enhanced atherosclerosis.[47] This drug has very different effects on the lipid profile because of its androgenic nature; in particular, HDL cholesterol is reduced, as are triglycerides. The effects on clotting factors are also generally in the opposite direction to those observed with estrogen; in particular, tibolone raises antithrombin III. Although tamoxifen is generally used for its antiestrogen properties, it is also an partial estrogen agonist or selective estrogen receptor modulator (SERM). Some data from randomized studies in breast cancer have suggested a reduction in heart disease risk,[48] although large cohort studies from the US have disputed this finding. Tamoxifen clearly increases the risk of venous thromboembolism, much like estrogen.[49] The only SERM to be evaluated in the context of a randomized controlled trial is raloxifene in the RUTH study in which no effect on cardiovascular risk was observed.[50]

TREATING CARDIOVASCULAR DISEASE

A bias against women is often proposed for the under-recognition and undertreatment of women with coronary heart disease. However, it is very difficult to ascertain whether this is a genuine bias against women or whether other factors such as the difference in age and the difference in probabilities of heart disease make the whole business of detection and treatment more complicated.

One factor that may influence presentation is a reluctance of women to consider cardiac disease to be a significant threat. Amongst female college students in the US, more than double the number of survey respondents considered cancer to be the prime cause of death amongst women, in sharp contrast to men, where nearly all respondents correctly identified heart disease.[51] Whereas this perceived risk is reasonably accurate for cancer, it greatly underestimates the risk from heart disease. The failure to perceive the threat of heart disease amongst women is true across all age groups, including women over 65.[52]

In addition to the pitfalls of diagnosing heart disease in women, physicians remain less likely to suspect coronary heart disease. This fact has been amply demonstrated using structured patients narratives relayed by actors of both genders; here, it was shown that women were 40% less likely to be put forward for coronary angiography despite identical stories.[53]

Clinical trials

A significant problem occurs when attempting to extrapolate the evidence base to women over 70 and that is that elderly women have been extensively and significantly under-represented in the clinical trial literature that guides current practice in cardiology. In a large meta-analysis of patients enrolled in 214 post-MI trials, only 20% were women. Moreover, over 60% of trials excluded persons over the age of 75 years. Studies with age-based exclusions had a smaller percentage of women compared with those without such exclusions (18% vs 23%).[54] Five percent of studies excluded women entirely. Similarly, and most strikingly in the statin studies up to 1999 for secondary prevention of heart disease, only 23% of the 31 683 participants were female and none were over age 75![55] In primary prevention studies, the findings were even more dramatic, with only 10% of studies enrolling women. Therefore, only in studies with no prespecified age exclusions or in trials conducted in the elderly do significant numbers of women become eligible. Even though the exclusion of women from trials calls into question whether the current evidence base can be generalized, it should not be used as an excuse for under-treatment, not treating women appropriately, or even withholding treatment.

Treatment outcomes in the elderly and in women

Revascularization

There has long been a suggestion that women are worse than men undergoing coronary revascularization strategies. In truth, surgical coronary revascularization becomes increasingly hazardous with increasing age, particularly over the age of 80 in both genders. As coronary disease of advancing age is more frequent in women than in men, this is an issue that significantly affects women. Despite this bias in opinion, the TIME study demonstrated that surgical revascularization in the elderly does not result in an excess mortality compared with medical treatment. Furthermore, the proportion of patients with improved symptoms was significantly higher in those treated surgically. Therefore, the interventions for revascularization of elderly men and women should be judged on a case-by-case basis, taking into consideration other comorbidities, especially diabetes, as well as the level of symptomatic impairment.[56]

Percutaneous coronary intervention

Most angioplasty cohorts demonstrate that women are older: the mean age is 60 and ≥65 in men and women, respectively. Studies of balloon angioplasty clearly demonstrate that, overall, women have a worse outcome at the time of the procedure, with a significantly higher in-hospital mortality.[57]

However, after correction for comorbid risk factors, there was less difference between the genders. Although age, diabetes, and hypertension are important, it appears that body surface area, a good marker for coronary artery size, is perhaps the most important predictor of mortality. Another difference is, that compared with men, is that a much higher proportion of women present for emergency rather than planned angioplasty, thus increasing the procedural risk. Long-term follow-up demonstrates that survival rates after angioplasty are similar after allowing for the difference in age. Similarly, clinical and angiographic restenosis with either angioplasty alone (Figure 4.4) or stenting is gender-independent.

The advent of intracoronary stenting appears to have diminished the importance of gender in predicting mortality. This probably reflects the large reduction in procedural complications. The impact of drug-eluting stents on the smaller-diameter arteries in women remains to be determined.

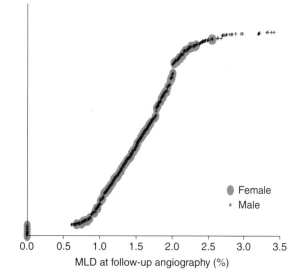

Figure 4.4 Cumulative distribution of minimum lumen diameter (MLD; representing the extent of coronary restenosis following simple balloon angioplasty) at 6-month follow-up angiography for men and women. (Unpublished data from the FLARE study.)

In one area in particular, women appear not to have benefited from coronary intervention, and that is as part of an early invasive strategy for acute coronary syndromes. Recent trials have established overall that in patients presenting with an acute coronary syndrome, i.e. unstable angina or a non-Q wave MI, an early aggressive revascularization strategy is more beneficial than the traditional wait-and-see approach. However, women have not benefited from such intervention and the reasons are unclear.[58] For example, women in the RITA 3 trials were older, and presented on average with less advanced disease. Under these circumstances, the potential benefits of intervention might be less. Interestingly, in the RITA study, virtually no women underwent bypass surgery as the revascularization strategy compared with men.[58] As most studies show a prognostic advantage of bypass over angioplasty, this may also have influenced the results. Nevertheless, in the absence of a purely female-based randomized controlled trial, the lack of benefit in women remains of an unclear etiology, and women should continue to be treated according to the overall results of the study.

Coronary bypass surgery

As with angioplasty, early reports suggested that women fared worse than men following bypass surgery, but here again this observation appears to be strongly related to the size of the coronary artery. Moreover, many of the original cohorts that demonstrated the mortality benefit of coronary surgery excluded both women as well as patients over 65; with such deficits, the evidence void in both these groups is obvious. Furthermore, with the increased use of multivessel stenting, the age at which coronary surgery is performed as well as the complexity of the underlying disease is increasing. Recent evidence suggests that with advanced surgical techniques, such as the extensive use of arterial conduits, the adverse effects of gender may now be of an historical nature.[59]

Outcome at the extremes of age

Scant data exist on intervention at the extremes of age. Data gleaned from large observational cohorts and synthesized into the risk scoring schemes for cardiac surgery consistently demonstrate that age over 80 increases surgical risks significantly. Nevertheless, the risks of surgery are sometimes overstated. For example, according to the logistic EuroSCORE for cardiac surgery, the combination of female gender and age 80 constitutes an operative mortality of just 5%.[60] The result using the alternative Parsonnet score is rather worse at 9%, but this is without allowing for any other comorbidities, which are significantly more prevalent in this age group. Less is known about percutaneous intervention due to the lack of a suitable risk model. The only randomized data from the TIME study demonstrated patients had improved quality of life but no difference in mortality at long-term follow-up for both coronary and valve surgery.[61]

Thrombolysis

Coronary thrombolysis is pivotal in the early treatment of acute MI in order to reduce subsequent mortality. A major body of literature demonstrates that women are less likely to receive thrombolytic therapy and more likely to receive it slowly. In a cohort of 1059 admissions with MI, women were less likely to receive thrombolysis, although total thrombolysis percentage in this study were low.[62] This lower rate of thrombolysis translated into a higher in-hospital mortality. Furthermore, women receive fewer other secondary prevention measures such as aspirin and beta blockade.[63]

Rehabilitation

It has been consistently demonstrated that women are less likely to attend cardiac rehabilitation.

Part of this appears to be a referral bias against women; however, the move towards automatic referral in recent years may have reduced this disparity. Two main reasons for this have been proposed: reticence in referral by clinicians and reduced attendance by women. Certainly there is more reticence amongst clinicians referring in for rehabilitation, but once women do attend they are equally likely to benefit.[65]

Other sequelae of vascular disease

The long-term sequelae of coronary disease, in particular, are not always fully appreciated, especially in the elderly. Depression is a very frequent comorbidity amongst survivors of MI, and there is a direct association between depressive symptoms and cardiovascular outcome.[66] Lack of recovery is often therefore inappropriately attributed to diminishing heart function, although the two are interrelated and the problem of undertreatment is only compounded by the perceived cardiotoxicity of some antidepressants. This perception is not accurate and, by and large, selective serotonin reuptake inhibitors (SSRIs) may be used safely and without undue risk of promoting arrhythmias.[67] Apart from depression, sexual function is often severely affected by the diagnosis of vascular disease. Although this becomes obvious in the male, female sexual dysfunction is more difficult to establish. A free and open discussion with an appropriately trained counsellor may often disclose unfounded fears about the dangers of sexual activity (see Chapter 16).

Stroke

A significant proportion of the burden of atherosclerosis in women is as a result of cerebrovascular disease rather than primary cardiovascular disease. This is often underappreciated and, as a result, women represent an undertreated population. As there is often a considerable overlap between the two entities, and stroke can be disabling and debilitating, most mortality in stroke survivors is due to MI. Men with high-grade carotid artery stenosis are at a considerably higher risk of a worse prognostic outcome than their female counterparts.[68] At the extreme of age, however, female gender predicts a doubling of the incidence of stroke, presumably as the male population has dwindled somewhat by this point.

Many of the demographic differences between men and women presenting with stroke are similar to those associated with coronary heart disease. In a larger European registry, women were nearly 5 years older than men, with a mean age of very nearly 75.[69] Furthermore, similar to MI, women had more diabetes and hypertension as well as atrial fibrillation. The presentation in women tends to be more severe, with a higher proportion of women experiencing coma, paralysis, and urinary incontinence. Carotid surgery was less likely to be performed in women. This may be in part because while 'rehabilitative' interventions such as speech therapy and physiotherapy were equally provided, investigations into the nature and cause of the event such as CT scanning, carotid ultrasound, and echocardiography were less frequently performed. The end result is that, even after correction for comorbidities, female gender predicts a higher long-term level of disability and handicap, although after correction mortality is gender-independent.

CONCLUSIONS

It is logical to ask what broad patient-centered inferences can be drawn from the evidence into how coronary disease affects women over 70? Most coronary disease in women will occur over the age of 65 and by age 75 there is very little difference in incidence between men and women. The reason for this remains obscure, and previous assumptions about the protective effects of sex hormones can no longer be accepted with a high degree of confidence. The simple truth is that women and healthcare professionals are unwilling to ascribe symptoms to coronary heart disease and therefore less likely to either present or refer for onward investigation and treatment. This circumstance is not helped by the non-standard presentation of women, particularly those with acute presentations that may lead to misleading diagnoses. Women with or at risk of heart disease benefit from preventive medicine such as blood pressure and lipid control to an equal extent as their male counterparts and therefore, vascular disease in women should be treated aggressively.

Remembering that as the absolute risk of cardiac events rises, then the attributable benefits of treatment also increase. Women are not more 'fragile' than men and should not be discriminated against for either revascularization or reperfusion therapies.

The time for excuses about the difficulties of diagnosis and treatment of women with established and suspected heart disease has passed, and what is needed on an urgent basis is a new 'gender-specific' way of thinking about cardiovascular disease, from prevention to bypass and everything in between.

REFERENCES

1. British Heart Foundation: www.bhf.org.uk.
2. American Heart Association: www.americanheart.org.
3. Kannel WB, McGee DL. Diabetes and glucose tolerance as risk factors for cardiovascular disease: the Framingham study. Diabetes Care 1979; 2(2): 120–6.
4. Austin M, Hokanson J, Edwards K. Hypertriglyceridemia as a cardiovascular risk factor. Am J Cardiol 1998; 81(4A): 7B–12B.
5. Njolstad I, Arnesen E, Lund-Larsen P. Smoking, serum lipids, blood pressure and sex differences in myocardial infarction. Circulation 1996; 92: 450–6.
6. Howard BV, Van Horn L, Hsia J, et al. Low-fat dietary pattern and risk of cardiovascular disease: the Women's Health Initiative Randomized Controlled Dietary Modification Trial. JAMA 2006; 295: 655–66.
7. Kaplan JR, Adams MR, Anthony MS, et al. Dominant social status and contraceptive hormone treatment inhibit atherogenesis in premenopausal monkeys. Arterioscler Thromb Vasc Biol 1995; 15(12): 2094–100.
8. McSweeney JC, Cody M, O'Sullivan P, et al. Women's early warning symptoms of acute myocardial infarction. Circulation 2003; 108(21): 2619–23.
9. Wu EB, Hodson F, Chambers JB. A simple score for predicting coronary artery disease in patients with chest pain. QJM 2005; 98(11): 803–11.
10. Daly C, Clemens F, Lopez Sendon JL. Gender differences in the management and clinical outcome of stable angina. Circulation 2006; 113: 490–8.
11. Kwok Y, Kim C, Grady D, Segal M, Redberg R. Meta-analysis of exercise testing to detect coronary artery disease in women. Am J Cardiol 1999; 83(5): 660–6.
12. Sketch M, Mohiuddin S, Lynch J, Zencka A, Runco V. Significant sex differences in the correlation of electrocardiographic exercise testing and coronary arteriograms. Am J Cardiol 1975; 36: 169–74.
13. Ho YL, Wu CC, Huang PJ, et al. Assessment of coronary artery disease in women by dobutamine stress echocardiography: comparison with stress thallium-201 single-photon emission computed tomography and exercise electrocardiography. Am Heart J 1998; 135(4): 655–62.
14. Funabashi N, Misumi K, Ohnishi H, Asano M, Komuro I. Clinical value of MDCT in the diagnosis of coronary artery disease in patients with a low pretest likelihood of significant disease. AJR Am J Roentgenol 2006; 186(6) 1659–68.

15. Lerner D, Kannel W. Patterns of coronary heart disease morbidity and mortality in the sexes: a 26 year follow-up of the Framingham population. Am Heart J 1986; 111: 383–90.

16. Effects of estrogen or estrogen/progestin regimens on heart disease risk factors in postmenopausal women. The Postmenopausal Estrogen/Progestin Interventions (PEPI) Trial. The Writing Group for the PEPI Trial. JAMA 1995; 273: 199–208.

17. Walsh BW, Schiff I, Rosner B, et al. Effects of postmenopausal estrogen replacement on the concentrations and metabolism of plasma lipoproteins. N Engl J Med 1991; 325(17): 1196–204.

18. Godsland IF. Effects of postmenopausal hormone replacement therapy on lipid, lipoprotein, and apolipoprotein (a) concentrations: analysis of studies published from 1974–2000. Fertil Steril 2001; 75(5): 898–915.

19. Koh Koh K, Mincemoyer R, Bui M, et al. Effects of hormone replacement therapy on fibrinolysis in postmenopausal women. N Engl J Med 1997; 336: 683–90.

20. Bonduki C, Lourenco D, Baracat E, et al. Effects of estrogen-progestin hormonal replacement therapy on plasma antithrombin III of postmenopausal women. Acta Obstet Gynecol Scand 1998; 77: 330–3.

21. Cushman M, Kuller LH, Prentice R, et al. Women's Health Initiative Investigators. Estrogen plus progestin and risk of venous thrombosis. JAMA 2004; 292: 1573–80.

22. Collins P, Rosano G, Sarrel P, et al. 17 beta-estradiol attenuates acetylcholine-induced coronary arterial constriction in women but not men with coronary artery disease. Circulation 1995; 92(1): 24–30.

23. Ridker PM, Hennekens CH, Buring JE, Rifai N. C-reactive protein and other markers of inflammation in the prediction of cardiovascular disease in women. N Engl J Med 2000; 342: 836–43.

24. Cushman M, Legault C, Barrett-Connor E, et al. Effect of postmenopausal hormones on inflammation-sensitive proteins: the Postmenopausal Estrogen/Progestin Interventions (PEPI) Study. Circulation 1999; 100: 717–22.

25. Pradhan AD, Manson JE, Rossouw JE, et al. Inflammatory biomarkers, hormone replacement therapy, and incident coronary heart disease: prospective analysis from the Women's Health Initiative observational study. JAMA 2002; 288: 980–7.

26. Lawlor DA, Ebrahim S, Davey Smith G. Role of endogenous oestrogen in aetiology of coronary heart disease: analysis of age related trends in coronary heart disease and breast cancer in England and Wales and Japan. BMJ 2002; 325: 311–12.

27. Gordon T, Kannel WB, Hjortland MC, McNamara PM. Menopause and coronary heart disease. The Framingham Study. Ann Intern Med 1978; 89(2): 157–61.

28. Tuomainen TP, Punnonen K, Nyyssonen K, Salonen JT. Association between body iron stores and the risk of acute myocardial infarction in men. Circulation 1998; 97(15): 1461–6.

29. Tzonou A, Lagiou P, Trichopoulou A, Tsoutsos V, Trichopoulos D. Dietary iron and coronary heart disease risk: a study from Greece. Am J Epidemiol 1998; 147(2): 161–6.

30. Liao Y, Cooper RS, McGee DL. Iron status and coronary heart disease: negative findings from the NHANES I epidemiologic follow-up study. Am J Epidemiol 1994; 139(7): 704–12.

31. Haynes SG, Feinleib M, Kannel WB. The relationship of psychosocial factors to coronary heart disease in the Framingham Study. III. Eight-year incidence of coronary heart disease. Am J Epidemiol 1980; 111(1): 37–58.

32. Stampfer MJ, Colditz GA. Estrogen replacement therapy and coronary heart disease: a quantitative assessment of the epidemiologic evidence. Prev Med 1991; 20: 47–63.

33. Grodstein F, Stampfer M, Manson J, et al. Postmenopausal estrogen and progestin use and the risk of cardiovascular disease. N Engl J Med 1996; 335: 453–61.

34. Rossouw JE, Anderson GL, Prentice RL. Risks and benefits of estrogen plus progestin in healthy postmenopausal women: principal results. From the Women's Health Initiative randomized controlled trial. JAMA 2002; 288(3): 321–33.

35. The Women's Health Initiative Steering Committee. Effects of conjugated equine estrogen

in postmenopausal women with hysterectomy: the Women's Health Initiative randomized controlled trial. JAMA 2004; 291: 1701–12.

36. Hulley S, Grady D, Bush T, et al. Randomized trial of estrogen plus progestin for secondary prevention of coronary heart disease in post-menopausal women. Heart and Estrogen/progestin Replacement Study research group. JAMA 1998; 280(7): 605–13.

37. Grady D, Herrington D, Bittner V, et al. HERS Research Group. Cardiovascular disease outcomes during 6.8 years of hormone therapy: Heart and Estrogen/progestin Replacement Study follow-up (HERS II). JAMA 2002; 288(1): 49–57.

38. Cherry N, Gilmour K, Hannaford P, et al. ESPRIT team. Oestrogen therapy for prevention of reinfarction in postmenopausal women: a randomised placebo controlled trial. Lancet 2002; 360(9350): 2001–8.

39. Viscoli CM, Brass LM, Kernan WN, et al. A clinical trial of estrogen-replacement therapy after ischemic stroke. N Engl J Med 2001; 345(17): 1243–9.

40. Clarke SC, Kelleher J, Lloyd-Jones H, Slack M, Schofield PM. A study of hormone replacement therapy in postmenopausal women with ischaemic heart disease: the Papworth HRT atherosclerosis study. BJOG 2002; 109(9): 1056–62.

41. Manson JE, Hsia J, Johnson KC, et al. Women's Health Initiative Investigators. Estrogen plus progestin and the risk of coronary heart disease. N Engl J Med 2003; 349: 523–34.

42. Hsai J, Langer RD, Manson JE, et al. Conjugated equine estrogens and coronary heart disease. Arch Intern Med 2006; 166: 357–65.

43. Grodstein F, Manson JE, Stampfer MJ. Hormone therapy and coronary heart disease: the role of time since menopause and age at hormone initiation. J Women's Health 2006; 15: 35–44.

44. Prentice RL, Langer RD, Stefanick ML, et al. Combined analysis of Women's Health Initiative observational and clinical trial data on post-menopausal hormone treatment and cardiovascular disease. Am J Epidemiol 2006; 163: 589–99.

45. Lloyd G, Patel N, McGing E, et al. Acute effects of hormone replacement with tibolone on myocardial ischaemia in women with angina. Int J Clin Pract 1998; 52: 155–7.

46. Campisi R, Camilletti J, Mele A, et al. Tibolone improves myocardial perfusion in postmenopausal women with ischemic heart disease: an open-label exploratory pilot study. J Am Coll Cardiol 2006; 47(3): 559–64.

47. Bots ML, Evans GW, Riley W, et al. OPAL Investigators. The effect of tibolone and continuous combined conjugated equine oestrogens plus medroxyprogesterone acetate on progression of carotid intima-media thickness: the Osteoporosis Prevention and Arterial effects of tiboLone (OPAL) study. Eur Heart J 2006; 27(6): 746–55.

48. Rutqvist LE, Mattsson A. Cardiac and thromboembolic morbidity among postmenopausal women with early-stage breast cancer in a randomized trial of adjuvant tamoxifen. The Stockholm Breast Cancer Study Group. J Natl Cancer Inst 1993; 85: 1398–406.

49. Costantino J, Kuller L, Ives D, Fisher B, Dignam J. Coronary heart disease mortality and adjuvant tamoxifen therapy. J Natl Cancer Inst 1997; 89: 776–82.

50. Barrett-Connor E, Mosca L, Collins P, et al. Raloxifene Use for The Heart (RUTH) Trial Investigators. Effects of raloxifene on cardiovascular events and breast cancer in postmenopausal women. N Engl J Med 2006; 355(2): 125–37.

51. Collins KM, Dantico M, Shearer NB, Mossman KL. Heart disease awareness among college students. J Community Health 2004; 29(5): 405–20.

52. Mosca L, Jones WK, King KB, et al. Awareness, perception, and knowledge of heart disease risk and prevention among women in the United States. American Heart Association Women's Heart Disease and Stroke Campaign Task Force. Arch Fam Med 2000; 9(6): 506–15.

53. Sculman K, Berlin J, Harless W, et al. The effect of race and sex on physicians' recommendations for cardiac catheterization. N Engl J Med 1999; 340: 618–26.

54. Gurwitz JH, Col NF, Avorn J. The exclusion of the elderly and women from clinical trials in acute myocardial infarction. JAMA 1992; 268(11): 1417–22.

55. Bandyopadhyay S, Bayer AJ, O'Mahony MS. Age and gender bias in statin trials. QJM 2001; 94(3): 127–32.

56. TIME Investigators. Trial of invasive versus medical therapy in elderly patients with chronic symptomatic coronary-artery disease (TIME): a randomised trial. Lancet 2001; 358(9286): 951–7.

57. Kelsey SF, James M, Holubkov AL, et al. Results of percutaneous transluminal coronary angioplasty in women. 1985–1986 National Heart, Lung, and Blood Institute's Coronary Angioplasty Registry. Circulation 1993; 87(3): 720–7.

58. Clayton TC, Pocock SJ, Henderson RA, et al. Do men benefit more than women from an interventional strategy in patients with unstable angina or non-ST-elevation myocardial infarction? The impact of gender in the RITA 3 trial. Eur Heart J 2004; 25(18): 1641–50.

59. Guru V, Fremes SE, Austin PC, Blackstone EH, Tu JV. Gender differences in outcomes after hospital discharge from coronary artery bypass grafting. Circulation 2006; 113(4): 507–16.

60. Roques F, Michel P, Goldstone AR, Nashef SA. The logistic EuroSCORE. Eur Heart J 2003; 24(9): 882–3.

61. Pfisterer M; Trial of Invasive versus Medical therapy in Elderly patients Investigators. Long-term outcome in elderly patients with chronic angina managed invasively versus by optimized medical therapy: four-year follow-up of the randomized Trial of Invasive versus Medical therapy in Elderly patients (TIME). Circulation 2004; 110(10): 1213–18.

62. Mahon N, McKenna C, Codd M, et al. Gender differences in the management and outcome of acute myocardial infarction in unselected patients in the thrombolytic era. Am J Cardiol 2000; 85: 921–6.

63. Gottlieb S, Harpaz D, Shotan A, et al. Sex differences in management and outcome after acute myocardial infarction in the 1990s: a prospective observational community-based study. Israeli Thrombolytic Survey Group. Circulation 2000; 102(20): 2484–90.

64. Rees K, Victory J, Beswick AD, et al. Cardiac rehabilitation in the UK: uptake among under-represented groups. Heart 2005; 91(3): 375–6.

65. Balady GJ, Jette D, Scheer J, Downing J. Changes in exercise capacity following cardiac rehabilitation in patients stratified according to age and gender. Results of the Massachusetts Association of Cardiovascular and Pulmonary Rehabilitation Multicenter Database. J Cardiopulm Rehabil 1996; 16(1): 38–46.

66. de Jonge P, Ormel J, van den Brink RH, et al. Symptom dimensions of depression following myocardial infarction and their relationship with somatic health status and cardiovascular prognosis. Am J Psychiatry 2006; 163(1): 138–44.

67. Glassman AH, O'Connor CM, Califf RM, et al. Sertraline Antidepressant Heart Attack Randomized Trial (SADHEART) Group. Sertraline treatment of major depression in patients with acute MI or unstable angina. JAMA 2002; 288(6): 701–9.

68. Dick P, Sherif C, Sabeti S, et al. Gender differences in outcome of conservatively treated patients with asymptomatic high grade carotid stenosis. Stroke 2005; 36(6): 1178–83.

69. Di Carlo A, Lamassa M, Baldereschi M, et al; European BIOMED Study of Stroke Care Group. Sex differences in the clinical presentation, resource use, and 3-month outcome of acute stroke in Europe: data from a multicenter multinational hospital-based registry. Stroke 2003; 34(5): 1114–19.

Dementia, capacity, and consent

5

Susan Welsh and Thomas R Dening

INTRODUCTION

Dementia is a disease of the brain, usually chronic or progressive in nature, with disturbances of 'multiple higher cortical functions including impairments in memory, thinking, orientation, comprehension, calculation, learning capacity, language and judgement.'[1] As it occurs predominantly in later life, it is a condition that will commonly affect women over 70; either the woman herself may have dementia or she may be a carer for someone with the disease (as a partner, friend, or relative).

This chapter covers the epidemiology, clinical features, and treatment of dementia, as well as providing guidance about issues of capacity and consent.

EPIDEMIOLOGY

Prevalence rates for dementia vary between studies, but approximately 3–5% of people aged ≥65 years old are affected,[2,3] rising exponentially with age. After 65, prevalence figures double approximately every 5 years, with incidence rates rising with age, particularly above the age of 75 years, from 7.4 per 1000 person years at age 65–69 to 84.9 per 1000 person years at age 85 and above.[4]

Given the extent of aging within the global population, the number of cases worldwide will increase dramatically, both in developed countries

(from 12 to 20 million between 2000 and 2050) and even more so in developing countries (from 13 to 84 million over the same period).[5] By 2025, around 75% of the estimated 1200 million individuals aged 60 and over will be living in developing countries.[6] These individuals will also be affected by high rates of comorbid physical and mental health problems, especially heart disease, diabetes, and depression. A considerable body of research exists in this area, including that of the 10/66 Dementia Research Group, which was established to encourage good-quality research into dementia.[7] Several developing nations have collaborated and research centers have been established in India, China, South East Asia, Latin America, the Caribbean, and Africa, to provide information about aspects of dementia across the globe, including its differential impact on women. Differences in prevalence rates between and within countries, however, can only be interpreted with confidence if assessment procedures are standardized and are culturally sensitive.

Even in developed countries, little systematic effort exists to identify cases of dementia, and the prevalence of cognitive impairment is often underestimated by general practitioners (GPs). In one study, UK GPs had identified only 58% of cases of dementia within their practices, and only 20% of these were known to local psychiatrists.[8]

CLINICAL FEATURES

Textbook definitions of dementia describe its effect on higher cortical functions as detailed in the Introduction, but in order to make a diagnosis of dementia, changes in emotional and social functioning are also required. Additionally, deteriorations in activities of daily living (ADLs), such as washing, dressing, eating, personal hygiene, and continence are required. Disturbances of consciousness are generally said to be absent, in order to distinguish the disorder from delirium. Nonetheless, states of altered consciousness do occur in some forms of dementia: e.g. vascular dementia and dementia with Lewy bodies. Dementia usually has a progressive course, although some patients remain stable without significant decline, often for several years. In clinical settings, a certain degree of flexibility is essential for diagnosis.

The commonest subtypes of dementia are Alzheimer's disease (the most important), vascular dementia, dementia with Lewy bodies, and several focal disorders, including frontotemporal dementia. Additionally, rarer conditions such as Pick's disease, Huntington's disease, human immunodeficiency virus (HIV), and Creutzfeldt–Jakob disease (CJD) may also cause dementia.[1]

Alzheimer's disease

Alzheimer's disease is the most common form of dementia, affecting approximately 50–70% of cases.[9] In 1907 Alzheimer reported the case of Auguste D, a 51-year-old woman with progressive cognitive impairment, delusions, and hallucinations,[10] and Kraepelin gave the disease its eponymous title 3 years later.[11]

The original autopsy findings revealed what are today recognized as the classical histological features: i.e. intracellular amyloid plaques and extracellular neurofibrillary tangles.[10] Modern work has demonstrated that reduced temporoparietal and hippocampal cortical activity of choline acetyltransferase are the principal neurochemical

findings, and these changes correlate with loss of cholinergic neurons in the nucleus basalis of Meynert.[12] Loss of locus coeruleus noradrenergic neurons and dorsal raphe serotonergic neurons has also been reported.[13]

Alzheimer's disease typically follows an insidious course, with memory impairment usually the first recognizable change, followed by a gradual decline in important ADLs, including self-care, shopping, food preparation, and management of household finances. Subsequently, disorders of speech and language (dysphasia) are seen, along with dyspraxias and agnosias. Eventually the person may become immobile and incontinent, requiring considerable help with personal care.

The two main international classification systems, International Classification of Diseases (ICD, 10th edition)[1] and the Diagnostic and Statistical Manual (DSM, 4th edition),[14] provide broadly similar diagnostic criteria. For research purposes, the National Institute of Neurologic, Communicative Disorders and Stroke – Alzheimer's Disease and Related Disorders Association (NINCDS-ADRDA)[15] criteria are the most extensively used.

Vascular dementia

Cerebrovascular disease is common and is often found alongside other pathology such as Alzheimer's disease. Vascular disease alone accounts for approximately 20%[16] of dementia cases. Furthermore, some degree of vascular pathology is found in approximately 40% of autopsy cases of dementia,[17] mirroring clinical experience of diagnostic overlap with Alzheimer's disease in many individuals.

Vascular dementia (VaD) presents a similar clinical picture to other forms of dementia, but a more abrupt, stepwise course is allegedly more typical of vascular pathology. Insight also tends to be better preserved, as are personality and episodic memory, compared with Alzheimer's disease. Disease of large vessels may be evidenced by focal lesions affecting motor and sensory tracts, such as exaggerated deep tendon reflexes, focal neurological weakness or rigidity. However, diffuse small-vessel disease is more often significant, producing lacunar infarcts and white matter changes. As a result, the clinical picture has more 'subcortical' features than Alzheimer's disease, including depressed mood, somatic complaints, and 'patchiness' of cognitive deficits along with generalized slowness, parkinsonian features, and emotional changes (apathy and/or emotional lability). Features of a dysexecutive syndrome, i.e. problems with initiation of tasks, poor planning, organizing, sequencing, set-shifting, abstracting, and attentional impairments, are common.

The most widely used diagnostic criteria are those of the National Institute of Neurologic Disorders and Stroke and the Association Internationale pour la Recherche et l'Enseignement en Neurosciences (NINDS-AIREN).[18]

Dementia with Lewy bodies

Dementia with Lewy bodies (DLB) has risen to prominence in recent years, with prevalence estimates of approximately 15%[16] of cases of dementia. It is characterized by a clinical syndrome of fluctuating, often rapidly progressive, cognitive impairment, visual hallucinations, and parkinsonian symptoms. Falls and visuospatial impairments are also common. Consensus criteria for diagnosis are available, based on the three main features listed above.[19] Brainstem or cortical Lewy bodies are considered essential for pathological diagnosis, although the majority of DLB cases (75%) also exhibit amyloid plaques, a pathological feature more commonly associated with Alzheimer's disease.[20] The relationship of Parkinson's disease and DLB reflects a common molecular pathology, i.e. the presence of Lewy bodies. In practice, the differential diagnosis between Parkinson's disease dementia and DLB is made upon the basis of whether the motor or the cognitive symptoms appear first. Visual hallucinations

are more indicative of DLB if they arise in the early stages of the dementia.[21]

Alongside the extrapyramidal disturbance, patients may be very sensitive to the side effects of antipsychotic drugs, which must be used with caution in any patient with dementia, but especially in DLB. However, DLB often responds well to treatment with acetylcholinesterase inhibitors (see below).

Frontotemporal dementia

The prevalence of frontotemporal dementia (FTD) almost equals that of Alzheimer's disease in the 45–64 age group,[22] with predominant pathology affecting either the frontal lobes or temporal lobes (latter known as semantic dementia). Frontotemporal dementia is a mixed group of disorders, including some with classical pathology of Pick's disease and others with symptoms of motor neuron disease. Clinically, the picture is influenced by whether frontal or temporal areas are mainly affected, the frontal variant presenting with behavioral changes, and temporal disease affecting semantic memory and producing progressive aphasia. In FTD there is no cholinergic deficit, but serotonin receptors are lost from the frontal and temporal cortices. The Lund–Manchester criteria for diagnosis claims to differentiate 100% of FTD and Alzheimer's disease patients.[23]

Summary characteristics of the commonest dementia subtypes in women over 70 are given in Table 5.1.

Mild cognitive impairment

Identifying individuals at risk of developing dementia in the early stages is obviously important, as this offers opportunities for early treatment or even prevention. Various terms have been used for the pre-dementia state, of which mild cognitive impairment (MCI) is currently the most favored. The criterion for MCI is memory impairment that

63

Table 5.1 Clinical features of dementia

	Percentage cause of cases of dementia	Course	Features
Alzheimer's disease	50–70	Insidious	Memory decline Decline in ADLs Dysphasias Dyspraxias Agnosias Immobility/incontinence (at terminal stage)
Vascular dementia	20	Can be abrupt and stepwise	Depression Somatic complaints Generalized slowness 'Patchy' cognitive deficits Dysexecutive syndrome
Dementia with Lewy bodies	15	Fluctuating Often rapidly progressive	Cognitive impairment Visual hallucinations Parkinsonian symptoms Falls

ADL, activity of daily living.

falls short of a diagnosis of dementia, although debate continues as to its boundaries with the memory changes of 'normal' aging. Individuals who have MCI have an increased risk of developing dementia, and Petersen's proposal, that MCI is the 'earliest point in the cognitive decline'[24] of someone destined to develop Alzheimer's disease, finds support in a number of recent studies that show deficits in verbal recall which precede a clinical diagnosis by 6 years.[25]

ASSESSMENT

Medical aspects

The essential elements of a preliminary clinical assessment of memory impairment are shown in Table 5.2. Because of the nature of dementia, it is important to obtain collateral history from an informant who knows the patient well.

Several medical conditions may cause cognitive impairment, including vascular, endocrine, neurodegenerative, vitamin deficiencies, systemic disease, neurological disorders, infection, and alcohol/drug misuse. Therefore, it is particularly important to exclude these in any woman over 70 with suspected dementia, using the investigations listed in Table 5.2, although in practice truly reversible dementia is rare.

An important diagnostic difficulty lies in differentiating dementia from delirium, although the two can coexist. Commonly a patient will present with features of delirium superimposed on a preexisting dementia. Respiratory tract and urinary tract infections (especially in women) and iatrogenic (medication) problems are the commonest causes of delirium.

Depression is the commonest reversible cause of cognitive impairment (see Chapter 6). It is also a common comorbid condition, with up to 20%

Table 5.2 Clinical and laboratory assessment of memory impairment

---

History of presenting complaint

Systems review
Psychiatric history
Medication history
Substance use/abuse
Family history
Past medical history
Collateral history from an informant
Mental state examination

Physical examination (including neurological examination)

Blood tests – full blood count, urea and
electrolytes, liver function tests, glucose,
vitamin B_{12} and folate (to exclude pernicious anaemia),
thyroid function tests (to exclude hypothyroidism),
erythrocyte sedimentation rate, calcium, and cholesterol
CT scan/MRI (to exclude space-occupying lesion,
normal pressure hydrocephalus, subdural hematoma)
Syphilis serology – as indicated
ECG – as indicated

---

of individuals with dementia showing significant depressive symptoms.[26] Indeed, diffuse microvascular pathology may predispose to both cognitive impairment and depression.[27] Thus, the overlap between depression and cognitive impairment is a complex issue. For example, it is well established that depression affects motivation and attention, but growing evidence also points to neuropsychological deficits that may be specific to patients with first episode late-life depression and which persist after the resolution of the depressive symptoms.[28] Pseudodementia is a term used to describe the reversible forms of cognitive impairment, most commonly applied to depression.

Neuropsychological assessment

Neuropsychological assessment serves as a diagnostic aid, and provides a profile of a patient's performance, demonstrating specific domains of impairment as well as relative sparing. This assists in appropriate diagnosis and management and is a useful means of evaluating treatment efficacy. Several different batteries of tests are available, of which the Mini-Mental State Examination (MMSE)[29] is the most widely used in clinical settings. This 10-minute bedside screening instrument provides a global index of cognitive impairment and needs to be supplemented by other information. The cut-off between normal and pathological is 23 or 24 out of a total score of 30.

The MMSE unfortunately demonstrates poor sensitivity to very mild dementia and, moreover, is also highly influenced by premorbid educational achievement, comorbid psychiatric conditions, and motivation. In a community study, 86% of individuals with dementia scored ≤23, with 92% of 'normals' scoring ≥24.[30] As a screening measure for dementia in general, it is more heavily weighted towards episodic memory (which is more impaired in Alzheimer's disease), than towards tests of frontal executive function, which are more suggestive of vascular dementia or FTD.

More comprehensive testing requires more detailed assessment tools, including the Cambridge Cognitive Examination (CAMCOG)[31] which covers seven areas of cognitive function, including orientation, language, memory, attention, calculation, praxis, abstract thinking and perception, or the Clinical Dementia Rating (CDR) scale.[32] The CDR uses a range of cognitive tests and informant data to generate scores: 0, indicates no dementia; 0.5, questionable dementia; 1, mild disease; 2, moderate illness; 3, severe illness.

In developing countries, low levels of education, literacy, and numeracy can distort results and lead to unimpaired persons (more particularly women) being falsely diagnosed with dementia. Tests such as the MMSE have stringent literacy requirements and individuals from poorer backgrounds may have lower scores. Use of westernized tests and informant questionnaires in the developing world may be culturally inappropriate.

Ideally, full neuropsychological testing by a clinical psychologist would be possible for every patient but this generally takes about 3 hours to complete and is thus resource-intensive.

Neuroimaging

Computed tomography (CT) is probably sufficient to detect most reversible or treatable causes of dementia, particularly those amenable to surgical interventions, e.g. cerebral neoplasia, subdural hematomas, and normal pressure hydrocephalus. Magnetic resonance imaging (MRI) is more sensitive than CT at showing white matter changes, and single-photon emission computed tomography (SPECT) may be helpful in identifying focal lesions, e.g. in FTD. In vascular dementia, cortical infarcts are shown; also infarcts in the basal ganglia and thalamus, multiple lacunae, and extensive white matter change.

Much work has examined the prospects for early diagnosis of dementia based on imaging of medial temporal lobe structures, especially the hippocampus.[33] Although subtle changes can be identified early on, or even before symptoms develop, this approach currently remains too insensitive for routine practice or for screening purposes.

GENETICS

Pedigrees with autosomal dominant inheritance of Alzheimer's disease have been recognized for many years. Three gene loci that may cause early-onset disease (<65 years) have been identified. Mutations occur in the amyloid precursor protein gene located on chromosome 21, and presenilin genes 1 and 2 on chromosomes 14 and 1, respectively.[34] In addition, the apolipoprotein E (ApoE) locus on chromosome 19 is associated with late-onset illness, i.e. possession of the ApoE ε4 allele is associated with increased risk of developing Alzheimer's disease, particularly in those homozygous for the gene,[35] whereas ApoE ε2 allele may confer protection.[36] However, for the majority of older people with dementia, genetic testing is not clinically useful either in making the diagnosis or in predicting future risk. ApoE ε4 testing is neither sensitive nor specific enough to make or exclude the diagnosis of Alzheimer's disease.

BEHAVIORAL AND PSYCHOLOGICAL SYMPTOMS OF DEMENTIA

Dementia is not only a disorder of cognition but also one that causes profound changes in other aspects of mental functioning, including mood and behavior. The so-called behavioral and psychological symptoms of dementia (BPSD)[37] occur in at least 40% of cases, with some studies suggesting lifetime rates as high as 80–90%.[38] These symptoms decrease quality of life for patients and caregivers alike, commonly account for the greatest burden of care, and are cited as common reasons for patients to move into institutional settings. Such symptoms include delusions and hallucinations, agitation, depression, irritability, euphoria, disinhibition, as well as apathy, aberrant motor behavior, night-time disturbance, appetite and/or eating abnormalities.

The Neuropsychiatric Inventory (NPI)[39] is the most widely used instrument for rating these symptoms and for assessing response to treatments. Apathy, depression, and aberrant motor behavior were the most frequent and severe symptoms identified in a recent study.[38] Psychotic symptoms, in particular delusions, tend to occur in the moderate stages of the illness, with low persistence over time. Antipsychotic drugs are modestly effective in treating psychotic symptoms and behaviors such as agitation and aggression,[40] but there is much concern about their safety and about excessive prescribing. Evidence for efficacy of antidepressants is also lacking.[41] Apart perhaps from visual hallucinations in DLB, there is no consistent relationship between the underlying illness causing dementia and the BPSD that may occur. Unlike the inexorable decline seen in cognitive and functional abilities, BPSD fluctuate in their presence and intensity over the course of the illness, though some, most notably aggressive behavior, may persist until near death. See Table 5.3 for a summary of all treatments for dementia (including BPSD).

Table 5.3   Pharmacological interventions in dementia

Class	Examples	Common uses	Comments
Cholinesterase inhibitors	Donepezil Galantamine Rivastigmine	Mild to moderate AD (and DLB) for symptomatic management of cognitive and non-cognitive symptoms	Started under specialist advice usually on a trial basis to assess efficacy and tolerability
N-methyl-D-aspartate (NMDA) receptor antagonist	Memantine	Moderate to severe AD	Used under specialist advice. Patients may deteriorate less slowly; usually reserved for people with advanced dementia who are living at home
Antidepressants	Selective serotonin reuptake inhibitors (SSRIs)	Depressive symptoms Emotional lability	Avoid tricylic antidepressants because of side effects, e.g. falls. Emotional lability may respond in days
Antipsychotics	Atypical (e.g. risperidone 0.5–1 mg/day), conventional (haloperidol 0.5–1 mg/day)	Psychotic symptoms Severe agitation/aggression	Risperidone and olanzapine are associated with increased risk of cerebrovascular accidents. Haloperidol can cause significant extrapyramidal side effects. All antipsychotics should be avoided in DLB
Clomethiazole	Clomethiazole	Sleep disturbance	Use selectively and on short-term basis
Benzodiazepine	Clonazepam	Myoclonic jerks	
Trazodone	Low-dose trazodone	Sleep disturbance, agitation	
Cardiovascular medications		To manage vascular risk factors	Important intervention for VaD

AD, Alzheimer's disease; VaD, vascular dementia; DLB, dementia with Lewy bodies.
Adapted from: Keith L, Rees M, Mander T, eds. Menopause, Postmenopause and Ageing. London: Royal Society of Medicine Press; 2005.

CARERS

The needs of carers have been repeatedly high-lighted, e.g. by the UK Audit Commission[42] and in the American Psychiatric Association's practice guidelines.[43] UK policy explicitly emphasizes the needs of carers as an integral part of services provided for older people.[44] Survival and quality of life of the person with dementia is linked to the psychological and physical well-being of the caregiver. Assessment of dementia therefore also requires consideration of the carer, and in some cases carers may need assessment in their own right: e.g. if they are very stressed or even clinically depressed by their duties, as would be the case if the patient is a partner or relative. Programs to provide education and support for carers can be effective in reducing carer stress.[45]

In the developing regions studied by the 10/66 group, most people with dementia were women and so too were their carers, usually either older women caring for their husbands or younger women caring for a parent.[46] This caring role was associated with substantial psychological strain and high rates of psychiatric morbidity. In addition, many carers in these areas were socio-economically disadvantaged, as they had either given up their own jobs or reduced their working hours to cope with this new and demanding role. Dementia thus contributes to a well-recognized cycle of poverty, educational disadvantage, and gender inequality in these areas, and creates additional barriers to social and economic prosperity that will continue into old age.

ELDER ABUSE

Older people with dementia suffer more physical illness and, consequently, are more often dependent on help from others, which can make them vulnerable to exploitation and abuse physically, financially, psychologically, and even sexually. Professionals must be alert to possible evidence of behavioral and physical symptoms of abuse. Patients may appear fearful of family members and reluctant to respond when questioned by professionals. A survey of 126 patients in a geriatric psychiatry service suggested that 16% had been subject to abuse.[47]

TREATMENT INTERVENTIONS

Social and psychological support

It is beyond the scope of this chapter to discuss the full range of services and support available to people with dementia and to their carers. Such services include help with personal care, day care provision, respite stays in hospital or residential environments, and also assistance with benefits and allowances. Specific psychological approaches such as reality orientation and behavior modification techniques may be useful.

Pharmacological interventions

Acetylcholinesterase inhibitors (AChEIs) are used in the treatment of Alzheimer's disease because of the impaired cholinergic transmission that is a hallmark of the illness. Currently three drugs are available worldwide: donepezil (Aricept), rivastigmine (Exelon), and galantamine (Reminyl). The clinical use of these medicines in the UK is guided by the National Institute for Health and Clinical Excellence (NICE).[48] Patterns of response to these treatments suggest that they benefit both cognitive and non-cognitive symptoms.[49] Gender and ApoE ε4 status do not serve as reliable predictors of treatment response. Whether the modest benefits of AChEIs are cost-effective in improving function and/or reducing carer stress, or in delaying institutional care, remain an area of some controversy. Drugs used for treatment of dementia are detailed in Table 5.3.

CAPACITY AND CONSENT

In the latter 20th century, requirements of informed consent became widespread in Western societies, justified by the obligation of respect for autonomy, which is recognized as the most important principle of contemporary bioethics. Respect for autonomy finds its roots in the liberal, moral, and political tradition of the importance of individual freedom of choice.[50] Because medical procedures that involve touching a patient are potentially a trespass or assault unless done with legal authority, patient consent is necessary to provide that authority.

Capacity assessment

Capacity is one of three components of valid consent – it must be given *voluntarily* by an *appropriately informed* person who has the *capacity* to consent. The nature and purpose of the treatment must be explained fully, together with possible side effects, and possible consequences of not having treatment. Assessment of capacity is a matter of clinical judgment, guided by professional practice and subject to legal requirements. It is part of everyday clinical practice. In medicolegal literature the terms competence and capacity are often used interchangeably, although 'competence' is the term favored in ethical literature with 'capacity' used in the legal sphere (in English Law). Capacity should be assessed in relation to the particular decision or activity. In each instance a decision should be a product of the patient's mind, not that of the doctor. It is ultimately for a Court to decide whether or not an individual is capable of making a particular decision, i.e. is competent to consent.

In the United Kingdom, the following three-stage test forms the criteria for any capacity assessment:

To have capacity an individual will possess the ability to:

- Comprehend and retain information material to the decision as to the likely consequences of having or not having the treatment
- Believe it
- Weigh the information in the balance in order to make a decision.[51]

The US has similar criteria for informed consent. The 'Four abilities model' of Grisso et al[52] closely mirrors the UK criteria for capacity assessment, including the ability to understand, appreciate, reason, and express a choice. Understanding refers to comprehending the meaning of what one is told, appreciation refers to forming beliefs about how that information relates to the self. Reasoning indicates putting the information together in an acceptable way.

The ability to make informed choices may be diminished by perceptual difficulties, such as impaired hearing or vision, aphasia, dysarthria, or bradykinesia, all of which may complicate the assessment process and lead to inappropriate labels of incompetence. Presenting materials in multiple formats and media, e.g. books (including large print), videos (adjustable volume), and use of clinical vignettes can facilitate better understanding. More than one session may be needed. As capacities for memory, judgment, reasoning, and planning diminish, patients with dementia lose decision-making capacity in every sphere of life. Examples include the capacity to drive, to manage finances, to execute advance directives, to consent to medical treatment, and ultimately to manage one's personal affairs. The situation may be worsened by comorbid depression or delirium. Marson et al[53] investigated the agreement of physician judgments of capacity to consent and found that there was high agreement among normal controls, i.e. 98%, but only 56% agreement for patients with mild Alzheimer's disease. Better inter-rater reliability was achieved for moderate to severe illness, and with the use of a structured capacity interview process. Although competency is ultimately a legal status, physicians and other healthcare professionals make judgments on a daily basis. In clinical settings, such judgments are rarely subject to judicial review. Despite conflicting measures of competency assessment, one overriding universal agreement was that executive function is the key to decision-making capacity rather than diagnostic labels or even measures of severity of dementia. Measures of semantic memory, simple reasoning, and short-term memory were key predictors of competency loss in patients with Alzheimer's disease, as judged by experienced physicians using specific legal standards.[54]

Several capacity assessment tools have been promoted specifically to assist with decisions about treatment or research treatment, including the MacArthur Competence Assessment Tool for Treatment (MacCAT-T), developed by Grisso and colleagues,[55] and the Capacity to Consent to Treatment Instrument.[56] Authors of both caution that these instruments can contribute to, but do not substitute for, an individual assessment and interpretation. Each instrument presents a hypothetical diagnosis and treatment alternatives, and asks the individual to demonstrate his/her capacity to understand and appreciate diagnostic and treatment information and to explain the reasoning behind choosing one treatment alternative over another. Methods for evaluating and rating these four legal standards are specified.

The law and incompetent adults

At present, the law in England and Wales states that no person can consent on behalf of another adult. If an adult lacks competence to consent to a medical procedure, the decision rests on a clinician's assessment of 'best interests'. 'Best interests' means treatment that is necessary to save life, or to ensure improvement or prevent deterioration in that person's health.[57] If competence fluctuates, routine procedures should be delayed to allow the person to make a competent decision about

accepting or rejecting the proposed intervention. It is good practice to consult relatives and others concerned with the care of the patient (but they cannot give or withhold consent).

Certain difficult decisions may require a declaration from the court, as the final arbiter, that the treatment is indeed in the patient's 'best interests'. Courts have established that unreasonable, even irrational views do not make patients incompetent.[58] Capacity is a matter of degree and fact, to be established in the circumstances of each patient, and each treatment proposal, and is often disputable. Capacity can be temporary, permanent, or fluctuating. Moreover, levels of competence must be adjusted to the consequences of acting on the decision. As the consequences for well-being become less substantial, the level of capacity required for competence should be decreased.[51] In other words, the level of capacity required to refuse a lifesaving treatment would be considerably greater than that required to accept a routine test. Competence thus varies with risk and even if a person is deemed competent to consent to treatment it does not follow that the patient is competent to refuse it, and vice versa.

The law in England and Wales is set to change in 2007, with the introduction of the Mental Capacity Act 2005.[59] Similar legislation exists in Scotland – the Adults with Incapacity (Scotland) Act 2000[60] – so this will bring the whole of the UK broadly into line with many other countries.

The Mental Capacity Act is founded upon five key principles:

1. A presumption of capacity – every adult has the right to make his or her own decisions and must be assumed to have capacity to do so unless it is proved otherwise.

2. The right for individuals to be supported to make their own decisions – people must be given all appropriate

help before anyone concludes that they cannot make their own decisions.

3. That individuals must retain the right to make what might be seen as eccentric or unwise decisions.

4. Best interests – anything done for or on behalf of people without capacity must be in their best interests.

5. Least restrictive intervention – anything done for or on behalf of people without capacity should be the least restrictive of their basic rights and freedoms.[61]

The Act covers all decisions on personal welfare, including financial, social, and medical issues, with statutory provision for substitute decision-making through creation of a Lasting Power of Attorney (before the onset of incapacity), or by Court-appointed Deputies. The legislation will be supported by appropriate bodies, and will include statutory provision for advocacy and for advance directives. It will become a criminal offence to ill-treat or neglect a person lacking capacity. Treatment for mental illness continues to be governed by the Mental Health Act 1983.

Advance directives, or living wills, are underpinned by the ethical imperative of respect for autonomy. Their aim is to extend the patient's autonomy into the future, in the face of subsequent incompetence. However, they have limited usefulness as they can fail to accurately anticipate the precise circumstances of future illness and, moreover, apply only to advanced refusals of treatment. In the US, the use of living wills was incorporated in California's Natural Death Act 1977, and superseded by the Patient Self-Determination Act (PSDA) 1990, which from 1991, has required all state facilities to provide adult patients with information relating to their legal right to make decisions about medical care, including the right to create an advance directive.[62]

Proxy decision-makers are expected to make choices based on what they believe the person would have wanted (prior competent choice), based on an understanding of the patient's values (substituted judgment standard). In the absence of this, a best interests standard is used by the proxy. Debates have centered on how much value to attach to the opinions of the person with dementia in order to determine what is good for them and which opinions should be relied upon: whether the wishes of the 'then self' or the 'now-self' should take precedence, or indeed whether a narrative perspective of both prior and current wishes and values should be considered.[63]

In the US, certain 'extraordinary' treatments also require court approval – e.g. sterilization, psychosurgery, electroconvulsive treatment, and in some states the administration of antipsychotic medication.

Consent for research

Research involving people who lack capacity, including those with dementia, is the subject of heated ethical debate. For example, not to offer equal opportunities to benefit from new treatments may be unfairly discriminatory, but efforts to secure autonomous decision-making in the form of surrogacy, etc., are difficult enough even for therapeutic interventions, and even more so in relation to research. Over the past 50 years, international bioethics associations have slowly liberalized guidelines for the participation of incompetent adults in research. Thus, the 5th revision of the Declaration of Helsinki (2000)[64] permits such research even without the prospect of direct benefit to the individual, if future patients could benefit. The prevailing view is that research on persons unable to give autonomous consent should be directly related to either the condition responsible for their incapacity or a special medical or social need produced by their incapacity. A study involving incapable subjects should be rejected if the desired scientific data can be obtained from a less-disabled group.[65]

Consensus recommendations for Institutional Review Boards and Investigators in the US, presented by the Alzheimer's Association,[66] have recently recommended permitting proxies to enroll individuals with dementia in research involving minimal risk and only if the person assents to the procedures. However, this remains controversial as some proxies may attribute inadequate significance to burdens they will not personally experience.[65] Where risks are judged as greater than minimal, the study must confer direct benefit to the person or the knowledge potentially gained from the research must be substantial. In the UK, similar principles are endorsed in the new Mental Capacity Act,[61] with approval via local Research Ethics Committees.

CONCLUSION

Expansion of the elderly population means that dementia will become increasingly important for healthcare professionals in all specialties

treating older women, as the condition may go unrecognized, or professionals may fail to appreciate the role of being a carer for someone with dementia. Women with dementia may be unable to give valid consent to accept a proposed medical intervention or to refuse it and carers may make healthcare choices influenced by a commitment to their carer role. In highlighting the main features of dementia and the range of problems this illness poses for patients and carers alike, we hope to have demonstrated the challenge of caring for older women who may be facing such difficulties, often with little support.

In clinical terms there remain considerable challenges in this area, along with increased recognition of the heterogeneity of dementia. Diagnostic and therapeutic possibilities are increasing, and recent advances in the understanding of the molecular biology and genetics of dementia will assisting in the future development of novel effective treatments. We also face ethical challenges, with judiciaries worldwide beginning to grasp, and respond to, the enormity of the task involved in protecting this most vulnerable population. In both of these areas, healthcare professionals will undoubtedly be at the forefront of progress.

REFERENCES

1. World Health Organization. International Classification of Diseases and Health Related Problems, 10th revision. Geneva: World Health Organization; 1992.
2. Copeland JR, Dewey ME, Wood N. Range of mental illness among the elderly in the community. Prevalence in Liverpool using the AGE-CAT package. Br J Psychiatry 1987; 150: 815–23.
3. Lyketsos CG, Steinberg M, Tschanz JT, et al. Mental and behavioural disturbances in dementia: findings from the Cache County Study on Memory in Aging. Am J Psychiatry 2000; 157: 708–14.
4. Matthews F, Brayne C; Medical Research Council Cognitive Function and Ageing Study Investigators. The incidence of dementia in England and Wales: findings from the five identical sites of the MRC CFA Study. PLoS Med 2005; 2(8): e193. http:/medicine. plosjournals.org.
5. Wimo A, Winblad B, Aguerro-Torres H, von Strauss E. The magnitude of dementia occurrence in the world. Alzheimer Dis Assoc Disord 2003; 17: 63–7.

6.   World Health Organization. Active Ageing: A Policy Framework, Geneva: WHO; 2002.

7.   Prince M, Graham N, Brodaty H, et al. Alzheimer's Disease International's 10/66 Dementia research group – one model for action research in developing countries. Int J Geriatr Psychiatry 2004; 19: 178–81.

8.   O'Connor DW, Pollitt PA, Hyde JB, et al. Do general practitioners miss dementia in elderly patients? BMJ 1998; 297: 1107–10.

9.   Cummings JL, Benson DF. Dementia: definition, prevalence, classification and approach to diagnosis. In: Cummings JL, Benson DF, eds. Dementia: A Clinical Approach. Boston: Butterworth-Heinemann; 1992.

10. Alzheimer A. Über eine eigenartige Erkrankung der Hirnrinde. Allgemeine Zeitschrift für Psychiatrie und Psychisch-Gerichtlich Medizine 1907; 64: 146–8.

11. Kraepelin E. Psychiatrie: ein Lehrbuch für Studierende und Ärzte. Leipzig: Johann Ambrosius Barth; 1910.

12. Proctor AW. Neurochemical correlates of dementia. Neurodegeneration 1996; 5: 403–7.

13. Forstl H, Burns A, Luthert P, et al. Clinical and neuropathological correlates of depression in Alzheimer's disease. Psychol Med 1992; 22: 877–84.

14. American Psychiatric Association. Diagnostic and Statistical Manual of Mental Disorders, 4th edn. Washington, DC: American Psychiatric Association; 1994.

15. McKhann G, Drachman D, Folstein M, et al. Clinical diagnosis of Alzheimer's disease. Report of the NINCDS-ADRDA Work Group under the auspices of the Department of Health and Human Service Task forces on Alzheimer's Disease. Neurology 1984; 34: 939–44.

16. Alzheimer's Society Demography Policy Position Report. www.Alzheimers.org.uk 2004.

17. Kalaria RN, Ballard C. Overlap between pathology of Alzheimer's disease and vascular dementia. Alzheimer Dis Assoc Disord 1999; 13(Suppl 3): S115–23.

18. Roman GC, Tatemichi T, Erkinjuntti T, et al. Vascular dementia: diagnostic criteria for research studies. Report of the NINDS-AIREN International Workshop. Neurology 1993; 43: 250–60.

19. McKeith IG, Galasko D, Kosaka K, et al. Consensus guidelines for the clinical and pathologic diagnosis of dementia with Lewy bodies (DLB): report of the consortium on DLB international workshop. Neurology 1996; 47: 1113–24.

20. Hansen L, Salmon D, Galasko D, et al. The Lewy body variant of Alzheimer's disease: a clinical and pathological entity. Neurology 1990; 40: 1–8.

21. Ballard C, Holmes C, McKeith IG, et al. Psychiatric morbidity in dementia with Lewy bodies: a prospective clinical and neuropathological comparative study with Alzheimer's disease. Am J Psychiatry 1999; 156: 1039–45.

22. Ratnavalli E, Brayne C, Dawson K, et al. The prevalence of frontotemporal dementia. Neurology 2002; 58: 1615–21.

23. Lund and Manchester Groups. Clinical and neuropathological criteria for fronto-temporal dementia. J Neurol Neurosurg Psychiatry 1990; 57: 416–18.

24. Petersen R. Mild Cognitive Impairment Clinical Trials. Nature Rev Drug Discovery 2003; 2: 646–53.

25. Fox NC, Warrington EK, Seiffer AL, et al. Presymptomatic cognitive deficits in individuals at risk of familial Alzheimer's disease. Brain 1998; 121: 1631–9.

26. Ballard GC, Bannister C, Oyebode F. Depression in dementia sufferers. Int J Geriatr Psychiatry 1996; 11: 507–15.

27. O'Brien J, Ames D, Schwietzer I. White matter changes in depression and Alzheimer's disease: a review of magnetic resonance imaging studies. Int J Geriatr Psychiatry 1996; 11: 681–94.

28. Abas MA, Sahakian BJ, Levy R. Neuropsychological deficits and CT scan changes in elderly depressives. Psychol Med 1990; 20: 507–20.

29. Folstein MF, Folstein SE, McHugh PR. "Mini-mental state". A practical method for grading the cognitive state of patients for the clinician. J Psychiatr Res 1975; 12: 189–98.

30. O'Connor DW, Pollitt PA, Hyde JB, et al. The reliability and validity of the Mini-Mental State in a British community survey. J Psychiatr Res 1989; 1: 87–96.

31. Roth M, Tym E, Mountjoy CQ, et al. CAMDEX: a standardised instrument for the diagnosis of mental disorder in the elderly with special reference to the early detection of dementia. Br J Psychiatry 1986; 149: 698–709.

32. Hughes CP, Berg L, Danziger WL, et al. A new clinical scale for the staging of dementia. Br J Psychiatry 1982; 140: 556–72.

33. Jack CRJ, Petersen RC, Yue CX, et al. Medial temporal atrophy on MRI in normal ageing and very mild Alzheimer's disease. Neurology 1997; 49: 786–94.

34. Hardy J. Amyloid, the presenilins and Alzheimer's disease. Trends Neuroscie 1997; 20: 154–9.

35. Corder EH, Saunders AM, Strittmatter WJ, et al. Gene dose of apolipoprotein E type 4 allele and the risk of Alzheimer's disease in late onset families. Science 1993; 261: 921–3.

36. Corder EH, Saunders AM, Risch NJ, et al. Protective effect of apolipoprotein E type 2 allele for late onset Alzheimer disease. Nat Genet 1994; 7: 180–4.

37. Finkel SI, Costa e Silva J, Cohen G, et al. Behavioral and psychological signs and symptoms of dementia: a consensus statement on current knowledge and implications for research and treatment. Int Psychogeriatr 1996; 8 (Suppl 3): 497–500.

38. Aalten P, de Vugt ME, Jaspers N, et al. The course of neuropsychiatric symptoms in dementia. Part 1: findings from the two year longitudinal Maasbed study. Int J Geriatr Psychiatry 2005; 20: 523–30.

39. Cummings JL, Mega M, Gray K, et al. The neuropsychiatric inventory: comprehensive assessment of psychopathology in dementia. Neurology 1994; 44: 2308–14.

40. Lonergan E, Luxenberg J, Colford J. Haloperidol for agitation in dementia. The Cochrane Library, issue 3. Chichester: John Wiley and Sons; 2004.

41. Bains J, Birks JS, Dening TR. Antidepressants for treating depression in dementia. The Cochrane Library, issue 3. Chichester: John Wiley and Sons; 2004.

42. Audit Commission. Forget- Me-Not. London: MWL Print Group; 2002.

43. American Psychiatric Association. Practice guideline for the treatment of patients with Alzheimer's disease and other dementias of late life. Am J Psychiatry 1997; 154 (Suppl.): 1–39.

44. Department of Health. National Service Framework for Older People. London: Department of Health; 2001.

45. Brodaty H, Gresham M. Effect of a training programme to reduce stress in carers of patients with dementia. BMJ 1989; 299: 1375–9.

46. The 10/66 Dementia Research Group. Care arrangements for people with dementia in developing countries. Int J Geriatr Psychiatry 2004; 19: 170–7.

47. Vida S, Monks RC, Des Rosiers SP. Prevalence and correlates of elder abuse and neglect in a geriatric psychiatry service. Can J Psychiatry 2002; 47: 459–67.

48. Alzheimer's disease – donepezil, rivastigmine, galantamine and memantine: www.nice.org.uk.

49. Doody RS, Stevens JC, Beck C, et al. Practice parameter: management of dementia (an evidence-based review). Report of the Quality Standards Subcommittee of the American Academy of Neurology. Neurology 2001; 56: 1154–66.

50. Beauchamp TL, Childress JF. Principles of Biomedical Ethics, 4th edn. Oxford: Oxford University Press; 1994.

51. Re C (adult: refusal of treatment) [1994] 1 All ER 819.

52. Grisso T, Appelbaum PS. Assessing Competence to Consent to Treatment; a Guide for Physicians and Other Health Professionals. New York: Oxford University Press; 1998.

53. Marson DC, McInturff B, Hawkins L, et al. Consistency of physician judgements of capacity to consent in mild Alzheimer's disease. J Am Geriatr Soc 1997; 45: 453–7.

54. Earnst KS, Marson DC, Harrell LE. Cognitive models of physicians' legal standard and personal judgements of competency in patients

with Alzheimer's disease. J Am Geriatr Soc 2000; 48: 919–27.

55. Grisso T, Appelbaum PS, Hill-Fotouhi C. The MacCAT-T: a clinical tool to assess patients' capacities to make treatment decisions. Psychiatr Serv 1997; 48: 1415–19.

56. Marson DC, Ingram KK, Cody HA, et al. Assessing the competency of patients with Alzheimer's disease under different legal standards. Arch Neurol 1995; 52: 949–54.

57. Re F (Mental Patient: Sterilisation) [1990] 2 AC 1.

58. Re MB (Medical Treatment) [1997] 2 FLR 426.

59. Mental Capacity Act: www.dca.gov.uk/menincap/legis.htm.

60. Adults with Incapacity (Scotland) Act 2000: http://www.opsi.gov.uk/legislation/scotland/acts2000/20000004.htm.

61. Mental Capacity Act 2005 – summary: www.dca.gov.uk/menincap/bill-summary.htm.

62. 42 U.S.C. 1395 cc (a) 910 et. seq (as amended November 1990).

63. Fellows LK. Competency and consent in dementia. J Am Geriatr Soc 1998; 46: 922–6.

64. World Medical Association. Declaration of Helsinki. Ferney-Voltaire: WMA; 1964 (and subsequent amendments).

65. Dresser R. Mentally disabled research subjects. The enduring policy issues. JAMA 1996; 276: 67–72.

66. Alzheimer's Association. Research consent for cognitively impaired adults, recommendations for Institutional Review Boards and Investigators. Alzheimer Dis Assoc Disord 2004; 18: 171–5.

Depression and mood changes

6

Sarah Cullum, Susan Tucker, and Thomas R Dening

INTRODUCTION

Depression is the most common mental health problem experienced by older women. Although everyone may feel sad or lonely at times, depressive illness in later life is qualitatively and quantitatively different. True depression is a serious and disabling condition that can affect every aspect of a person's functioning, leading to personal and family distress, exacerbation of physical and cognitive disorders, greater use of health and social care resources, and increased mortality from both natural causes and suicide.

Factors predisposing to depression in old age include female gender, physical ill health, life/loss events, social isolation, and poverty. As depression is not a normal or inevitable response to aging, its detection is important. Although particular challenges surround assessing and treating elderly depressed women, good grounds for therapeutic optimism also exist.

As life expectancy improves, health professionals will see increasing numbers of older women, many of whom have long-standing chronic illnesses and/or multiple pathologies. Given the high prevalence of depression in such a population, clinicians should be alert to the possibility that depression may be causing or exacerbating other conditions. This chapter should help the reader develop his or her familiarity with depression in the elderly woman. Consideration is given to the presentation, prevalence, risk, assessment, treatment, and outcome in a range of common settings. The emphasis is on practical advice, and case studies illustrate the issues discussed.

Although this book focuses on 'women over 70', much of the research concerned with depression in 'the elderly' has looked at people aged 65, 60, or even 55 plus. As findings from younger adults cannot (and probably should not) necessarily be extrapolated to older adults, wherever possible, we have limited our sources to work in which the majority of the study population were aged at ≥65 years old. Because only a small proportion of this literature specifically addresses depression in older *women,* we must necessarily talk about older *people* in a number of instances.

DEFINITIONS OF DEPRESSION

The term 'depression' describes a broad and heterogenous group of mood disturbances ranging from transient feelings of lowered mood to a major mental illness with features such as weight loss and insomnia. It can be conceptualized either as a syndrome in which certain diagnostic criteria must be met to achieve the status of a 'case', or as a continuum of depressive symptoms that range from mild to severe. Depression may appear for the first time in later life for many older women, but for others it may also be the recurrence of a chronic disorder that originated earlier in life for others.

Standard diagnostic criteria for depression, using the International Classification of Diseases,

10th edn, guidelines[1] (ICD-10; see Table 6.1) emphasize the qualitative differences between depressed mood and ordinary feelings of sadness. Various specified symptoms, both psychological and physical, are crucial to making a diagnosis. However, in practice, a simple symptom count does not really reflect the degree of distress or functional impairment experienced by an older person; rather, a focus on the personal and social needs of the individual is more likely to be helpful. As a general rule, if depressive symptoms are sufficient to interfere with daily life, intervention should be considered. Although depression may occur as part of a bipolar manic-depressive disorder, unipolar depression is much more common and is the focus of this chapter.

EPIDEMIOLOGY OF DEPRESSION

Epidemiological studies of depression in later life generally consider morbidity in four specific settings: the community, primary care setting, hospital, and care homes. Consensus supports the commonplace nature of depression in older people, but prevalence rates vary according to the definition of depression and the nature of the population sampled. For example, studies making discrete psychiatric diagnoses persistently show lower rates of depression than those reporting the presence of depressive symptoms.

Despite geographical and cross-cultural differences, about 2% of elderly people living at home have a major depressive illness, whereas 12–15% have significant depressive symptoms.[2,3] Women are more likely to be depressed than men, and various studies report gender ratios of roughly 1.5:1 or 2:1.[2,4] This gender imbalance carries over into the primary care setting, where up to 6–9% of older people have depressive disorder,[5] although primary care studies are scarce.[6]

Still higher prevalence rates are seen in hospital settings. Studies suggest that around 15–25% of older hospital patients suffer with major depression[7] and more than a third display clinically significant depressive symptoms.[8] Higher rates are reported in care homes,[6] where the true prevalence may be even greater, as a large proportion of this population have dementia, which can complicate, or take precedence over, the diagnosis of depression (see Chapter 5).

Numerous factors contribute to these high prevalence levels and to differences between

Table 6.1 ICD-10 criteria for depressive disorder

At least two of the following symptoms must be present:

- depressed mood that is definitely abnormal for the individual, present for most of the day and almost every day, largely uninfluenced by circumstance, and sustained for at least 2 weeks
- loss of interest or pleasure in activities that are normally pleasurable
- decreased energy or increased fatigability

An additional symptom or symptoms from the following list should be present, to give a total of at least four:

- loss of self-confidence or self-esteem
- unreasonable feelings of self-reproach or excessive or inappropriate guilt
- recurrent thoughts of death or suicide, or any suicidal behavior
- complaints or evidence of diminished ability to think or concentrate, such as indecisiveness or vacillation
- change in psychomotor activity, with agitation or retardation (either subjective or objective)
- sleep disturbance of any type
- change in appetite (decrease or increase) with corresponding weight change

settings and countries. Biological and social variables are important, and depression in elderly women often has multiple causes:

- *A family history of depression* is a significant risk factor for people whose depression originated in younger adulthood.[6] However, genetic factors appear to be less influential in older than in younger people.[9]
- *Physical ill health.* Although the etiological pathway is unclear and, in some disorders, causality may be bidirectional, a number of conditions, including thyroid disorder, stroke, dementia, cancer, cardiovascular disorders, and Parkinson's disease, have been associated with a higher prevalence of depression in older women.[10] Deep white matter lesions seen on magnetic resonance imaging (MRI) may be a specific risk factor in first-onset depression in old age.[11] As might be expected, greater severity of physical disorder and greater functional disability may provoke a depressive disorder, which may in turn increase the degree of disability associated with the original impairment.[12]
- *Socioeconomic factors* including poverty (poor income, housing, and education) and social isolation (low levels of social contact and/or support) are associated with late-life depression.[5,13] Women caregivers are particularly at risk, especially those who care for people with behavioral problems.[6]
- *Life events,* particularly when they involve loss, such as the death of a loved one or a severe deterioration in health, may precipitate depression.[14] Although many bereaved women adjust well to their changed situation, and the effect of bereavement on the development of a depressive disorder is no different between men and women, traditional widowhood practices in some countries pose a significant threat to a woman's well-being.[15]

- *Female gender.* Women are more likely to become depressed than men. Although part of the difference may be due to biological factors, including reproductive function,[16] gender mainly acts as an intermediary variable, determining exposure to the above social/life event risk factors (older women are more likely to be poor, lonely, carers, or widowed than older men).[13,15]
- *Medication.* A number of drugs, including beta-blockers, levadopa, corticosteroids, gastrointestinal drugs, and antipsychotics, have been shown to cause, provoke, or sustain depression.[17]

PRESENTATION

The features of depression in older individuals are generally very similar to those seen in the rest of the population and an older woman with depression will typically display several of the symptoms listed in Table 6.1. The experience of depressed mood and/or loss of pleasure are central, but diurnal variation is common, with the person's mood usually lowest in the morning and lifting towards evening. Of interest, older people make fewer complaints of depressed mood than younger adults and the individual herself may not perceive her spirits to be low.[6]

An older woman with depression might look tired, sad, or disinterested and speak slowly, pausing before replying to questions, initiating little conversation, and/or speaking in a monotonous tone. Her speech content may be sad or even morbid, and lack depth and detail, while she may have obvious difficulty concentrating. Marked physical complaints are often present, including somatic symptoms such as disturbed sleep, lack of energy, and aches and pains, as well as hypochondriacal complaints and anxiety.[6] The extent to which depression presents differently in older men and women has yet to be clarified, but some work suggests that elderly women are particularly likely to experience appetite and weight loss.[18]

Changes in behavior are frequent, and an older woman with depression will often move slowly and make poor eye contact (although some patients with an agitated depression will be restless and unable to sit still). It is not unusual for the person to have withdrawn from previously enjoyed leisure activities, or to find that domestic tasks are 'too much of an effort'. If psychotic symptoms also occur, they are generally congruent with mood, e.g. delusions of poverty, guilt, or imminent disaster. Auditory hallucinations, if they occur, are often derogatory or accusatory, which the woman may think is justified because she believes she is a 'bad person'.

Inter-relationships between depression and physical illness are important in many ways. For example, symptoms such as insomnia, weight loss, and fatigue may overlap. Depression can also adversely affect both the presentation and prognosis of a concomitant physical disorder, exacerbating pain, increasing medical complications, slowing recovery, and increasing mortality. Depression in the presence of dementia is also complex. Behavioral disturbances, notably agitation, aggression, and refusal to eat, are common presenting problems, and depression in dementia can lead to poorer cognitive functioning, communication skills, and performance on instrumental activities of daily living.[19] Case studies 1 gives some examples about the presentation of depression in older women. As should now be obvious, a thorough assessment is necessary in each case in which depression is suspected.

Finally, we must draw attention to the importance of an older person presenting with ideas and/or acts of self-harm. Thoughts of life not being worth living are relatively common, but active thoughts of suicide, or suicidal plans, are less so. Among older people, acts of deliberate self-harm are more likely to be associated with depressive illness and rates of completed suicide

Case studies 1: examples of the presentation of depression in elderly women

Mrs A

Mrs A is a 72-year-old lady who lives with her chronically ill husband. When seen at home by a community nurse she looks tired and drawn and makes no attempt to join in conversation. Upon direct questioning, she speaks only briefly and appears to have difficulty concentrating. She does, however, acknowledge that she is sleeping poorly, waking around 4 a.m., and that she has no energy. Further questioning reveals that Mrs A has little appetite and has lost 3 kg in the space of a month, while even her garden, her 'first love', is not giving her pleasure. She describes her mood as 'down'.

Mrs B

Mrs B is an 81-year-old widow who repeatedly presents to her primary care physician complaining of problems with her digestion. She describes an 'obstruction' in her throat and an 'unsettled tummy'. According to her daughter, she has recently eaten no more than a couple of mouthfuls before complaining of nausea and pushing the plate aside. When asked directly about her mood, Mrs B states that it is 'alright', and reiterates concerns about her physical health. In further conversation, however, it becomes apparent that she has gradually withdrawn from all her usual social activities, and that she is spending a lot of time ruminating on her late husband's death, which she unrealistically believes she could have prevented.

Miss C

Miss C is an 89-year-old lady who lives in a nursing home. She has a known diagnosis of Alzheimer's disease. Staff describe a clear change in her presentation over a 4-week period. Whereas she had previously been acceptant of assistance with personal care, and seemed to enjoy contact with staff and family visitors, she now fails to acknowledge the latter and often hits out when approached. Observed from a distance, Miss C is seen sitting in an armchair, head bowed. She appears agitated, frequently changing her position and wringing her hands, and does not respond to her name.

are relatively high, albeit greater among men than women.[10] Older people rarely take manipulative overdoses and a previous suicide attempt is the single factor most predictive of suicide, so even when an act of self-harm appears trivial this must be treated seriously.[6]

IDENTIFICATION

Older individuals with depression consult their doctors up to two or three times more often than the non-depressed, offering plenty of opportunities for identification. However, despite its high prevalence, depression in the elderly is often missed. Factors contributing to underdetection involve both clinicians *and* older people themselves. Doctor factors include the misplaced belief that low mood is an understandable response to ageing and the complex overlap of depression with other medical and cognitive disorders that compete for attention and make diagnosis difficult.[10,20] Patient factors include lack of awareness that depression is a distinct and treatable illness and the perceived stigma of mental illness. An additional factor is the authoritarian nature of communication between health workers and female patients in many parts of the world that makes it difficult for women to disclose emotional distress.[21] Regardless, in general, women are more likely than men to seek help and to be prescribed antidepressant medication.[21]

Several practice guidelines recommend the use of validated screening instruments to improve the detection of depression in high-risk populations such as hospital patients and care home residents.[3,22] Even though screening tools are not diagnostic, they provide a helpful framework for discussion, and scores within a certain range indicate the likelihood of depression. The Geriatric Depression Scale (GDS),[23] in its full 30-item or shortened versions, is most widely used. These valid and reliable self-report questionnaires with their simple yes/no formats focus on the psychological, rather than the physical, symptoms of depression. Although GDS ratings remain valid in people with mild or moderate cognitive impairment,[24] interviewer-administered instruments are more likely to detect depression in more severe dementia, of which the Cornell Scale[25] is perhaps best known.

Used alone, screening tools have little impact on the recognition of depression,[26] and any suspected depression must be followed by a thorough psychiatric assessment. This is particularly important in view of the absence of any specific test for depression. As in all areas of medicine, a full history and an examination of both physical and mental state are mandatory. The main areas to be covered in the history are shown in Table 6.2. Corroboratory information should be obtained from a close relative/carer as well as the woman herself, as low mood may prevent the individual from giving a full account of herself, but the same may be said for cognitive, hearing, and/or visual impairments. It is perhaps stating the obvious to say that older people assessed in hospital or care homes should be seen in a private setting free of distractions; the unfortunate reality is that this does not always happen.

A careful description of the presenting problems and their onset forms the foundation of a good assessment. Factors precipitating or predisposing to depressive disorder should be thoroughly

Table 6.2 Elements of a psychiatric history

The presenting complaint and its history

Family history:

- family history of psychiatric disorder

Personal history:

- pregnancy and birth
- early development
- childhood
- schooling and higher education
- occupations
- sexual history
- marriage and cohabitation
- children
- tobacco, drug, and alcohol use
- forensic history

Previous medical history

Previous psychiatric history (including any postnatal disorder):

- duration
- severity
- treatment (successes and failures)

Present medication:

- compliance
- ability to self administer

Premorbid personality

Activities of daily living:

- personal hygiene
- mobility
- domestic activities
- leisure activities
- driving

Current living conditions

Current social circumstances and support

---

explored (including apparently trivial stressors such as the death of a favourite pet) and the relative contribution of physical, social, and psychological variables should be considered, as all may influence subsequent care. Any family or personal history of affective disorder must be identified, and prior treatments that have proved successful/unsuccessful ascertained. A history of life events, including a full medical history, must also be collected, and the individual should be asked about their medication (particularly potentially depressogenic ones) and use of alcohol/illegal drugs (which can predispose to depressive symptoms and/or be used in an attempt to self-medicate a pre-existing depression). Premorbid personality can be assessed by asking how the person has coped with previous life difficulties and whether they are usually 'a worrier'.

The practitioner must also inquire in detail about the older woman's daily life activities, as recent changes in behavior, such as the withdrawal from social activities or uncharacteristic neglect of the home, may be particularly indicative of depression. Information about the woman's social support network (both formal and informal) should also be obtained, both to throw light on current functioning and to give some indication of potential future support. Although grief is not a psychiatric disorder, it is worth noting that bereavement sometimes antedates a depressive illness, and the anniversary of a bereavement is a time of particular vulnerability. Depression should be suspected if the woman has suicidal thoughts, persistent and pervasive feelings of guilt, maintains grief by keeping everything unchanged ('mummification') and/or presents with marked functional disability.

The mental state examination (Table 6.3) is a systematic record of observations about the person that permits an insight into their internal world and reflects how they are coping. Particular questions should be asked about any loss of enjoyment/interest and depressive thoughts such as hopelessness, worthlessness, or guilt. These are particularly important in view of older people's tendency to minimize feelings of sadness whereas other depressive symptoms that might be clarified include the extent of any sleep disturbance (difficulty getting to sleep, early morning wakening, or hypersomnia), appetite changes, or loss of libido. The issue of suicidal ideas and acts can be addressed by starting with an open question, such as 'Have you ever thought

Table 6.3 Elements of a mental state examination

Appearance (of the person, and, if they are at home,
    their house)
Behavior
Speech (quantity, tone, rate, and content)
Mood
Thought content (including obsessional phenomena
    and delusions)
Disturbances of perception (hallucinations and illusions)
Cognitive function (including attention, concentration,
    orientation, and memory)
Insight

life was not worth living?'. If the answer is yes,
then going on to ask more probing questions,
such as 'Have you ever felt so bad that you
thought about trying to end your life?', 'Have you
thought how you might do it?', and 'How close
have you been to carrying out these actions?'

A screening measure of cognitive function,
such as the Mini-Mental State Examination
(MMSE),[27] is also useful to distinguish depression
from dementia (see Chapter 5). A high score on
the MMSE will usually exclude dementia. A
low score should be treated with caution as it
may due to physical illness causing poor concentration and/or mild confusion, or to pseudodementia (depression presenting with confusion
and forgetfulness that may be mistaken for a
dementing illness, but has a shorter time course).
More common is the occurrence of depression in
dementia: although a person with dementia may
find it difficult to explain how they are feeling,
the close observation of their behavior and the
report of an informant can be especially helpful.

A careful physical examination is required to
establish whether a systemic disorder might be
causing the depressive symptoms and to identify
any comorbid physical illness. It is not easy to
decide whether symptoms are due to a depressive or
physical disorder, as illustrated in Case studies 2.
However, presentation with a number of psychological and/or cognitive features of depression,

*Case studies 2: examples of diagnostic difficulties
in the assessment of depression*

Mrs D

Mrs D is an 80-year-old woman who has been
married to her childhood sweetheart for
62 years. In recent weeks she has become
tremulous and slow in her movements, and
upon examination she has increased tone, shuf-
fling gait, and an expressionless face. The initial
diagnosis is Parkinson's disease, but her husband
reports that he has terminal cancer and that
since Mrs D was told this she has become more
withdrawn, not wishing to socialize with their
friends, eating less, and losing weight. She has
also suggested that they make a suicide pact as
he is unlikely to survive and she does not want
to live without him. Following treatment with
antidepressants, both her depression and the
physical signs of Parkinson's disease improve.

Mrs E

Mrs E is a 78-year-old lady who was admitted
to a medical ward with a urinary tract infection. She is referred to the liaison psychiatrist
for assessment of her mental state, and found
to be low in mood with disturbed sleep and
appetite and suicidal ideas. Her transfer to the
psychiatric unit is delayed due to MRSA
infection and she is nursed in isolation for a
further 6 weeks. By the time she reaches the
psychiatric ward, Mrs E is refusing food and
fluids, needs help with all activities of daily
living, and scores within the range for
dementia on a cognitive rating scale. However, staff suspect pseudodementia and she
recovers her usual function and returns home
after treatment with ECT.

Miss F

Miss F is 72-year-old lady who has a long
history of recurrent depressive disorder that

has required treatment with ECT. On this occasion she presents with anxiety, hyperventilation, occasional diarrhea, disturbed sleep, loss of appetite, and the belief that she has an incurable disease and is going to die. On routine investigation she is found to be slightly anemic, but her main problem is thought to be recurrence of her depressive illness. She is started on antidepressant therapy, which helps her sleep, but she continues to feel anxious and the diarrhea persists. Her stools prove fecal occult blood positive and a subsequent gastroendoscopy reveals stomach cancer.

somatic symptoms disproportionate to known pathology, the emergence of new symptoms in the context of chronic disease (e.g. early morning wakening), and/or recent changes in pain threshold may be signs of a depressive disorder.

Routine laboratory investigations include a complete blood count, vitamin B_{12}, folate, plasma viscosity, urea and electrolytes, and liver and thyroid function tests. Depending on the clinical picture and history, other investigations such as bone chemistry, cholesterol, glucose, and syphilis serology may be deemed necessary. Abnormal results may indicate the cause of the depression (and any treatable organic cause *must* be excluded), but more commonly reflect poor nutrition and weight loss secondary to depression and self-neglect (see Chapter 8). In certain instances, a chest X-ray, electroencephalogram, or a lumbar puncture (usually for neurosyphilis) will be required, and if there has been a rapid onset of symptoms and/or neurological signs of head injury/brain disorder are present, a skull X-ray, computed tomography (CT) scan, MRI, or single-photon emission computed tomography (SPECT) scan of the brain might also be required.

MANAGEMENT

Even when depression is detected, the response, in terms of the provision of medication, psychological therapies, and/or social support is often inadequate.[3] However, age is not an adverse predictor of response to treatment[10,28] and the treatment of depressive symptoms leads to better medical and psychological prognoses, regardless of whether the onset of symptoms is primarily medical or psychological.[29] As with any medical disorder, the aim of treatment is to reduce morbidity and mortality. Thus, the goals of treatment of depressive disorder include the prevention of suicide, the reduction of depressive symptoms, the prevention of relapse and recurrence, and the improvement of daily functioning and quality of life.

Most older individuals with depression benefit from a multifactorial, multidisciplinary approach that takes account of their psychosocial *and* physical situation.[3,22,30] One of the first decisions to be made is whether referral to a specialist is necessary. Factors that favor urgent referral to a psychiatrist include the active presence of suicidal ideas or plans, psychotic symptoms, marked agitation, or self-neglect. Referral is also appropriate if the woman has had a previous lifetime episode of mania (as treatment of her current depressive disorder may precipitate another swing into mania), has had a previous episode of depression in the last year, or has failed to respond to various treatment strategies as well as when the diagnosis is in doubt.[6,22]

In formulating management plans, the clinician should discuss the alternatives with the woman and take into account any past or family history of depression, previous response to treatment (if applicable), and the predisposing factors identified at assessment. Depressogenic medication should be discontinued where possible, and any underlying or coexistent physical disorder optimized. Other general measures include the provision of advice about nutrition, sleep hygiene, anxiety management, and exercise,[30] although some combination of antidepressants and/or psychological therapies will also usually be needed. Where concerns exist about the woman's social situation, an energetic approach to improve her social circumstances and a social work assessment may prove invaluable.

Physical treatments

Whereas antidepressant drugs alone will relieve the depression of some women, the prescription of medication is usually part of a wider treatment plan. One of the main challenges for the effective use of antidepressants is the high rate of non-compliance present in both younger and older adults. Older people may be confused by complex regimens, perhaps forget to take the tablets, cannot open containers, or simply do not want to take the medicine (but omit to tell their doctor for fear of causing offence). Strategies to optimize compliance include the use of calendar blister packs or dosette boxes, once-daily medication, non-childproof containers, and education that specifically addresses the individual's concerns. The woman might be reassured that depression is an illness and not a sign of weakness or incipient dementia, for example, or that antidepressants are not addictive. At the same time, all older people prescribed antidepressants should be informed about the delay in onset of effect, likely side effects, and possible discontinuation symptoms of antidepressant medication.[22]

Table 6.4[31] shows the different classes of antidepressants and their associated side effects. Relatively few trials of antidepressants include representative samples of older people, but a recent Cochrane review concluded that tricyclic antidepressants (TCAs), selective serotonin reuptake inhibitors (SSRIs), and monoamine oxidase inhibitors (MAOIs) are all equally efficacious in people aged 60 plus, with a response rate of around 50–60%.[28] No one medication is ideal, or suitable for every person, although in view of its favorable side-effect profile and relative safety, the SSRI citalopram is often recommended as a first-line treatment.[22] However, mirtazapine may be a better choice for people with insomnia or poor appetite.[32] Additional night sedation may be required in the initial weeks of any treatment, but the benefits must be balanced against the risk of falls (see Chapter 3).

In general, three main factors guide the clinician's choice of drug:

- *Tolerability*. Adverse side effects of antidepressants occur more often in older individuals and have a more deleterious effect. Orthostatic hypotension, the most common side effect of the older TCAs, may lead to a fall/hip fracture in older women, and the anticholinergic, cardiovascular, and sedative side effects of these drugs can also be of concern. Newer compounds are generally better tolerated, but the most frequently used of these, the SSRIs, can cause hyponatremia, leading to acute confusion and convulsions.[32]
- *Drug interactions*. The likelihood that an older woman will be taking multiple medications makes it particularly important to consider drug interactions, the potential for which is increased by age-related changes in pharmacokinetics due to impaired renal and hepatic function (see Chapter 9).
- *Lethality in overdose*. TCAs are generally more lethal in overdose than SSRIs. However, several reports suggest that a metabolite of citalopram may be cardiotoxic in overdose.[32]

The important message is that the prescription of antidepressants must be tailored to the individual, and the general rule must be 'start low, go slow'. Therapeutic levels must be achieved,

Table 6.4 Antidepressants: classes, side effects, and contraindications

Class	Examples	Adverse effects	Contraindications
Tricyclic antidepressants (TCAs)	Amitriptyline Imipramine Lofepramine Dothiepin Clomipramine	Confusion, blurred vision, constipation, urinary retention, orthostatic hypotension, cardiac arrhythmias, reduced seizure threshold, sedation (more with amitriptyline, less with lofepramine)	Prostatism, narrow angle glaucoma, post-myocardial infarction, heart block
Selective serotonin reuptake inhibitors (SSRIs)	Fluoxetine Citalopram Paroxetine Sertraline	Nausea, diarrhea, headache, agitation, (particularly fluoxetine), sedation, decrease of seizure threshold. Weight loss & rash with fluoxetine. Withdrawal syndrome with anxiety & dizziness (especially with paroxetine). Decreased libido & anorgasmia. Occasionally hyponatraemia. Occasionally extrapyramidal side effects	MAOIs
Monoamine oxidase inhibitors (MAOIs)	Phenelzine Tranylcypromine Isocarboxazid	Confusion, weight gain, hypotension, constipation, urinary retention, sedation, hepatotoxicity, edema, leukopenia, psychosis, hypertensive crisis unless tyramine-containing foods avoided	Cardiovascular disease, diabetes, pheochromocytoma, liver disease
Reversible inhibitor of MAO-A (RIMA)	Moclobemide	Sleep disturbances, nausea, agitation, confusion. Hypertension reported (may be related to tyramine ingestion)	
Serotonin and norepinephrine reuptake inhibitor (SNRI)	Venlafaxine	Nausea, insomnia, dry mouth, somnolence, dizziness, sweating, nervousness, headache, sexual dysfunction, hypertension at high doses, withdrawal syndrome	MAOIs; hepatic or renal impairment (use lower doses)
Norepinephrine and specific serotonin antidepressant (NASSA)	Mirtazapine	Sedation, increased appetite, weight gain, edema, rarely blood dyscrasias, convulsions, myoclonus. Nausea and sexual dysfunction are uncommon	
Atypical	Trazodone	Sedation, dizziness, postural hypotension, nausea, low cardiotoxicity, priapism	

Adapted from Katona and Livingston.[31]

however, and although the dosages required in older women may be lower than for younger adults, this is often not the case. As response to treatment in the elderly often takes longer than in younger adults, whichever drug is chosen should not be considered ineffective until the woman has received the full therapeutic dose for at least 6 weeks, and sometimes up to 12 weeks. If no response is seen to a full therapeutic trial, the patient should be reassessed to ensure that depressive disorder is the correct diagnosis. The next step is to try another antidepressant, either from the same or from a different class,[22] but clinicians must be aware of interactions between antidepressants when contemplating medication change. If the second medication also shows little or no response, referral to a psychiatrist, who may try alternative strategies such as augmentation with lithium or, in more resistant/severe cases, electroconvulsive therapy (ECT), is indicated. ECT is an extremely effective treatment for depression in later life, with recovery rates of around 80%,[33] but the risks associated with anesthesia mean that it is now less widely used.

Psychological therapies

In both mild and moderate depression, psychological treatment specifically focused on depression (such as problem-solving therapy, brief cognitive behavior therapy, and counseling) of 6–8 sessions over 10–12 weeks should be considered.[3,22] Put simply, psychological therapies aim to change one or more of a person's cognitions (beliefs and attitudes), behaviors and emotions, thus enhancing their ability to cope. The theory and provision of psychological therapies for the elderly have been slow to develop, primarily due to negative impressions about their applicability to the elderly.[34] However, recent evidence suggests that a range of cognitive, behavioral, and interpersonal therapies can be helpful in the treatment of older people with depression, either alone or in combination with medication:[30]

- *Cognitive and cognitive behavior therapy* gives primacy to the role of cognitions in the development of depression.
- *Behavior therapy* stresses the relationship between activity and mood.
- *Interpersonal psychotherapy* gives primacy to the importance of relationship problems as a source of depression and focuses on the treatment of one or more the following disturbances in current relationships: abnormal grief, interpersonal disputes, role transition, and interpersonal deficits (the lack of skills to develop and sustain relationships).

It is perhaps worth stressing that, whichever approach is adopted, working with older adults usually also involves working with their families or caregivers. Indeed, the need to take a family systems approach and to involve significant others is one of the modifications recommended when using psychological therapies with older as opposed to younger people. Other suggested adaptations include providing more education about the nature of depression and the purpose/process of therapy; working at a slower pace; setting concrete goals; and making greater use of reinforcement strategies such as writing things down and repetition.[29,35]

The treatment of depression in physical illness and dementia

The treatment of depression in physical illness is essentially the same as for depression alone, although the possible interaction of antidepressant medication with other drugs, their adverse side effects, and contraindications to treatment need special consideration. Some of the common problems encountered are summarized in Table 6.5.

Table 6.5 Considerations in the treatment of depression in physical illness and dementia

Condition	Treatment
Cardiovascular disease	Use SSRIs in preference to TCAs, which prolong Q-Tc interval
Recent MI	Avoid ADs for 2 months and then use SSRIs if possible
Heart failure	Avoid ADs that cause postural hypotension: TCAs, trazodone, and venlafaxine. May augment effect of antihypertensives, but venlafaxine may exacerbate hypertension. Use SSRIs
Arrhythmias	SSRIs are relatively safe
Warfarin (used in AF)	ADs may interact adversely with warfarin metabolism
	Citalopram least likely to affect INR
Renal failure	TCAs: use divided doses. SSRIs: citalopram can be given at normal doses, but paroxetine and fluoxetine at reduced doses. Venlafaxine: reduced dose in mild/moderate renal failure and avoided in severe renal failure
Liver failure	Most ADs have extensive hepatic metabolism and should be given in reduced doses. Safest TCA is imipramine and safest SSRIs are paroxetine and citalopram
Parkinson's disease	TCAs may improve motor symptoms, but may reduce absorption of levodopa and worsen symptoms. SSRIs may cause tremor; paroxetine and fluoxetine may worsen extrapyramidal symptoms. MAOIs may trigger hypertensive crisis in people on levodopa
Epilepsy	If depression develops postictally or subictally, modify anticonvulsant treatment. Some anticonvulsants may exacerbate depression, some may alleviate (carbamazepine, valproate). SSRIs relatively safe. TCAs may reduce seizure threshold
Stroke	TCAs may cause acute confusional state due to anticholinergic action; may also decrease seizure threshold. Citalopram effective in treatment of depression and 'emotional incontinence' associated with stroke. Aspirin may increase free plasma concentrations of TCAs, SSRIs, and trazodone
Dementia	TCAs may cause acute confusional state due to anticholinergic action. Citalopram may improve recent memory and orientation as well as improve mood and reduce panic

ADs, antidepressants; AF, atrial fibrillation; INR, international normalized ratio; MI, myocardial infarction; MAOIs, monoamine oxidase inhibitors; TCAs, tricyclic antidepressants; SSRIs, selective serotonin reuptake inhibitors.

However, management challenges should not prevent the depressed person with physical illness from receiving complete treatment.

Decisions about the management of depression in patients with dementia are based on the same principles, although there is less evidence to support the various treatment strategies.

Nevertheless, improvements in mood and associated behavioral disturbances have been reported with medication and behavior therapies.[36] Psychosocial interventions undertaken in collaboration with care home staff can be effective in treating elderly depressed care home residents with dementia.[37] Sadly, these are often not available.

Maintenance treatment

Current guidelines suggest that antidepressants should be continued for at least 6 months after the woman has recovered from a first episode of depression, and for 2 years if there has been more than one episode in the last few years or if the depression has lasted more than 2 years.[3,22] However, the impact of relapse on an elderly person with a limited life span is a reasonable argument for longer, possibly lifelong treatment. This eventually needs to be balanced against the risks of overtreatment and the adverse effects of antidepressant medication (particularly cardiovascular risks), whereas the use of psychotherapy offers an effective alternative form of prophylaxis.[38]

Prevention of relapse

The importance of treating early and adequately cannot be underestimated. Although depression is prone to relapse, recurrence, and chronicity, most older people recover if given appropriate treatment. One review of the prognosis of depression in old age[39] showed that of older people receiving inpatient treatment for their depression, 60% recovered and either remained well or had relapses or recurrences from which they also recovered. In contrast, patients living in the community had a worse outcome at 2 years (despite having less severe depressive disorder), with 27% remaining depressed and just 34% recovered. Direct comparison is difficult, as rates of antidepressant prescribing were lower in this population. Poor outcome is associated with physical illness severity, cerebral pathology, and the severity and chronicity of the depressive illness.[6]

PREVENTION OF DEPRESSION

Strategies to prevent depression aim to buffer older women from the biological, psychological, and social risk factors that may precipitate the disease. Some interventions are appropriate for high-risk groups such as counseling for the recently bereaved or exercise groups for care home residents.[40] More general measures that may be helpful include prompt treatment of any physical disorder, avoiding polypharmacy, and promotion of an active and healthy lifestyle, including sleep and diet. Referral to voluntary or statutory agencies who can provide social contact, formal help, or advice may also be beneficial, but given that one of the most important factors protecting against the development of depression is the feeling that one is supported, simply taking the time to really listen to older women might be one of the most helpful things the care provider can do.[21]

MENTAL HEALTH SERVICES FOR OLDER PEOPLE

The discussions of depression and dementia in this book clearly show that mental health problems are common in older people and their effects are wide ranging, both in terms of social issues and healthcare outcomes. Indeed, the most recent policy guidance for England is entitled Everybody's Business.[41]

Although most mental health problems are managed in primary care and the general community, specialist mental health services have an important role in supporting primary and social care and in the management of more complex or difficult cases. Specialist old age psychiatry originated in the UK between the 1940s and 1970s, and the model has now spread internationally. By 2003, at least 40 countries had some form of specific provision for this patient group. The World Health Organization provides a list of service principles,[42] although there are variations between countries, depending on the available levels of resources and on other factors, e.g. the role of neurologists or geriatric physicians in treating dementia.

Specialist old age psychiatry services[43] generally consist of multidisciplinary community
teams, memory clinics, inpatient beds, and other
facilities, including day care and respite care, as
well as consultation–liaison services to general
hospital services. Community teams usually
comprise psychiatrists, community psychiatric
nurses, occupational therapists, psychologists,
and social workers, along with support staff, and
these providers usually cover a defined geographical catchment area.

In practice, services emphasize the importance of supporting older people and their carers
at home where possible. Integrated partnership
working with carers, primary care, and social
care providers is vital for services to function
successfully. Certain groups within the population require particular attention, including people from minority ethnic backgrounds, people
with learning disabilities, inhabitants of rural
communities, older people in prison, and older
lesbian and gay people. Gender issues are very

important too: not only do women constitute
the majority of older people, but they are more
likely to live alone, to present with mental
health problems, and to be resident in care
homes. More detailed accounts of service issues,
including the evidence for their efficacy, are
available elsewhere.[44,45]

CONCLUSION

Depression has a greater impact on health-related
quality of life than many chronic medical disorders such as lung disease, arthritis, hypertension,
and diabetes.[46,47] Depression is, fortunately, emi-
nently treatable, and studies have shown that
treatment of depression not only improves mental
health outcomes but also affects physical health
and quality of life in a positive manner.[48–50] It is
hoped that this chapter will have encouraged the
reader to play an active part in the early detection
and management of depression.

REFERENCES

1. World Health Organization. The ICD 10 Classification of Mental and Behavioural Disorders, 10th edn. Geneva: World Health Organization; 1992.
2. Copeland JR, Beekman AT, Dewey ME, et al. Depression in Europe. Geographical distribution among older people. Br J Psychiatry 1999; 174: 312–21.
3. National Institutes of Health. Diagnosis and treatment of depression in late life. NIH consensus statement. 1991. http://consensus.nih.gov/1991/1991DepressionLateLife086html.htm.
4. Weissman MM, Leaf PJ, Tischler GL, et al. Affective disorders in five United States communities. Psychol Med 1988; 18(1): 141–53.
5. Blazer DG. Depression in late life: review and commentary. J Gerontol A Biol Sci Med Sci 2003; 58(3): 249–65.
6. World Psychiatric Association. WPA International Committee for Prevention and Treatment of Depression. Depressive Disorder in Older Persons. New York: NCM Publishers; 1999. http://www.wpanet.org/sectorial/edu4.html.
7. Cullum S, Tucker S, Todd C, Brayne C. Screening for depression in older medical inpatients. Int J Geriatr Psychiatry 2006; 21(5): 469–76.
8. Koenig HG, Blazer DG. Epidemiology of geriatric affective disorders. Clin Geriatr Med 1992; 8(2): 235–51.
9. Brodaty H, Luscombe G, Parker G, et al. Early and late onset depression in old age: different aetiologies, same phenomenology. J Affect Disord 2001; 66(2–3): 225–36.
10. Alexopoulos GS. Depression in the elderly. Lancet 2005; 365(9475): 1961–70.

11. O'Brien J, Desmond P, Ames D, et al. A magnetic resonance imaging study of white matter lesions in depression and Alzheimer's disease. Br J Psychiatry 1996; 168(4): 477–85.

12. Prince MJ, Harwood RH, Blizard RA, et al. Impairment, disability and handicap as risk factors for depression in old age. The Gospel Oak Project V. Psychol Med 1997; 27(2): 311–21.

13. Beekman AT, Copeland JR, Prince MJ. Review of community prevalence of depression in later life. Br J Psychiatry 1999; 174: 307–11.

14. Cole MG, Dendukuri N. Risk factors for depression among elderly community subjects: a systematic review and meta-analysis. Am J Psychiatry 2003; 160(6): 1147-56.

15. World Health Organization. Women, Ageing and Health. Fact Sheet No. 252. 2000. http://www.who.int/mediacentre/factsheets/fs252/en/print.html.

16. Kornstein SG. The evaluation and management of depression in women across the life span. J Clin Psychiatry 2001; 62(Suppl 24): 11–17.

17. Dhondt T, Derksen P, Hooijer C, et al. Depressogenic medication as an aetiological factor in major depression: an analysis in a clinical population of depressed elderly people. Int J Geriatr Psychiatry 1999; 14(10): 875–81.

18. Kockler M, Heun R. Gender differences of depressive symptoms in depressed and nondepressed elderly persons. Int J Geriatr Psychiatry 2002; 17(1): 65–72.

19. Ballard C, Bannister C, Oyebode F. Depression in dementia sufferers. Int J Geriatr Psychiatry 1996; 11(6): 507–15.

20. Alexopoulos GS. Interventions for depressed elderly primary care patients. Int J Geriatr Psychiatry 2001; 16(6): 553–9.

21. World Health Organization. Gender and Women's Mental Health. 2005. http://www.who.int/mental_health/prevention/genderwomen/en/print.html.

22. National Institute for Clinical Excellence. Depression: Management of Depression in Primary and Secondary Care. Clinical Guideline 23: 2004.

23. Yesavage JA, Brink TL, Rose TL, et al. Development and validation of a geriatric depression screening scale: a preliminary report. J Psychiatr Res 1983; 17(1): 37–9.

24. Burke WJ, Houston MJ, Boust SJ, et al. Use of the Geriatric Depression Scale in dementia of the Alzheimer type. J Am Geriatr Soc 1989; 37(9): 856–60.

25. Alexopoulos GS, Abrams RC, Young RC, et al. Cornell Scale for Depression in Dementia. Biol Psychiatry 1988; 23(3): 271–84.

26. Gilbody S, House A, Sheldon T. Screening and case finding instruments for depression. Cochrane Database Syst Rev 2005; (4): CD002792.

27. Folstein MF, Folstein SE, McHugh PR. "Mini-mental state". A practical method for grading the cognitive state of patients for the clinician. J Psychiatr Res 1975; 12: 189–98.

28. Wilson K, Mottram P, Sivanranthan A, et al. Antidepressant versus placebo for depressed elderly. Cochrane Database Syst Rev 2001; (2): CD000561.

29. Zarit S, Zarit J. Mental Disorders in Older Adults. Fundamentals of assessment and treatment. New York: Guilford Press; 1998.

30. Frazer CJ, Christensen H, Griffiths KM. Effectiveness of treatments for depression in older people. Med J Aust 2005; 182(12): 627–32.

31. Katona C, Livingston G. Drug Treatment in Old Age Psychiatry. London: Martin Dunitz; 2003.

32. Taylor D, Paton C, Kerwin R. The Maudsley Prescribing Guidelines, 7th edn. London: Martin Dunitz; 2003.

33. Mulsant BH, Rosen J, Thornton JE, et al. A prospective naturalistic study of electroconvulsive therapy in late-life depression. J Geriatr Psychiatry Neurol 1991; 4(1): 3–13.

34. Hepple J. Psychotherapies with older people: an overview. Adv Psychiatri Treat 2004; 10: 371–7.

35. Karel MJ, Hinrichsen G. Treatment of depression in late life: psychotherapeutic interventions. Clin Psychol Rev 2000; 20(6): 707–29.

36. Rosenberg P, Onyike C, Katz I, et al. Clinical application of operationalized criteria for 'Depression of Alzheimer's Disease'. Int J Geriatr Psychiatry 2005; 20(2): 119–27.

37. Llewellyn-Jones RH, Baikie KA, Smithers H, et al. Multifaceted shared care intervention for late life depression in residential care: randomised controlled trial. BMJ 1999; 319(7211): 676–82.

38. Ong Y, Martineau F, Lloyd C, et al. A support group for the depressed elderly. Int J Geriatr Psychiatry 1987; 2(2): 119–23.

39. Cole MG, Bellavance F. The prognosis of depression in old age. Am J Geriatr Psychiatry 1997; 5(1): 4–14.

40. McMurdo ME, Rennie L. A controlled trial of exercise by residents of old people's homes. Age Ageing 1993; 22(1): 11–15.

41. Department of Health, Care Services Improvement Partnership. Everybody's Business. Integrated Mental Health Service for Older Adults: A Service Development Guide. London: Department of Health; 2005.

42. World Health Organization. Organization of Care in Psychiatry of the Elderly: A Technical Consensus Statement. Geneva: WHO/WPA; 1997.

43. Challis D, Reilly S, Hughes J, et al. Policy, organisation and practice of specialist old age psychiatry in England. Int J Geriatr Psychiatry 2002; 17(11): 1018–26.

44. Bartels SJ, Dums AR, Oxman TE, et al. Evidence-based practices in geriatric mental health care: an overview of systematic reviews and meta-analyses. Psychiatr Clin North Am 2003; 26(4): 971–90.

45. Draper B, Melding P, Brodaty H, eds. Psychogeriatric Service Delivery: An International Perspective. Oxford: Oxford University Press; 2005.

46. Wells KB, Stewart A, Hays RD, et al. The functioning and well-being of depressed patients. Results from the Medical Outcomes Study. JAMA 1989; 262(7): 914–19.

47. Hays RD, Wells KB, Sherbourne CD, et al. Functioning and well-being outcomes of patients with depression compared with chronic general medical illnesses. Arch Gen Psychiatry 1995; 52(1): 11–19.

48. Unutzer J, Katon W, Callahan CM, et al. Collaborative care management of late-life depression in the primary care setting: a randomized controlled trial. JAMA 2002; 288(22): 2836–45.

49. Bruce ML, Ten Have TR, Reynolds CF III, et al. Reducing suicidal ideation and depressive symptoms in depressed older primary care patients: a randomized controlled trial. JAMA 2004; 291(9): 1081–91.

50. Lin EH, Katon W, Von Korff M, et al. Effect of improving depression care on pain and functional outcomes among older adults with arthritis: a randomized controlled trial. JAMA 2003; 290(18): 2428–9.

Urogenital aging

7

Roger P Goldberg

BACKGROUND

Steadily increasing numbers of women over age 70, at least in the developed world, have brought about an increasing appreciation of urogenital aging and its role in a woman's overall function and quality of life. In the US alone, the population of women aged 65 or over is projected to double over the next 25 years, and this age stratum is expected to account for nearly a quarter of the total US population by 2040.[1] In Europe, women presently constitute about 60% of the population over age 70 and one-fifth of the total population.[1] Regardless of their place of residence, women over 70 are increasingly seeking answers for urogenital problems that routinely were dismissed as 'inevitable' by former generations of women and their doctors.

Urogenital aging is associated with a cluster of potential symptoms, which can impact urinary, genital, and/or sexual functioning. By age 65, for example, one out of every three women suffers some degree of urinary incontinence, and millions choose an operation to relieve what can be in some instances a socially debilitating symptom. Others experience irritative lower urinary tract symptoms without actual leakage, but with nocturia and urgency significantly impacting quality of life. By age 70, up to 11% of the general female population will have undergone major surgery for either incontinence or prolapse (another major condition associated with urogenital aging) – a number roughly equal to the lifetime risk of breast cancer. Aside from

bladder dysfunction and prolapse, other age-related changes include vulvovaginal atrophy and sexual dysfunction. Dyspareunia represents but one of the most common reasons prompting women to seek local hormone therapy after menopause, and is often accompanied by other aspects of sexual dysfunction, which are covered in a separate chapter of this book (see Chapter 16). In terms of public health, disorders associated with urogenital aging account for substantial medical, economic, and social burdens. For example, Luber et al reported that mature age groups generate 10 times the number of urogynecology consults per 1000 woman-years, compared with their younger counterparts.[2]

Although these various 'issues' associated with female urogenital aging attract less attention than impotence (the major urogenital aging problem in men), in recent years women's health providers have begun to more consistently screen for urogenital disorders and have had the opportunity to offer therapies that may vastly enhance quality of life. This chapter provides a brief overview of key symptoms and conditions relating to urogenital aging that play an important role in the general healthcare of women over 70.

HYPOESTROGENISM AND UROGENITAL ATROPHY

The permanent and natural decline in endogenous estrogen during the decades after menopause has important implications for the lower urinary tract and vagina – both of which share a common embryology, and both of which remain highly sensitive to estrogen throughout the woman's life. Although from 10 to 40% of the postmenopausal female population are believed to have symptoms of urogenital atrophy, the percentage of women receiving effective hormonal therapy remains low.[3]

Estrogen receptors exist in the bladder and urethra, distal vagina, and pelvic floor muscles.[4,5] In fact, the concentration of estrogen receptors is roughly similar in the urethra and distal vagina.[6] Therefore, it should not be surprising that lack of estrogen after menopause, in addition to causing vaginitis, dryness, and dyspareunia, may also result in urinary urgency, nocturia, and dysuria. During the postmenopausal years, estrogen deficiency leads to decreased connective tissue density, thinning of the vaginal and urethral epithelium, and decreased urogenital vascularity.[7] It is postulated that hypoestrogenism affects the sensory threshold of the urinary tract in elderly patients, leading to decreased functional bladder capacities.[8] Alpha receptors localized in the urethral sphincter are thought to help muscle tone; estrogen receptors are also present in the squamous epithelium of the proximal and distal urethra, vagina, and trigone. Through these various receptors, estrogens may assist continence by increasing urethral resistance, bladder sensory threshold, perfusion of the urethral vascular bed, and adrenoreceptor sensitivity in urethral smooth muscle.

Symptoms

The symptoms of urogenital atrophy are often vague in older women. Patients may report any combination of vulvovaginal dryness and pruritus, dyspareunia, urinary urgency, frequency, and/or nocturia. Assessment of urogenital atrophy is mainly clinical – with typical findings including loss of lubrication and increased friability, and sensitivity to examination, as well as thinning of the labia and loss of interlabial fold, and the presence of a urethral caruncle. During the early stages of atrophy, scattered small petechiae may be visible throughout the vaginal epithelium and may be associated with a thin, clear discharge. Assessment of vaginal pH, which can be performed with a simple indicator strip, typically reveals no distinct shift from normal acidity. Genital tract inflammation or infections with *Monilia, Trichomonas*, herpes, or human papillomavirus (HPV) may increase afferent sensation and lead to irritative voiding symptoms. Testing for these conditions should be performed based on the clinical presentation. Heavy vaginal discharge may be confused with urinary incontinence. Although not generally necessary in clinical practice, a vaginal smear analyzed for karyotypic index may reveal fewer superficial cells in relation to the total population of squamous cells. Decreased estrogen levels may trigger a shift in vaginal flora from non-uropathogens (lactobacilli) to uropathogens – one of several possible reasons for increased urinary tract infections among hypoestrogenic postmenopausal women.

It is worth emphasizing that although we try whenever possible to consider urogenital symptoms and disorders in terms of a single, discrete condition relating to either the lower urinary tract or vulvovaginal area, this is not always possible. In actual practice, urological and genital symptoms often overlap in confusing ways. Therefore, the proper clinical approach for evaluating a urogenital complaint should provide a routine assessment of both the 'uro' and 'genital' elements in an efficient but complete manner. For example, the estrogen status of the vulva and vagina should be carefully assessed in any woman presenting with bladder or urethral symptoms, as postmenopausal hypoestrogenic atrophic changes throughout the urogenital tissues may contribute to irritative lower urinary tract symptoms and increased rate of atrophic (sterile) and bacterial cystitis.

Estrogen replacement

Treatment of urogenital atrophy centers on the use of local hormone replacement therapy (HRT). A number of clinical trials have established the efficacy of this approach for treating urogenital symptoms.[9–11] Other studies also indicate that vaginal estrogen (including intravaginal estriol and the vaginal ring) may be effective in reducing the risk of recurrent urinary tract infections in postmenopausal women.[12,13] However, oral and transdermal systemic estrogens may not represent an appropriate choice for first-line therapy, because of an unfavorable risk/benefit profile, which was revealed by the Women's Health Initiative, and their poorer efficacy.[14] Local forms of treatment arguably offer the 'best of both worlds' – i.e. an efficacy on urogenital symptoms that is superior to systemic forms of therapy, along with an inherently more favorable safety profile.

Exogenous estrogens increase the presence of intermediate and superficial cells in vagina, bladder, and urethra of postmenopausal women. Estradiol reduces the amplitude and frequency of spontaneous detrusor contractions.[15] The majority of evidence obtained from patients with an 'overactive bladder' suggests that local estrogen therapy has the potential to improve urinary urgency, frequency, nocturia, and dysuria but not incontinence.[11] However, postmenopausal oral HRT may increase the risk of developing urinary incontinence perhaps by disrupting already biomechanically deficient collagen.[14,16,17] For this reason, in 2004 the American College of Obstetricians and Gynecologists formally stated that oral estrogens cannot be recommended as treatment for any type of urinary incontinence, and further cautioned that oral therapy may exacerbate symptoms. Other authors have cautioned that these findings do not exclude the possibility that systemic estrogens could theoretically be effective in preventing stress incontinence and treating urge incontinence.[18] Nevertheless, ongoing concerns over the long-term use of systemic estrogen will undoubtedly limit its use for the foreseeable future.

A Cochrane review of 16 randomized trials concluded that vaginal estrogen therapy is safe and effective for the treatment of vaginal atrophy.[19] Creams, pessaries, tablets, and the estradiol vaginal ring were reported as being equally effective in treating the symptoms of vaginal atrophy. Adverse events were found to be rare, although the authors did note the possibility of higher rates of vaginal bleeding and breast pain with use of higher doses of conjugated equine estrogen cream when compared with estradiol tablets. It seems clear that the following, currently available preparations are safe and generally well tolerated. When used at standard doses, even the upper limits of serum estradiol levels are within the normal menopausal range:

- Vaginal estrogen cream/pessaries:
  conjugated estrogens
  estradiol
  estriol
- Vaginal tablet:
  estradiol, low dose
- Slow-release vaginal ring:
  estradiol, low dose

UROGENITAL AGING: IMPACT ON LOWER URINARY TRACT SYMPTOMS

Irritative voiding symptoms and incontinence are two of the most important manifestations of urogenital aging. Aging may adversely affect neurological control of micturition, urinary tract structure, tissue repair, elasticity of tissue, and nerve degeneration. The prevalence of incontinence increases from approximately 13% in women 18–23 years old to 56% in the elderly.[20–22] Studies of community-dwelling women aged ≥60 years old from various populations in Europe and the US indicate prevalence rates averaging 32–38%.[23,24] In 1995, the direct and indirect costs of urinary incontinence were estimated around $26 billion for individuals over age 65 in the US.[25]

The most common cause of urinary leakage in women, and especially younger women, is stress urinary incontinence (SUI) − defined as involuntary leakage during effort or exertion. With age, rates of stress incontinence increase and become less clearly related to a woman's obstetrical history as urethral closure pressures and functional length decrease.[26] However, for women over 70, irritative voiding and urge urinary incontinence (UUI) often represent more bothersome symptoms. This age-dependent condition is defined as involuntary leakage of urine accompanied by or immediately preceded by urgency. The most common changes observed with advancing age, in addition to a decline in pelvic floor muscle strength, include reduced maximum bladder capacity, increased urgency, frequency, and decreased 'warning time', reduced urinary flow rate, and postvoid fullness. On the structural and ultrastructural level, certain changes in the detrusor muscle appear consistently in the elderly and evolve over time, leading some investigators, including Elbadawi et al, to propose that age-related detrusor instability be categorized as a specific and distinct entity.[27] Through the much broader clinical 'lens' of quality of life, other studies suggest that *urge incontinence* tends to have a greater impact in older women than *stress incontinence*, as the unpredictability of accidents becomes a major barrier for women trying to maintain an active social routine. Therefore, urge symptoms should receive careful attention when the healthcare professional tries to positively impact the urogenital health of women over 70.

Irritative voiding and 'overactive bladder' in older women

Overactive bladder (OAB) is particularly common in postmenopausal women. In particular, the so-called 'dry' OAB (urgency, frequency, and nocturia, *without* incontinence episodes) is often a direct result of urogenital aging. Hypoestrogenism, atrophic cystourethritis, and genital prolapse are a few of the age-dependent changes that underlie this association. One validated telephone survey reported an overall OAB female prevalence of 16.9%, separated into 7.6% 'dry' and 9.3% 'wet' (urgency and frequency *with* incontinence episodes).[28] Prevalence rates are often underreported due to stigma and embarrassment, or to a sense that the condition is inevitable and untreatable. As a result, only 60% of OAB patients inform their healthcare provider of their problems.[29,30]

In recent years, it has become clear that the direct and indirect costs of age-related lower urinary tract dysfunction are staggering. In one conservative estimate by Hu et al, the total economic costs of OAB were found to exceed US$12 billion in 2000 in the US.[31] Beyond the economic toll, the true consequences of this condition lie in the heavy psychological and social burdens endured by affected individuals.

The physiology of OAB has been the subject of much recent interest and some disagreement. Sometimes, a discrete disease process initiates a cascade of events leading to overactive vesical function − and the prevalence of many of these underlying conditions increases with age. Examples include anatomic and inflammatory sources such as urethrotrigonitis, urolithiasis, bladder outlet obstruction following surgery or advanced pelvic organ prolapse, and neoplasia. Older women are also more prone to neurological triggers for irritative voiding, including cerebrovascular accidents, intracranial lesions, or parkinsonism. Notwithstanding such discrete medical conditions the fact remains that roughly 90% are idiopathic, without a clear underlying cause.[32] OAB is estimated to exist in up to 61% of incontinent nursing home patients.[33] In the elderly, a significant percentage of women with detrusor overactivity also have impaired contractility of the detrusor muscle.

Among women over 70, as previously mentioned, hypoestrogenism may play a role with regard to urgency and frequency symptoms. Urgency and frequency symptoms may, in turn, sometimes dramatically resolve with local estrogen-based therapy. Pelvic organ prolapse may also play a contributory role by partially obstructing the bladder neck, leading to bladder trabeculations and the onset of OAB symptoms – an obstructive mechanism similar to that of benign prostatic hyperplasia in men, which also leads to OAB symptoms.

Women with irritative lower urinary tract symptoms are often plagued by a constellation of symptoms that leave them uncomfortable, embarrassed, and ashamed, and an individual's self-esteem and body image may be profoundly altered by chronic wetness, skin irritation, and odor, or the need for absorbent products. Among women over 70, the social implications of OAB can become even more profound, as urge incontinence becomes a common reason underlying nursing home admissions.[34] It also limits other activities, as was found in one study of 2190 patients over 55 years in which women with incontinence spent less time walking, communicating with friends and family by telephone or email, working for pay, using a computer, and engaging in personal grooming and hygiene than similar continent women.[35]

Further, many patients with symptoms of urogenital aging begin to adopt alternative coping strategies to compensate for urinary urgency symptoms. For example, patients with urgency and incontinence may restrict their wardrobe to dark clothing in order to hide urine stains, avoid sexual intimacy, reduce oral fluid intake, limit travel to those locations where they know where bathrooms are available (bathroom mapping), or choose seats near bathrooms.[36]

Recently, evidence has come forward that irritative voiding symptoms have a statistically significant correlation with falls and fractures in older women (see Chapter 3). Brown et al reported that community-dwelling women with urge incontinence (>1 event per week) were at a significant increased risk for falls (odds ratio [OR] = 1.26; 95% CI 1.14–1.40) and fractures (non-spine non-traumatic fracture relative hazard = 1.34; 95% CI 1.06–1.69).[37] Also, individuals with daily urge incontinence were at a 35% increased risk of falls compared with controls.[37] This finding is supported by Wagner et al, who, in a subanalysis of data from the NOBLE dataset, found that individuals with OAB had more than twice the odds of being injured in a fall than people without OAB (OR = 2.26), as well as a trend towards higher rates of bony fracture (OR = 1.53).[38] Frequent trips to the bathroom throughout the night in patients with OAB-related nocturia most likely play an important role. Considering the higher prevalence of OAB in older women with decreased bone mass, these secondary effects relating to safety and fracture risk should be considered when assessing the public health impact of urogenital aging.

Evaluation of the lower urinary tract

Evaluation of bladder symptoms in older women begins with a general, followed by a urinary, medical history for systemic disease (neurological, cardiac, endocrine, renal). Patients with SUI typically complain of urinary leakage upon coughing, sneezing, or other activities that increase abdominal pressure. Risk factors for SUI include prior vaginal deliveries, menopause, vaginal surgery, radiation, pelvic injury, obesity, lung disease, smoking, strenuous exercise, and weight-bearing occupations. In contrast, patients with UUI complain of urine loss with a strong urge before reaching the toilet. Urge episodes may be provoked by environmental or psychological triggers, such as handwashing, the sound of running water, or reaching home ('latchkey urge'). As mentioned previously, many women over 70 have urinary frequency, urgency, and nocturia in the absence of incontinence episodes.

Women over 70 commonly take one or several medications for chronic or acute conditions unrelated to the urogenital tract. Because a number of these medications can exacerbate urogenital tract complaints, a careful review of medications should always take place. Table 7.1

details medications that potentially affect urogenital tract symptoms. Tamoxifen, taken by many women for the treatment and sometimes prevention of breast cancer, has antiestrogenic effects that are manifest in the urogenital tract with side effects ranging from mild vaginal dryness to severe vaginitis.

A self-completed bladder diary that records the frequency and volumes of micturition, number of incontinent episodes, associated symptoms, and fluid intake may be useful to help clarify the patient's history. Once the complete history is elicited, it is important to corroborate symptoms with signs and urodynamic diagnoses.

Table 7.1   Drugs that may affect the urogenital tract

Class of drugs	Side effect	Impact on urogenital function
Psychotropic agents: antidepressants and antipsychotics	Anticholinergic, sedation	Urinary retention
Sedatives/hypnotics	Sedation, muscle relaxation, confusion	Urinary retention
Caffeine, alcohol, diuretics		Urgency, frequency, polyuria
Narcotics	Sedation, delirium	Urinary retention, fecal impaction
ACE inhibitors	Cough	Aggravate pre-existing stress incontinence
Calcium channel blockers		Urinary retention, overflow incontinence
Anticholinergics	Dry mouth, constipation, sleepiness, or drowsiness	Urinary retention, overflow incontinence
Alpha-adrenergic agonists	Increased urethral tone	Urinary retention
Alpha-adrenergic blockers	Decreased urethral tone	Stress urinary incontinence
Beta-adrenergic agonists	Inhibited detrusor function	Urinary retention
Partial estrogen antagonists	Urogenital atrophy	Urgency, frequency, dysuria, dyspareunia

ACE, angiotensin-converting enzyme.

Among postmenopausal women, deficiencies in antidiuretic hormone levels or activity may lead to excessive night-time urine production ('reverse diuresis'). Simple comparison of daytime and night-time voided volumes may highlight this problem, defined as more than one-third of the 24-hour output occurring during the night-time. The use of synthetic desmopressin may be considered in these cases.

During the physical examination, particular attention should be paid to conditions that impact lower urinary tract function such as volume overload, venous insufficiency, or congestive heart failure. Ambulatory capacity and mental status should also be assessed to evaluate a patient's functional capability. It is important to bear in mind, particularly in elderly women, that incontinence is transient in up to one-third of community-dwelling elderly and up to one-half of acutely hospitalized patients.[39] The mnemonic DIAPPERS has been suggested as a simple means to recall the most common reversible causes of incontinence[40] (Table 7.2). If a neurological abnormality is suspected, urgent referral to a neurologist is imperative.

Assessment of urethral mobility with a 'Q-tip test' provides an accurate measure of urethral support. A deflection of the inserted lubricated cotton swab >30° above the horizontal suggests urethral hypermobility. Patients who exhibit SUI without hypermobility should be further evaluated for intrinsic urethral sphincter dysfunction. A basic evaluation to screen for advanced pelvic organ prolapse can be performed with a standard Sims' or Graves' speculum. In this manner, larger cystocele or rectocele defects can be visually appreciated; and, if present, referral to a specialist for further evaluation may be warranted. In some cases, it may remain unclear to what extent a woman's urogenital discomfort is attributable to the degree of prolapse objectively determined on examination. One diagnostic option in this circumstance is a 'pessary test', which involves inserting a vaginal pessary for a period of several weeks, and monitoring for improvement (or lack thereof) while the prolapse obstruction is partially relieved. Surgical repair of advanced prolapse provides rather unpredictable results on OAB symptoms – although it is safe to say that, for some women, the relief of mechanical bladder neck obstruction after pelvic reconstructive surgery results in significant improvement of urgency/frequency symptoms.

The supine empty stress test is a simple test to suggest intrinsic sphincter dysfunction. Once the patient has been catheterized, or if she has recently voided, she is asked to cough and perform a Valsalva maneuver three times in the supine position. This test has a 90% positive predictive value for intrinsic urethral sphincter dysfunction, a type of SUI that may significantly impact treatment recommendations and rates of cure.

Urinalysis is necessary to rule out infection and hematuria. Patients with urinary tract infections should be treated prior to further work-up of incontinence. Sterile microscopic hematuria may indicate bladder or upper urinary tract disorders. Patients with sterile hematuria on repeat clean catch specimens should be referred to a urologist or urogynecologist for evaluation of the bladder with cystourethroscopy as well as upper tract evaluation.

Table 7.2 Reversible causes of incontinence: **DIAPPERS**

Delirium or confusion

Infection, urinary symptoms

Atrophic genital tract changes (vaginitis or urethritis)

Pharmaceutical agents (see Table 7.1)

Psychological factors

Excess urine production (excess fluid intake, volume overload, hyperglycemia, or hypercalcemia)

Restricted mobility (chronic illness, injury, or restraint)

Stool impaction

Adapted from Resnick.[40]

Assessment of the postvoid residual urine quantity should be performed in all patients with incontinence, to rule out urinary retention and overflow. This can be undertaken with ultrasound or catheterization. Significant urinary retention is rare in women in the absence of advanced prolapse, neurological disorders, or prior urogenital tract surgery.

Urodynamic investigations usually include filling and voiding cystometry. In women with suspected UUI, changes in bladder pressure in response to bladder filling can be measured and thus help determine the presence of involuntary detrusor contractions. It also allows for the evaluation of bladder sensation, compliance, capacity, and control during the urine storage phase. If initial evaluation fails to fully define the etiology of an incontinent woman's problem, more sophisticated urodynamic testing is indicated.

MANAGING THE UROLOGICAL EFFECTS OF AGING

Helping a woman to reduce or eliminate incontinence episodes plays a key role in restoring her vulvovaginal comfort, quality of life, and sexual function. For women bothered by symptoms of 'dry' overactive bladder, the benefits to quality of life can be equally profound. Treatment options are detailed in Table 7.3.

Stress urinary incontinence

Treatments for SUI include pelvic floor exercises, biofeedback, pelvic floor electrical stimulation, vaginal continence devices, urethral obstructive devices, urethral bulking agents, and surgery.

Pelvic floor exercises

Pelvic floor exercises improve pelvic floor function by enhancing urethral resistance as a

Table 7.3 Treatments for incontinence

Treatments for stress urinary incontinence include:
- medications
- pelvic floor exercises
- biofeedback
- pelvic floor electrical stimulation
- vaginal continence devices
- urethral obstructive devices
- urethral bulking agents
- surgery

Treatment options for overactive bladder include:
- behavioral and dietary modifications
- pharmacological interventions
- pelvic floor electrical stimulation
- electromagnetic innervation
- sacral neuromodulation
- bladder augmentation
- diversion operations

result of increasing strength and endurance of the periurethral and paravaginal muscles. Such exercises lead to improvement of stress incontinence symptoms in 56–95% of patients, and for women with OAB the ability to strongly contract the pelvic floor muscles provides a valuable tool for urge suppression. Patients who are selected for treatment with pelvic floor exercises should be self-motivated and demonstrate an ability to isolate the correct muscles on pelvic examination. If patients are unable to isolate the correct muscles on their own, then pelvic floor exercises with 'biofeedback' are indicated. 'Biofeedback' with auditory and visual information regarding contraction of the pelvic floor muscles improve patient awareness and correct isolation of pelvic floor muscles.[41] Some studies indicate improvement as high as 87% with biofeedback.[42]

Some patients are unable to isolate their pelvic floor muscles, even with 'biofeedback'. Pelvic floor electrical stimulation is an alternative for these patients. These modalities isolate and contract the pelvic floor muscles for the patient and improve overall muscle tone. In the over-70 population, women with atrophic vaginal changes should be encouraged to pre-treat with local estrogen, before inserting and utilizing pelvic floor stimulation probes.

Drug therapy

Medications for the treatment of SUI include alpha-adrenergic agonists, which act on smooth muscle to increase resting urethral pressure. Increased risks of stroke and hypertension have been reported in some patients using these medications, however. Tricyclic antidepressants, such as imipramine and doxepin, have both anticholinergic and central alpha-adrenergic effects, making them suitable for the treatment of both SUI and UUI. Duloxetine is a new treatment for SUI. It is a dual serotonin and norepinephrine (noradrenaline) reuptake inhibitor that increases neural input to the urethral sphincter, thereby relieving the symptoms of SUI. It improves symptoms of SUI in about 50% of women. This medication has not been approved in all countries.[43]

Pessaries

Incontinence pessaries represent another treatment option for women seeking to avoid or postpone operative management. One study determined that 24% of women with SUI were subjectively cured using these devices.[44] External (FemAssist, CapSure) and internal (FemSoft) urethral occlusive devices are also available for SUI, but are not widely accepted. In women over 70, it is particularly important to assure that they have the dexterity and motivation to manage these devices properly and by themselves.

Surgery

Surgical options for SUI have improved markedly in recent years, and the latest minimally invasive approaches allow for short procedure times under local anesthesia, an important breakthrough for older women not interested in undergoing the morbidity and recuperation associated with the surgeries that were available in the past. Midurethral 'tension-free' slings using Prolene mesh have, over the past 7–8 years, steadily begun to dominate the surgical treatment of SUI.[45] These operations have the ability to achieve cure (dry) rates for SUI in 75–96% of cases. The newest tension-free Prolene slings can be set in place under local anesthesia in 20 minutes or less, on an outpatient basis. Their high efficacy and low risk appear to be establishing a new 'gold standard' for the surgical management of SUI, and these devices have become widely implemented as first-line surgical therapy worldwide. Recently, several 'next-generation' tension-free sling procedures have been introduced, with possible advantages in terms of technical ease and safety, further increasing the widespread interest in this mode of therapy for SUI. Patients with severe SUI without urethral hypermobility are generally not favorable surgical candidates, and may respond well to treatment with office-based periurethral bulking agents.[46]

In the over-70 age population, many women present with overlapping stress incontinence and urge symptoms. It is important for such patients to recognize that urgency and frequency symptoms may persist and require further medical or behavioral therapy, even if a full cure for SUI is achieved with the surgical intervention. SUI procedures vary in their efficacy for the treatment of concurrent OAB, and may sometimes even cause the new onset of overactive bladder symptoms.

Overactive bladder

Treatment options for OAB include behavioral and dietary modifications, medications, pelvic floor electrical stimulation, electromagnetic innervation, sacral neuromodulation, and bladder augmentation and diversion operations.

Treatments for OAB are primarily nonsurgical and include behavioral interventions, medications, and the use of various devices. The simplest behavioral interventions rely on monitoring and adjusting fluid intake and diet. The use of a bladder diary can provide valuable information pertaining to voiding habits and fluid intake. Limiting the use of caffeinated and alcoholic beverages and other foods known to increase urgency can improve symptoms.

Pelvic floor exercises

Bladder retraining represents a cost-free, risk-free strategy to discuss with women of all ages, including women over 70 who are bothered by OAB. In simplest terms, the intervention involves teaching the patient to resist and inhibit the sensation of urgency when it occurs, to delay micturition, and to establish cortical control over micturition. 'Bladder drills' utilize pelvic floor muscle contractions to inhibit detrusor contractions through the 'vesicoinhibitory pathways' (that suppress voluntary detrusor contractions at the termination of normal micturition) in combination with mental and physical distraction techniques. Strict voiding intervals are set, based on the frequency of incontinence episodes, and patients void only at proscribed time intervals. The intervals are slowly increased, depending on patient response. Cure rates may be as high as 18%, with a 51% reduction in incontinence episodes.[47]

Many postmenopausal women find it difficult to recruit the necessary muscles. In this case, biofeedback and pelvic floor physiotherapy can be offered – and may help to resolve urodynamic detrusor overactivity in 44% of women, using visual or auditory signals to guide women on correct and incorrect pelvic floor muscle

contractions.[41] Pelvic floor electrical stimulation is also effective for some cases of urge incontinence and detrusor overactivity, with cure rates ranging from 30 to 50%.

Drug therapy

Several medications are available for the treatment of OAB, and, in general, are safe for use in older women. Most of those drugs are anticholinergic agents that act to inhibit binding of acetylcholine to muscarinic receptors, thereby blocking involuntary detrusor contractions completely or decreasing their amplitude.[48,49] None offer pure selectivity for the lower urinary tract, and therefore all may trigger side effects in other organ systems: the most common side effects are dry mouth and constipation, both of which may limit compliance, especially in women over 70. Aside from efficacy, one should also carefully consider central nervous system (CNS) side effects, such as blurred vision, when treating older women.

Antimuscarinic agents remain the most popular family of medications for the treatment of overactive bladder, although tricyclic antidepressants such as imipramine and doxepin are occasionally used for their combined anticholinergic/ central adrenergic effects, which make them useful for mixed incontinence. The anticholinergics offer roughly a 60–80% reduction in incontinence episode frequency, and cure rates between 10 and 25%. Oxybutynin chloride is a relatively non-selective antimuscarinic agent with extensive use. The immediate-release form is effective, but nearly two-thirds of patients experience moderate to severe dry mouth. The extended-release oral formulation, and also the oxybutynin transdermal patch, demonstrate markedly improved side-effect profiles. Tolterodine was first approved in 1998 as an alternative to oxybutynin; head-to-head trials against extended-release oxybutynin demonstrated reasonable efficacy for this medication, but no dramatic differences when compared with the existing options. Trospium chloride is a newer, non-selective antimuscarinic agent that offers the possible benefit of not crossing the blood–brain barrier (according to animal studies), and low rates of CNS side effects make it a reasonable consideration when treating older women or those with ongoing CNS or dementia symptoms. Solifenacin succinate and darifenacin represent the newest additions to the overactive bladder market, and a prospective, double-blind study showed solifenacin to have greater efficacy than extended-release tolterodine.[50]

Surgery

Surgical therapy may be an option for some women, but bladder augmentation and urinary diversion are rarely ever necessary. The introduction of sacral neuromodulation has provided an alternative for patients unresponsive to medications, devices, and behavior modification. Under local anesthesia, a small quadripolar electrode lead is placed in the S3 foramina and connected to an external pulse generator for a 7–14-day testing period. If there is greater than 50% symptom reduction during this time, a subcutaneous programmable pulse generator is subsequently implanted in the subcutaneous tissue of the buttocks.

CONCLUSION

Because urogenital aging complicates urinary as well as genital functions, it represents an important factor influencing quality of life among women over 70. The majority of women experiencing either a loss of sexual function or persistent lower urinary tract symptoms unfortunately receive no treatment. The sequelae of urogenital aging can often be addressed without extensive testing. Treatment strategies include local hormone replacement, prevention of recurrent urinary tract infection, and management of prolapse and bladder dysfunction. Experimental work with new oral medications, injections, and topical agents should offer many new alternatives for treating the major types of age-related urogenital dysfunction in the future.

REFERENCES

1. U.S. Census Bureau. World Population Information. http://www.census.gov/ipc/www/world.html
2. Luber KM, Boero S, Choe JY. The demographics of pelvic floor disorders: current observations and future projections. Am J Obstet Gynecol 2001; 184: 1496–503.
3. Cardozo L, Bachmann G, McClish D, Fonda D, Birgenson L. Meta-analysis of estrogen in the management of urogenital atrophy in postmenopausal women: second report of the Hormones and Urogenital Therapy Committee. Obstet Gyencol 1998; 92: 722–7.
4. Blakeman PJ, Hilton P, Bulmer JN. Oestrogen and progesterone receptor expression in the female lower urinary tract, with reference to oestrogen status. BJU Int 2000; 86(1): 32–8.
5. Smith P, Heimer G, Norgren A, Ulmsten U. Localization of steroid hormone receptors in the pelvic muscles. Eur J Obstet Gynecol Reprod Biol 1993; 50(1): 83–5.
6. Iosif CS, Batra S, Ek A, Astedt B. Estrogen receptors in the human female lower urinary tract. Am J Obstet Gynecol 1981; 141: 817–20.
7. Bent AE, McLennan MT. Geriatric urogynecology. In: Ostergard DR, Bent AE, eds, 4th edn. Urogynecology and Urodynamics Theory and Practice. Baltimore: Williams & Wilkins; 1996: 441–62.

8. Sultana CJ, Walters MD. Estrogen and urinary incontinence in women. Maturitas 1994; 20: 129–38.

9. Nilsson K, Heimer G. Low-dose oestradiol in the treatment of urogenital oestrogen deficiency – a pharmacokinetic and pharmacodynamic study. Maturitas 1992; 15: 121–7.

10. Smith P, Heimer G, Lindskog M, Ulmsten U. Oestradiol-releasing vaginal ring for treatment of postmenopausal urogenital atrophy. Maturitas 1993; 16: 145–54.

11. Fantl JA, Cardozo L, McClish DK. Estrogen therapy in the management of urinary incontinence in postmenopausal women: a meta-analysis. First Report of the Hormones and Urogenital Committee. Obstet Gynecol 1994; 83: 12–18.

12. Raz R, Stamm WE. A controlled trial of intravaginal estriol in postmenopausal women with recurrent urinary tract infections. N Engl J Med 1993; 329: 753–6.

13. Rozenberg S, Pastijn A, Gevers R, Murillo D. Estrogen therapy in older patients with recurrent urinary tract infections: a review. Int J Fertil Womens Med 2004; 49: 71–4.

14. Hendrix SL, Cochrane BB, Nygaard IE. Effects of estrogen with and without progestin on urinary incontinence. JAMA 2005; 293: 935–48.

15. Shenfeld OZ, McCammon KA, Blackmore PF, Ratz PH. Rapid effects of estrogen and progesterone on tone and spontaneous rhythmic contractions of the rabbit bladder. Urol Res 1999; 27(5): 386–92.

16. Grodstein F, Lifford K, Resnick NM, et al. Postmenopausal hormone therapy and risk of developing urinary incontinence. Obstet Gynecol 2004; 103(2): 254–60.

17. Jackson S, James M, Abrams P. The effect of oestradiol on vaginal collagen metabolism in postmenopausal women with genuine stress incontinence. BJOG 2002; 109: 339–44.

18. DuBeau CE. Estrogen treatment for urinary incontinence: never, now, or in the future? JAMA 2005; 293: 998–1001.

19. Suckling J, Lethaby A, Kennedy R. Local oestrogen for vaginal atrophy in postmenopausal women. Cochrane Database Syst Rev 2003; CD001500.

20. Diokno AC, Brock BM, Brown MB, et al. Prevalence of urinary incontinence and other urological symptoms in the noninstitutionalized elderly. J Urol 1986; 136: 1022–5.

21. Lin HH, Torng PL, Sheu BC, Shau WY, Huang SC. Urodynamically age-specific prevalence of urinary incontinence in women with urinary symptoms. Neurourol Urodyn 2003; 22(1): 29–32.

22. Miller YD, Brown WJ, Russell A, Chiarelli P. Urinary incontinence across the lifespan. Neurourol Urodyn 2003; 22: 550–7.

23. Handa VL, Garrett E, Hendrix S, et al. Progression and remission of pelvic organ prolapse: a longitudinal study of menopausal women. Am J Obstet Gynecol 2004; 190: 27–32.

24. Diokno AC, Brock BM, Brown MB, Herzog AR. Prevalence of urinary incontinence and other urological symptoms in the noninstitutionalized elderly. J Urol 1986; 136: 1022–5.

25. Wagner TH, Hu TW. Economic costs of urinary incontinence in 1995. Urology 1998; 51: 355–61.

26. Rud T. Urethral pressure profile in continent women from childhood to old age. Acta Obstet Gynecol Scand 1980; 59: 331–5.

27. Elbadawi A, Yalla SV, Resnick NM. Structural basis of geriatric voiding dysfunction. IV. Bladder outlet obstruction. J Urol 1993; 150: 1668–80.

28. Stewart W, Herzog AR, Wein AJ, et al. Prevalence and impact of overactive bladder in the US: results from the NOBLE program. Neurourol Urodyn 2001; 20: 406.

29. Milsom I, Abrams P, Cardozo L, et al. How widespread are the symptoms of an overactive bladder and how are they managed? A population-based prevalence study. BJU Int 2001; 87(9): 760–6.

30. Ricci JA, Baggish JS, Hunt TL, et al. Coping strategies and health care-seeking behavior in a

US national sample of adults with symptoms suggestive of OAB. Clin Ther 2001; 23: 1245–59.

31. Hu T, Wagner TH, Bentkover JD, et al. Estimated economic costs of OAB in the United States. Urology 2003; 61: 1123–8.

32. Goldberg RP, Sand PK. Pathophysiology of the overactive bladder. Clin Obstet Gynecol 2002; 45(1): 182–92.

33. Resnick NM, Yalla SV, Laurino E. The pathophysiology of urinary incontinence among institutionalized elderly persons. N Engl J Med 1989; 320: 1–7.

34. Verdell L. Consumer Focus '99: A Survey. Spartanburg South Carolina: National Association for Continence; 1999.

35. Fultz NH, Fisher GG, Jenkins KR. Does urinary incontinence affect middle-aged and older women's time use and activity patterns? Obstet Gynecol 2004; 104(6): 1327–34.

36. Abrams P, Wein AJ. The impact of overactive bladder on patients and society, and current approaches to treatment. Institute for Medical Studies CME Activity; 2002.

37. Brown JS, Vittinghoff E, Wyman JF, et al. Urinary incontinence: does it increase risk for falls and fractures? Study of Osteoporotic Fractures Research Group. J Am Geriatr Soc 2000; 48: 721–5.

38. Wagner TH, Hu TW, Bentkover J, et al. Health-related consequences of overactive bladder. Am J Manag Care 2002; 8(19 Suppl): S598–607.

39. Resnick NM. Geriatric incontinence. Urol Clin North Am 1996; 23(1): 55–74.

40. Resnick NM. Urinary incontinence in the elderly. Med Grand Rounds 1984; 3: 281–90.

41. Gormley EA. Biofeedback and behavioral therapy for the management of female urinary incontinence. Urol Clin North Am 2002; 29: 551–7.

42. Burns PA, Pranikoff K, Nuchajski TH, et al. A comparison of effectiveness of biofeedback and pelvic muscle exercise treatment of stress urinary incontinence in older community-dwelling women. J Gerontol 1993; 48: 167–74.

43. Mariappan P, Ballantyne Z, N'Dow JM, Alhasso AA. Serotonin and noradrenaline reuptake inhibitors (SNRI) for stress urinary incontinence in adults. Cochrane Database Syst Rev 2005; (3): CD004742.

44. Robert M, Mainprize TC. Long-term assessment of the incontinence ring pessary for the treatment of stress incontinence. Int Urogynecol J 2002; 13(5): 326–9.

45. Atherton MJ, Stanton SL. The tension-free vaginal tape reviewed: an evidence-based review from inception to current status. BJOG 2005; 112: 534–46.

46. Pickard R, Reaper J, Wyness L, et al. Periurethral injection therapy for urinary incontinence in women. Cochrane Database Syst Rev 2003; (2): CD003881.

47. Nygaard IE, Kreder KJ, Lepic MM, et al. Efficacy of pelvic floor muscle exercises in women with stress, urge and mixed urinary incontinence. Am J Obstet Gynecol 1996; 174: 120–5.

48. Huggins ME, Bhatia NN, Ostergard DR. Urinary incontinence: newer pharmacotherapeutic trends. Curr Opin Obstet Gynecol 2003; 15(5): 419–27.

49. Slack RA, Jackson S. Non-surgical treatment for detrusor overactivity. J Br Menopause Soc 2006; 12(3): 109–14.

50. Chapple CR, Martinez-Garcia R, Selvaggi L, et al. For the STAR study group. A comparison of the efficacy and tolerability of solifenacin succinate and extended release tolterodine at treating overactive bladder syndrome: results of the STAR trial. Eur Urol 2005; 48: 464–70.

Section III
Management problems

Normative values of investigations in elderly women

8

Isabelle Bourdel-Marchasson and Franck Lamouliate

INTRODUCTION

The scientific basis for normative values used for health promotion and therapeutic guidelines for women over the age of 70 is poor to non-existent. Values are largely extrapolated from data obtained from individuals younger than 65 years and tend to include more men than women. As such, they may not address gender-specific issues. This chapter therefore examines commonly measured variables in the clinical care of elderly women. Changes with age, pitfalls in interpretation, and health implications are discussed.

BLOOD PRESSURE

The prevalence and incidence of cardiovascular disease (coronary heart disease and stroke) increase rapidly in women during and after the seventh decade.[1] Assessment of blood pressure (BP) in clinical practice should address two main issues – hypertension and orthostatic hypotension – although this latter variable is often overlooked. Blood pressure values change with age in both sexes, and hypertension is a major risk factor for cardiovascular disease, heart failure, and dementia. Before the age of 60 years, diastolic and systolic pressure increase simultaneously. Thereafter, diastolic pressure falls in contrast to systolic pressure, which rises and thus pulse pressure increases.[2] An increase in systolic pressure is observed in hypertensive as well as normotensive individuals. This change is related to an age-dependent increase in arterial stiffness, leading to loss of arterial wall elasticity. On the one hand, diastolic pressure decreases, owing to the lack of pressure restitution during diastole; on the other hand, systolic pressure increases, owing to the loss of cushioning of the systolic pressure peak. Pulse wave velocity is considered as the best measure of arterial stiffness but is not used in routine clinical practice.[2] A very important consequence of increased arterial stiffness is the development of orthostatic hypotension in aging individuals, which is a risk factor for falls (see Chapter 3).

Hypertension

Blood pressure trends are different in the two sexes. In premenopausal women, blood pressure is lower than in men. It catches up by the sixth decade, and frequently becomes slightly higher thereafter. After age 70, however, pulse pressure is higher in women than in men.[3] Smaller body height could explain the lower peripheral but not central systolic pressure in young women compared with men: systolic blood pressure amplification from central to peripheral arteries increases with body height and is therefore more pronounced in men.[4] Arterial elasticity is higher in young women than in men, possibly mediated by the relaxing effect of estrogen on arterial wall smooth muscle.[5] Thus, overall systolic BP is lower in young women. After the menopause, the effect of estrogen is lost and arterial stiffness and pulse pressure increase, so that after age 70, blood pressure levels are similar in both sexes.

Hypertension, as a major risk factor for stroke, coronary heart disease, and cognitive decline including Alzheimer's disease,[6] is thus a target for preventive medicine in elderly women. Furthermore, hypertension affects more elderly women than men.[7] An Italian population-based study has shown that hypertension affects 67.3% of women and 59.4% of men between the ages of 65 and 85.[7]

The diagnosis of hypertension should be based ideally on multiple measurements. Blood pressure should be measured in the recumbent position and checked three times before any therapeutic decision is made, except in cases of symptomatic hypertension. However, the accuracy of measurements performed during a single clinical physical examination is limited by the 'white-coat effect'. Other schemes to diagnose hypertension include the patient's own measurements after a 10-minute rest, with three estimations twice a day during 3 consecutive days, and 24-hour ambulatory blood pressure measurements. The white-coat effect varies with age and is common in young elderly women (65–75 years), but uncommon in those over 85, as shown by comparing 24-hour ambulatory and individual clinical measurements.[8] This latter study also showed that nocturnal blood pressure falls decline in the very elderly, especially in women. Given these disparities, 24-hour ambulatory measurements seem to be an effective screening tool for hypertension, avoiding overdiagnosis and also detecting nocturnal hypotension in young-old women.

Orthostatic hypotension

Orthostatic hypotension (OH) results from the failure to maintain blood pressure in the upright position. Although autonomic failure is the main cause for OH, arterial stiffness associated with aging is another causative mechanism.[9] This condition involves from 6 to 30% of elderly individuals in population-based studies and can be defined as a drop of 20 mmHg or more of systolic BP or 10 mmHg of diastolic pressure after 1–3 minutes of standing.[10] In the study which cites these parameters, the main risks for systolic hypotension were male gender and diabetes and for diastolic hypotension were diuretic and calcium antagonist use, and dizziness when turning the neck, high systolic pressure, and low body weight. This same study pointed to OH as a strong predictor of cardiovascular deaths.[10] In addition, in day-to-day practice, OH is well known as a risk factor for falls[11] (see Chapter 3).

Given the risks cited above, clinical screening for OH is of great importance in elderly women. The use of a head-up tilt-table procedure is an accurate way to detect OH and to follow up the efficacy of corrective measures. OH is mostly associated with hypertension in the elderly, and 24-hour ambulatory BP measurements, combined with a position sensor, can detect both nocturnal hypertension and OH.

Goals for antihypertensive treatment in elderly women

Numerous data from randomized controlled trials have shown the benefit of treating hypertension and various guidelines have been developed. South African guidelines recommend that target BP for antihypertensive management should be systolic BP <140 mmHg, diastolic <90 mmHg, with minimal or no drug side effects.[12] Although lesser reduction will elicit benefit, this is not optimal. The reduction of BP in the elderly and in those with severe hypertension should be achieved gradually over 6 months to avoid precipitating acute cardiovascular events. Stricter BP control is required for patients with end-organ damage, coexisting risk factors, and comorbidity

Thus, in diabetes or renal failure the target is 130/80 mmHg; in congestive heart failure 120/75 mmHg; and in proteinuria >1 g/day, it is 125/80 mmHg.[12] In France it is recommended that guidelines used for young people should be applied until the age of 80.[13] Thereafter, owing to the lack of scientific evidence except for stroke prevention, the therapeutic goal should be balanced with the expected benefits on an individual basis. Thus, an evaluation of comorbidities, complications arising from hypertension, orthostatic hypotension, number of concomitant medications, quality of life, and life expectancy should direct specific therapeutic goals.

BODY MASS INDEX AND BODY COMPOSITION

Obesity as well as undernourishment (protein–energy malnutrition, PEM) are both important concerns in the aging population (see Chapter 14). Body mass index (BMI) is now widely used to evaluate obesity. It compares body weight (in kilograms) to height (in meters): BMI = weight/height^2. 'Normal' values are less than 24.9 kg/m^2, and 'overweight' between 25 and 29.9 kg/m^2. 'Obese' patients are subdivided into three classes: Class 1 = BMI 30–34.9 kg/m^2; Class 2 = BMI 35–39.9 kg/m^2; and the 'extreme obese' Class 3 = BMI ≥40 kg/m^2. Clinical assessment of body composition necessitates other anthropometric measures, including waist circumference, skin fold thickness (triceps), and limb circumference. The proportion of android (upper body) fat is greater in men than in women, and increases slowly with age.[14] Cardiovascular risk in adult females increases when waist circumference exceeds 88 cm, according to ATPIII criteria for metabolic syndrome.[15] In men, the cut-off point is set at 102 cm for waist circumference.

Estimation of body fat content can be achieved with anthropometric measures and, more accurately, bioelectric impedance analysis (BIA). However, the generally accepted reference standard, underwater weighing, is not used routinely in clinical practice. It is possible to estimate body fat mass using the following equation:

$$\text{Body fat (kg)} = 1.4\,\text{BMI} + 0.48T - 25.81$$

where T is the triceps skin fold (mm).[16] PEM is poorly described by BMI. Whereas a BMI of ≤18 is strongly suggestive of PEM, a substantial number of undernourished individuals have BMIs in the normal range. Kinetics of weight changes are better: a 5% unintentional weight loss during the past month is a strong indicator of undernourishment.

Obesity

Lifelong increases of BMI have been described in both physically active men and women, in a survey of 433 healthy individuals aged 18–94 years[17] (Figure 8.1). Mean BMI in healthy women >75 years old is close to 25, and thus in the 'overweight' range. Such findings suggest that normal weight could be different in elderly women than in their younger counterparts. However, a criticism of this study, as well others, is that it is cross-sectional and only surviving, mainly healthy, older subjects were examined. Longitudinal data of BMI over many decades are not yet available.

The prevalence of obesity in elderly Danish women is estimated to be about 15–20%, with no significant change during the past 30 years.[18] In the US it is estimated that the prevalence of obesity in adults aged ≥60 years old will increase from 32.0% in 2000 to 37.4% in 2010 (range 33.6–39.6%). The number of obese adults aged ≥60 will increase from 14.6 to 20.9 million (range 18.8–22.2 million).[19] However, interestingly in this study the prevalence of obesity fell to 20% in those aged over 80. Little is known about the prevalence of obesity in nursing home residents.

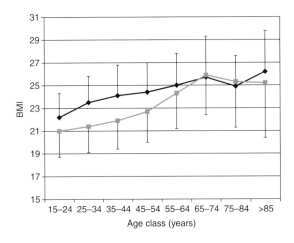

Figure 8.1 Body mass index (BMI) measures in 253 healthy men (♦) and 180 healthy women (■) aged 18–94 years old.[17]

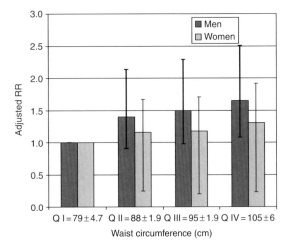

Figure 8.2 Waist circumference (in quartiles from Q I to Q IV) and 15-year risk for stroke in older women and men.[22] RR, relative risk.

In the US, obesity in newly admitted nursing home residents has increased from 15% in 1992 to more than 25% in 2002.[20]

Although the global impact of obesity in older women is not yet clearly defined, obesity is a risk factor for hypertension, cardiovascular disease, and diabetes. All these conditions are associated with increased disability. Obesity in middle-aged women (but not in men) is associated with an increased risk of dementia 27 years later.[21] However, the impact of obesity in later life was not ascertained in this study. In 70-year-old Europeans, high waist circumference (≥99 cm) and BMI ($\geq 28 \, kg/m^2$) are risks for stroke in older men but not women, even after adjustment for other cardiovascular risk factors (Figure 8.2).[22] In older type II diabetic patients, moderate excess weight (BMI $\geq 30.9 \, kg/m^2$) predicts a better survival, whereas obesity is a negative prognostic factor in patients younger than 65 years in older diabetics.[23]

Protein–energy malnutrition

At the opposite end of the spectrum, PEM is a very important concern in the elderly, particularly in hospitals and residential care homes.[24] The MNA (Mini Nutritional Assessment), is a simple, non-invasive, well-validated screening tool for malnutrition in elderly persons and is recommended for early detection of risk of malnutrition.[25] (Table 8.1). The MNA is an 18-item questionnaire comprising anthropometric measurement (BMI, mid-arm and calf circumference, and weight loss) combined with a questionnaire regarding dietary intake (number of meals consumed, food and fluid intake, and feeding autonomy), a global assessment (lifestyle, medication, mobility, presence of acute stress, and presence of dementia or depression), and a self-assessment (self-perception of health and nutrition). It correlates highly with clinical assessment and objective indicators of nutritional status (albumin level, BMI, energy intake and vitamin status). A low MNA score can predict hospital-stay outcomes in older patients and can be used to follow up changes in nutritional status. In more than 10 000 elderly persons, the prevalence of undernutrition assessed by the MNA is 1–5% in community-dwelling elderly persons and outpatients, 20% in hospitalized older patients, and 37% in institutionalized elderly patients.[25]

Table 8.1 The MNA scale

NESTLÉ NUTRITION SERVICES

Nestlé

Mini Nutritional Assessment
MNA®

Last name: First name: Sex: Date:

Age: Weight, kg: Height, cm: I.D. Number:

Complete the screen by filling in the boxes with the appropriate numbers.
Add the numbers for the screen. If score is 11 or less, continue with the assessment to gain a Malnutrition Indicator Score.

Screening

A Has food intake declined over the past 3 months due to loss of appetite, digestive problems, chewing or swallowing difficulties?
0 = severe loss of appetite
1 = moderate loss of appetite
2 = no loss of appetite

B Weight loss during last months
0 = weight loss greater than 3 kg (6.6 lbs)
1 = does not know
2 = weight loss between 1 and 3 kg (2.2 and 6.6 lbs)
3 = no weight loss

C Mobility
0 = bed or chair bound
1 = able to get out of bed/chair but does not go out
2 = goes out

D Has suffered psychological stress or acute disease in the past 3 months
0 = yes   2 = no

E Neuropsychological problems
0 = severe dementia or depression
1 = mild dementia
2 = no psychological problems

F Body Mass Index (BMI) (weight in kg)/(height in m)^2
0 = BMI less than 19
1 = BMI 19 to less than 21
2 = BMI 21 to less than 23
3 = BMI 23 or greater

Screening score (subtotal max. 14 points)

12 points or greater   Normal – not at risk no need to complete assessment
11 points or below   Possible malnutrition – continue assessment

Assessment

G Lives independently (not in a nursing home or hospital)
0 = no   1 = yes

H Takes more than 3 prescription drugs per day
0 = yes   1 = no

I Pressure sores or skin ulcers
0 = yes   1 = no

J How many full meals does the patient eat daily?
0 = 1 meal
1 = 2 meals
2 = 3 meals

K Selected consumption markers for protein intake
• At least one serving of dairy products (milk, cheese, yogurt) per day? yes ☐ no ☐
• Two or more serving of legumes or eggs per week? yes ☐ no ☐
• Meat, fish or poultry every day yes ☐ no ☐
0.0 = if 0 or 1 yes
0.5 = if 2 yes
1.0 = if 3 yes

L Consumes two or more servings of fruits or vegetables per day?
0 = no   1 = yes

M How much fluid (water, juice, coffee, tea, milk...) is consumed per day?
0.0 = less than 3 cups
0.5 = 3 to 5 cups
1.0 = more than 5 cups

N Mode of feeding
0 = unable to eat without assistance
1 = self-fed with some difficulty
2 = self-fed without any problem

O Self view of nutritional status
0 = view self as being malnourished
1 = is uncertain of nutritional state
2 = views self as having no nutritional problem

P In comparison with other people of the same age, how do they consider their health status?
0.0 = not as good
0.5 = does not know
1.0 = as good
2.0 = better

Q Mid-arm circumference (MAC) in cm
0.0 = MAC less than 21
0.5 = MAC 21 to 22
1.0 = MAC 22 or greater

R Calf circumference (CC) in cm
0 = CC less than 31   1 = CC 31 or greater

Assessment (max. 16 points)
Screening score
Total Assessment (max. 30 points)

Malnutrition Indicator Score

17 to 23.5 points   at risk of malnutrition ☐
Less than 17 points   malnourished ☐

Ref.: Guigoz Y, Vellas B and Garry PJ. 1994. Mini Nutritional Assessment: A practical assessment tool for grading the nutritional state of elderly patients. *Facts and Research in Gerontology.* Supplement #2:15–59.
Rubenstein LZ, Harker J, Guigoz Y and Vellas B. Comprehensive Geriatric Assessment (CGA) and the MNA: An Overview of CGA, Nutritional Assessment, and Development of a Shortened Version of the MNA. In: "Mini Nutritional Assessment (MNA): Research and Practice in the Elderly". Vellas B, Garry PJ and Guigoz Y, editors. Nestlé Nutrition Workshop Series. Clinical & Performance Programme, vol. 1. Karger, Bâle, in press.

® Société des Produits Nestlé S.A., Vevey, Switzerland, Trademark Owners

08.98 USA

Body composition and osteoporosis

Bone mineral density is correlated with body fat rather than muscle mass in women. In a study of 301 men and women aged ≥65, muscle is associated more closely than fat with bone mineral content (BMC) as well as with bone mineral density (BMD) in men.[26] In women, however, correlations of BMC with muscle are only slightly greater than those with fat, and correlations with BMD were consistently greater with fat than with muscle. In women, fat mass was associated significantly with BMC but muscle mass was not. The exception was for women taking estrogen, in whom neither fat nor muscle was associated significantly with adjusted BMC. Thus, body fatness may be more important than muscle in maintaining bone mineral content in elderly women not taking estrogen. Similar results were found in a larger study, confirming the correlation between fat mass and BMD in women and not in men.[27]

Body composition changes and functional status

Living independently for as long as possible is a major concern in the elderly. Weight loss has been proposed in elderly obese women with the purpose of maintaining mobility. However, such intervention should be considered with caution, partly because of the protective effect of fat mass on bone quality.

In a cohort of 2619 (1337 women) well-functioning older adults aged 70–79 years participating in the Health, Aging, and Body Composition (Health ABC) Study, obesity was associated with an increased risk of mobility impairment after 4 years.[28] However, those reporting weight loss and, in particular, unintentional weight loss, have the highest risk of functional limitation, which is higher than those reporting unintentional weight gain. In women,

weight loss consisted of 5% of initial lean mass and 12.7% fat mass, whereas weight gain consisted of 2.96% of initial lean mass and 13.7% initial fat mass. Thus, weight loss, even followed by weight gain, is likely to result in a fall in lean body mass.[29] In elderly women, a decrease of the lean to fat mass ratio is associated with an increased risk of functional limitation. Increased physical activity can reduce the decrease in muscle mass: a low-fat diet combined with exercise can limit the decrease in lean body mass during weight loss in older men and women.[30]

The age-related decrease in lean mass is mainly related to the decrease in muscle mass, which is now named sarcopenia. This is defined as a muscle mass lower than 2 standard deviations compared with a 40-year-old sex-matched population. Sarcopenia is, however, not only related to aging, but also physical activity, comorbidity, and nutritional status. Severe sarcopenia is associated with functional dependency.

Although the functional benefit of weight loss is doubtful in elderly women, no study has shown a benefit of weight gain in PEM without a concomitant increase in physical activity.

HEMATOLOGY

Complete blood counts are routinely performed as a screening investigation for a wide range of pathologies, regardless of the patient's age or gender. Both anemia and polycythemia are signs of underlying pathology and are associated with increased mortality.

Anemia

Anemia, defined as hemoglobin <12.0 g/dl in women and <13.0 g/dl in men, is a common condition in the elderly.[31] Its frequency is lower in women than in men, and increases with age as shown in a cross-sectional (Figure 8.3) as well

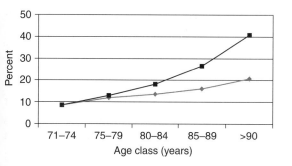

Figure 8.3 Prevalence of anemia in community-living elderly dwellers: ■, men (Hb <13.0 g/dl); ♦, women (Hb <12.0 g/dl).[31]

as in a longitudinal follow-up study (increase from 4.2% to 8.9% in 70-year-old women after 10 years).[31] In this review, Carmel proposed three etiological categories:

- anemias caused by diseases are more common in the elderly (such as cobalamin deficiency, chronic diseases or inflammation, and myelodysplastic syndrome)
- anemias without predilection for the elderly
- anemias from unknown causes.

Of the chronic conditions, impaired renal function, heart failure, and cancers justify a thorough examination. Basic investigations include mean corpuscular volume; white cell, platelet, and reticulocyte counts; serum iron, ferritin; creatinine clearance; and occult blood tests. In old age, an association between anemia and renal function is found when creatinine clearance (CC) is ≤30 ml/min.[32] Also age- and hemoglobin-adjusted erythropoietin levels are significantly reduced. Unfortunately, the high frequency of anemia in very old women can trivialize it and impede thorough investigation. This process is mandatory, as no data support the concept that anemia could solely be due to aging.

In the elderly, anemia is associated with poor outcomes, including disability and mortality, even after adjusting for demography, renal function,

and frailty.[33] Frailty was defined as fulfilling 3 of 5 criteria: unintentional 10% weight loss in 1 year; grip strength, timed walk, or activity level in the lowest quintile; and self-reported poor energy.

Anemia is also associated with an increased risk of falls in elderly community dwellers after adjustment on potential cofounders.[34] Recurrent falls are a condition with poor prognosis, associated with frailty and increased risk of institutionalization (see Chapter 3). In the InCHIANTI Italian cohort, anemia was also associated with depression, another condition associated with adverse outcomes (see Chapter 6).[35]

With the exception of anemia associated with heart failure, the effects of diagnosis and treatment of anemia in the elderly have not been investigated. Here, a combined intervention, including beta-blockers, angiotensin-converting enzyme (ACE) inhibitors, angiotensin receptor blockers, and erythropoietin injections to correct anemia, improves cardiac function.[36]

Polycythemia

Increased hemoglobin concentration or hematocrit >0.60% is suggestive of polycythemia, which can be confirmed by measuring red cell mass. The main differential diagnosis is relative erythrocytosis mainly due to dehydration with reduction of plasma volume. Polycythemia vera (PV) is a myeloproliferative disorder. The incidence of PV in adults varies from 1 to 3 per 100 000 person-years. Median age at diagnosis is about 60 years in women. Criteria for PV diagnosis are increased cell mass, normal arterial oxygen saturation (>92%), splenomegaly, and any of following: thrombocytosis, leukocytosis, raised alkaline phosphatase, cyanocobalamin or unsaturated cyanocobalamin binding capacity.[37]

Secondary polycythemia is much more frequent in the elderly and is mainly due to chronic hypoxia. In the acute care geriatric setting, anemia is so frequent that most patients with normal or slightly increased hemoglobin value are likely to be hypoxic.

The prognosis of increased hemoglobin concentration in older individuals is mainly related to the underlying hypoxia. In a prospective cohort study with 11.2 years of follow-up of 5888 community-dwelling men and women 65 years old, higher hemoglobin levels were associated with increased mortality.[33]

BIOCHEMISTRY

Creatinine and creatinine clearance

Numerous factors, including hypertension, diabetes, vascular diseases, drugs, and long-term exposure to toxics (cadmium, lead, silver), affect renal aging. In a large cross-sectional study, mean estimations of creatine clearance fell from 53.8 ml/min in young-old (65–74 years old) to 28.6 ml/min in old-old (more than 85 years old) women. The lowest values were found in those with hypertension, cardiovascular disease, and limitations in functional autonomy as well as those reporting use of diuretic or cardiovascular medications.[38]

Estimation of CC in the elderly is important. A CC lower than 40 ml/min is an independent risk factor for adverse drug events.[39] Another effect of poor renal function is impaired vitamin D metabolism. Decreased vitamin D status and calcium intake are associated with lower muscle strength, increased risk of falling, and a higher rate of fracture.[40] In a meta-analysis, vitamin D supplementation reduces the risk of falls among ambulatory or institutionalized older individuals with stable health by more than 20%.[41]

In the elderly, serum creatinine is a poor estimate of renal filtration capacity; therefore, it is more appropriate to estimate CC. Indeed, in older and undernourished individuals, serum creatinine is often in the normal range despite a decrease in glomerular filtration rate. In clinical practice, it is theoretically possible to measure CC using both serum creatinine and 24-hour urinary creatinine using the following formula:

$$CC = ([\text{urinary creatinine}] \times \text{urinary rate}) / [\text{serum creatinine}]$$

However, urinary creatinine measurements can be inaccurate because of factors such as incontinence or incomplete bladder emptying. Thus, estimations of CC using serum creatinine, age, and gender are now preferable (Table 8.2). The Cockcroft and Gault formula (CG) is widely used. However, this formula underestimates CC in patients older than 80 by about 20–30%.[42] The known inaccuracy of the formula in people with lower and higher weights has led to other formulas being devised. Two equations from the Modification of Diet in Renal Disease (MDRD) aim to be independent of body weight.[43]

The three formulas have been compared in 22 403 hospital inpatients aged ≥65 years old at time of discharge.[44] The study confirms that CGCC underestimates CC in underweight subjects and overestimates it in overweight ones. Large discrepancies with these three methods in individual patients were also found. Systematic underestimation of CC using the MDRD has also been shown in the elderly.[45] As the CGCC is simple to calculate, most trials use it to adjust drug dosages in accordance with renal excretion in the elderly.

Cholesterol

Cholesterol is one of the best-known targets for cardiovascular disease prevention. However, after the age of 75 the prognostic value of cholesterol changes (see Traissac et al[46] for review). Indeed the increasing comorbidities in the elderly modify the prognostic value of cardiovascular factors and, in particular, serum lipids.

Table 8.2 Estimation of creatinine clearance (CC)[42,43]

Cockcroft and Gault CC in ml/min

$((140 - age) \times weight/(72 - [serum\ creatinine])) \times 0.85$ if woman

weight in kg, serum creatinine in mg/dl.

$((140 - age) \times weight/[serum\ creatinine]) \times (1.04$ if woman, 1.23 if man)

weight in kg, serum creatinine in μmol/L.

MDRD 1 in ml/min/1.73 m^2

$((170 \times [serum\ creatinine]^{-0.999} \times (age)^{-0.176} \times [blood\ urinary\ nitrogen\ in\ mg/dl]^{-0.170} \times [serum\ albumin\ in\ g/dl]^{0.318}) \times (0.762$ if woman or 1.18 if black man)

serum creatinine in mg/dl, blood urinary nitrogen in mg/dl, serum albumin in mg/dl.

MDRD 2 in ml/min/1.73 m^2

$(186.3 \times [serum\ creatinine]^{-1.154} \times (age)^{-0.203}) \times 0.742$ if woman

serum creatinine in mg/dl.

$32788 \times [serum\ creatinine]^{-1.154} \times (age)^{-0.203}) \times 0.742$ if woman

serum creatinine in μmol/L.

Total plasma cholesterol decreases with age. In 60-year-old women in the European Working Party on High blood pressure in the Elderly (EWPHE) study, mean total cholesterol was 267 mg/dl and decreased to 245 mg/dl in those older than 85.[47] These results could have been the result of selection of individuals with a better prognosis but were confirmed by the 20-year follow-up of the Honolulu Heart Program, which included only men.[48]

In the old-old (>85 years old), the now well-known relationship between total cholesterol is reversed-J shaped. The highest mortality is seen in the lower cholesterol quartile and a secondary increase is seen in the highest quartile. However, the Established Populations for Epidemiologic Studies in the Elderly (EPESE) found a linear correlation between cholesterol and coronary mortality after multiple adjustments on sex, comorbidity, and malnutrition.[49] However, the highest quartile contained 20% men, and 60% were present in the lowest one. The Italian Longitudinal Study on Aging (ISLA) did not confirm that adjustments on comorbidity and nutrition status lead to a linear correlation. Highest mortality risk was associated with the lowest cholesterol values, with no difference between genders.[50] The Leiden 85+ study has shown that 10-year mortality was decreased in the highest quartile due to lower cancer and infection mortalities.[51] The highest mortality was found when both high-density lipoprotein (HDL) and low-density lipoprotein (LDL) cholesterol were low (<36 mg/dl and <106 mg/dl, respectively). Low HDL cholesterol is also associated in most studies with an increased risk of stroke in older subjects.[46]

The predictive value of lipoprotein Lp(a) for coronary heart disease was found in the ISLA study only in older individuals with diabetes or increased LDL cholesterol.[52] In healthy centenarians, Lp(a) was increased without any other lipid changes. In those older than 75 years, lipoprotein structure may differ from that found in individuals younger than 65 years.[53] Furthermore, association between decreased Lp(a) and increased cytokine (interleukin-6; IL-6) level suggests that chronic inflammatory syndrome influences Lp(a) plasma concentrations.[54]

A low cholesterol level at a particular time point does not mean that it has always been at that level for that individual. High cholesterol before 60, could have contributed to cardiovascular disease, still present 20 years later, whereas cholesterol, particularly HDL cholesterol, may have fallen due to the presence of inflammatory disease.

Serum albumin and markers of inflammation

Albumin

Serum albumin is the most abundant plasma protein, containing 585 amino acids (MW = 66 000 Da), with normal concentrations being close to 42 g/L. Its synthesis occurs in the liver at a slow rate (150 mg/kg/day) and reflects the total body amino acid pool.[55] Albumin contributes to 80% of maintenance of colloidal osmotic pressure. It transports organic molecules, drugs, and metals. Albumin has a large distribution volume, with 60% in the extravascular compartment.

Although albumin is characterized as a nutritional protein owing to the close relationship between its concentrations and total body nitrogen, the most important changes in its levels are seen in inflammatory conditions. In the hypermetabolic state, for example, the extravascular compartment expands and thus the distribution space for albumin is larger, resulting in decreased concentrations in both plasma and the extravascular space.[56]

The amplitude of the change is correlated with the severity of the inflammation, best evaluated by C-reactive protein (CRP) determination. Regression of inflammation reverses the processes and albumin concentrations rise. During the course of inflammation, a high demand for synthesis of inflammatory and visceral proteins, coupled with reduced dietary intake, lead to a decrease of total body nitrogen, mainly at the expense of muscle mass. Thus, after inflammation regresses, albumin concentrations do not return to baseline. Repeated episodes or chronic inflammation results in decreased albumin levels, and these are related to the severity and duration of the disease.

Albumin levels can now be used as a prognostic marker. Low albumin concentrations in older persons increase the risk of poor health outcomes, including functional decline. Thus in healthy 70–79 year olds, albumin levels lower than 38 g/L were predictive of 8-year functional decline and mortality. Furthermore, the highest risk was found in people whose cholesterol was below 167 mg/dl.[57] Also, albumin levels below the cut-off point of 38 g/L are predictive of 5-year loss of muscle mass.[58] In this study, the proportion of women was higher in the group with albumin levels <38 g/L (56.1%) than in those with albumin levels >42 g/L (46.2%). The physiological difference in muscle mass between the sexes renders women more vulnerable to the effects of inflammation and deprivation.

Markers of inflammation

A large number of changes, distant from the site or sites of inflammation and involving many organ systems, may accompany inflammation. Accordingly, these systemic changes have since been referred to as the acute-phase response even though they accompany both acute and chronic inflammatory disorders.[59] During the acute-phase response, levels of various protein such as CRP, are markedly increased. Conditions that commonly lead to substantial changes in the plasma concentrations of acute-phase proteins include infection, trauma, surgery, burns, tissue infarction, various immunologically mediated inflammatory conditions, and advanced cancer. Moderate or small changes occur after strenuous exercise, psychological stress, and in several psychiatric illnesses. The cytokines that are produced during, and participate in, inflammatory processes are the chief stimulators of the production of acute-phase proteins. These inflammation-associated cytokines include interleukins IL-6 and IL-1β and tumor necrosis factor-alpha (TNF-α).

CRP levels also change with age. Analysis of the National Health and Nutrition Examination Survey (NHANES), which includes a sample of 21 004 people, found that levels of CRP range from 0.1 to 296.0 mg/L, with a skewed distribution (mean = 4.3, median = 2.1).[60] The levels of CRP are higher among women than among men (median = 2.7 mg/L vs 1.6 mg/L) and increase with age (median = 1.4 mg/L among those 20–29 years old vs 2.7 mg/L among those ≥80 years old). Researchers have begun to use a CRP level of ≥2 mg/L as the threshold for defining high cardiovascular risk. With use of this threshold, 52% of the adult population in the US would be considered at high risk. The proportion of people with a level of ≥2 mg/L is substantial at all ages (e.g. 41% among those 20–29 years old vs 62% among those ≥80 years old).

The most important marker of chronic inflammation in the elderly is IL-6. High levels of IL-6 are associated with decrease in physical function in older women with various stages of disability (Women's Health and Aging Study).[61] Furthermore, in the Framingham Heart Study, IL-6 is a significant predictor of sarcopenia in women ($p = 0.02$), but not in men.[62]

Physical activity may decrease chronic inflammation. In a US study of 870 people aged 70–79 who were in the top third of community-dwelling older persons with respect to physical and cognitive functioning, high levels of recreational activity are associated with lower levels of the inflammatory markers IL-6 and CRP.[63]

Thus, in clinical practice, measurement of albumin and inflammatory markers have the potential to be indicators of functional decline.

CONCLUSIONS

In elderly women, the aim is to maintain autonomy and quality of life. So-called normal values of common variables used in clinical practice change with age. Others can be used as predictors of functional decline and are associated with increased mortality. However, it is important not to solely attribute abnormal levels simply to aging; underlying pathology needs to be excluded.

REFERENCES

1. Rothwell PM, Coull AJ, Silver LE, et al. Population-based study of event rate, incidence, case fatality, and mortality for all acute vascular events in all arterial territories (Oxford vascular study). Lancet 2005; 366: 1773–83.

2. Franklin SS. Ageing and hypertension: the assessment of blood pressure indices in predicting coronary heart disease. J Hypertens 1999; 17 (Suppl): S29–36.

3. Franklin SS, Gustin WT, Wong ND, et al. Hemodynamic patterns of age-related changes in blood pressure. The Framingham Heart Study. Circulation 1997; 96: 308–15.

4. London GM, Guerin AP, Pannier B, Marchais SJ, Stimpel M. Influence of sex on arterial hemodynamics and blood pressure. Role of body height. Hypertension 1995; 26: 514–19.

5. Mendelsohn ME, Karas RH. The protective effects of estrogen on the cardiovascular system. N Engl J Med 1999; 340: 1801–11.

6. Tzourio C, Dufouil C, Ducimetiere P, Alperovitch A. Cognitive decline in individuals with high blood pressure: a longitudinal study in the elderly. EVA Study Group. Epidemiology of Vascular Aging. Neurology 1999; 53: 1948–52.

7. The Italian Longitudinal Study on Aging Working Group. Prevalence of chronic diseases in older Italians: comparing self-reported and clinical diagnoses. Int J Epidemiol 1997; 26: 995–1002.

8. Fotherby MD, Potter JF. Twenty-four-hour ambulatory blood pressure in old and very old subjects. J Hypertens 1995; 13: 1742–6.

9. Boddaert J, Tamim H, Verny M, Belmin J. Arterial stiffness is associated with orthostatic hypotension in elderly subjects with history of falls. J Am Geriatr Soc 2004; 52: 568–72.

10. Luukinen H, Koski K, Laippala P, Kivela SL. Prognosis of diastolic and systolic orthostatic hypotension in older persons. Arch Intern Med 1999; 159: 273–80.

11. Fortinsky RH, Iannuzzi-Sucich M, Baker DI, et al. Fall-risk assessment and management in clinical practice: views from healthcare providers. J Am Geriatr Soc 2004; 52: 1522–6.

12. Milne FJ, Pinkney-Atkinson VJ. Hypertension guideline 2003 update. S Afr Med J 2004; 94: 209–16, 218, 220–5.

13. HAS. [Management of adults with essential hypertension.] http://www.anaes.fr ed., Haute autorité de Santé. [in French].

14. Ley CJ, Lees B, Stevenson JC. Sex- and menopause-associated changes in body-fat distribution. Am J Clin Nutr 1992; 55: 950–4.

15. Executive Summary of The Third Report of The National Cholesterol Education Program (NCEP) Expert Panel on Detection, Evaluation, And Treatment of High Blood Cholesterol In Adults (Adult Treatment Panel III). JAMA 2001; 285: 2486–97.

16. Chapman NC, Bannerman E, Cowen S, MacLennan WJ. The relationship of anthropometry and bio-electrical impedance to dual-energy X-ray absorptiometry in elderly men and women. Age Ageing 1998; 27: 363–7.

17. Kyle UG, Genton L, Hans D, et al. Age-related differences in fat-free mass, skeletal muscle, body cell mass and fat mass between 18 and 94 years. Eur J Clin Nutr 2001; 55: 663–72.

18. Heitmann BL, Stroger U, Mikkelsen KL, Holst C, Sorensen TI. Large heterogeneity of the obesity epidemic in Danish adults. Public Health Nutr 2004; 7: 453–60.

19. Arterburn DE, Crane PK, Sullivan SD. The coming epidemic of obesity in elderly Americans. J Am Geriatr Soc 2004; 52: 1907–12.

20. Lapane KL, Resnik L. Obesity in nursing homes: an escalating problem. J Am Geriatr Soc 2005; 53: 1386–91.

21. Whitmer RA, Gunderson EP, Barrett-Connor E, Quesenberry CP Jr, Yaffe K. Obesity in middle age and future risk of dementia: a 27 year longitudinal population based study. BMJ 2005; 330: 1360.

22. Dey DK, Rothenberg E, Sundh V, Bosaeus I, Steen B. Waist circumference, body mass index, and risk for stroke in older people: a 15 year longitudinal population study of 70-year-olds. J Am Geriatr Soc 2002; 50: 1510–18.

23. Zoppini G, Verlato G, Leuzinger C, et al. Body mass index and the risk of mortality in type II diabetic patients from Verona. Int J Obes Relat Metab Disord 2003; 27: 281–5.

24. Bourdel-Marchasson I, Barateau M, Sourgen C, et al. Prospective audits of quality of PEM recognition and nutritional support in critically ill elderly patients. Clin Nutr 1999; 18: 233–40.

25. Guigoz Y, Lauque S, Vellas BJ. Identifying the elderly at risk for malnutrition. The Mini Nutritional Assessment. Clin Geriatr Med 2002; 18: 737–57.

26. Baumgartner RN, Stauber PM, Koehler KM, Romero L, Garry PJ. Associations of fat and muscle masses with bone mineral in elderly men and women. Am J Clin Nutr 1996; 63: 365–72.

27. Taaffe DR, Cauley JA, Danielson M, et al. Race and sex effects on the association between muscle strength, soft tissue, and bone mineral

density in healthy elders: the Health, Aging, and Body Composition Study. J Bone Miner Res 2001; 16: 1343–52.

28. Lee JS, Kritchevsky SB, Tylavsky F, et al. Weight change, weight change intention, and the incidence of mobility limitation in well-functioning community-dwelling older adults. J Gerontol A Biol Sci Med Sci 2005; 60: 1007–12.

29. Newman AB, Lee JS, Visser M, et al. Weight change and the conservation of lean mass in old age: the Health, Aging and Body Composition Study. Am J Clin Nutr 2005; 82: 872–8; quiz 915–16.

30. Hays NP, Starling RD, Liu X, et al. Effects of an ad libitum low-fat, high-carbohydrate diet on body weight, body composition, and fat distribution in older men and women: a randomized controlled trial. Arch Intern Med 2004; 164: 210–17.

31. Carmel R. Anemia and aging: an overview of clinical, diagnostic and biological issues. Blood Rev 2001; 15: 9–18.

32. Ble A, Fink JC, Woodman RC, et al. Renal function, erythropoietin, and anemia of older persons: the InCHIANTI study. Arch Intern Med 2005; 165: 2222–7.

33. Zakai NA, Katz R, Hirsch C, et al. A prospective study of anemia status, hemoglobin concentration, and mortality in an elderly cohort: the Cardiovascular Health Study. Arch Intern Med 2005; 165: 2214–20.

34. Penninx BW, Pluijm SM, Lips P, et al. Late-life anemia is associated with increased risk of recurrent falls. J Am Geriatr Soc 2005; 53: 2106–11.

35. Onder G, Penninx BW, Cesari M, et al. Anemia is associated with depression in older adults: results from the InCHIANTI study. J Gerontol A Biol Sci Med Sci 2005; 60: 1168–72.

36. Hampl H, Hennig L, Rosenberger C, et al. Effects of optimized heart failure therapy and anemia correction with epoetin beta on left ventricular mass in hemodialysis patients. Am J Nephrol 2005; 25: 211–20.

37. van Genderen PJ, Troost MM. Polycythaemia vera and essential thrombocythaemia in the elderly. Drugs Aging 2000; 17: 107–19.

38. Salive ME, Jones CA, Guralnik JM, et al. Serum creatinine levels in older adults: relationship with health status and medications. Age Ageing 1995; 24: 142–50.

39. Evans RS, Lloyd JF, Stoddard GJ, Nebeker JR, Samore MH. Risk factors for adverse drug events: a 10-year analysis. Ann Pharmacother 2005; 39: 1161–8.

40. Dukas L, Schacht E, Stahelin HB. In elderly men and women treated for osteoporosis a low creatinine clearance of <65 ml/min is a risk factor for falls and fractures. Osteoporos Int 2005; 16: 1683–90.

41. Bischoff-Ferrari HA, Dawson-Hughes B, Willett WC, et al. Effect of vitamin D on falls: a meta-analysis. JAMA 2004; 291: 1999–2006.

42. Garg AX, Papaioannou A, Ferko N, et al. Estimating the prevalence of renal insufficiency in seniors requiring long-term care. Kidney Int 2004; 65: 649–53.

43. Levey AS, Bosch JP, Lewis JB, et al. A more accurate method to estimate glomerular filtration rate from serum creatinine: a new prediction equation. Modification of Diet in Renal Disease Study Group. Ann Intern Med 1999; 130: 461–70.

44. Pedone C, Corsonello A, Incalzi RA. Estimating renal function in older people: a comparison of three formulas. Age Ageing 2006; 35: 121–6.

45. Verhave JC, Fesler P, Ribstein J, du Cailar G, Mimran A. Estimation of renal function in subjects with normal serum creatinine levels: influence of age and body mass index. Am J Kidney Dis 2005; 46: 233–41.

46. Traissac T, Salzmann M, Rainfray M, Emeriau JP, Bourdel-Marchasson I. [What is the significance of cholesterol levels after the age of 75?] Presse Med 2005; 34: 1525–32. [in French]

47. Staessen JA, Birkenhager WH. Cognitive impairment and blood pressure: quo usque

tandem abutere patientia nostra? Hypertension 2004; 44: 612–13.

48. Schatz IJ, Masaki K, Yano K, et al. Cholesterol and all-cause mortality in elderly people from the Honolulu Heart Program: a cohort study. Lancet 2001; 358: 351–5.

49. Corti MC, Guralnik JM, Salive ME, et al. Clarifying the direct relation between total cholesterol levels and death from coronary heart disease in older persons. Ann Intern Med 1997; 126: 753–60.

50. Brescianini S, Maggi S, Farchi G, et al. Low total cholesterol and increased risk of dying: are low levels clinical warning signs in the elderly? Results from the Italian Longitudinal Study on Aging. J Am Geriatr Soc 2003; 51: 991–6.

51. Weverling-Rijnsburger AW, Blauw GJ, Lagaay AM, et al. Total cholesterol and risk of mortality in the oldest old. Lancet 1997; 350: 1119–23.

52. Solfrizzi V, Panza F, Colacicco AM, et al. Relation of lipoprotein(a) as coronary risk factor to type 2 diabetes mellitus and low-density lipoprotein cholesterol in patients > or =65 years of age (The Italian Longitudinal Study on Aging). Am J Cardiol 2002; 89: 825–9.

53. Thillet J, Doucet C, Chapman J, et al. Elevated lipoprotein(a) levels and small apo(a) isoforms are compatible with longevity: evidence from a large population of French centenarians. Atherosclerosis 1998; 136: 389–94.

54. Ariyo AA, Thach C, Tracy R. Lp(a) lipoprotein, vascular disease, and mortality in the elderly. N Engl J Med 2003; 349: 2108–15.

55. Melchior J-C, Thuiller F. Evaluation de l'état nutritionnel. In: Leverve X, Cosnes J, Erny P, Hasselman M, eds. Traité de Nutrition Artificielle de l'Adulte. Paris: SFNEP; 1998: 415–32.

56. Ruot B, Papet I, Bechereau F, et al. Increased albumin plasma efflux contributes to hypo-albuminemia only during early phase of sepsis in rats. Am J Physiol Regul Integr Comp Physiol 2003; 284: R707–13.

57. Reuben DB, Ix JH, Greendale GA, Seeman TE. The predictive value of combined hypoalbuminemia and hypocholesterolemia in high functioning community-dwelling older persons: MacArthur Studies of Successful Aging. J Am Geriatr Soc 1999; 47: 402–6.

58. Visser M, Kritchevsky SB, Newman AB, et al. Lower serum albumin concentration and change in muscle mass: the Health, Aging and Body Composition Study. Am J Clin Nutr 2005; 82: 531–7.

59. Gabay C, Kushner I. Acute-phase proteins and other systemic responses to inflammation. N Engl J Med 1999; 340: 448–54.

60. Woloshin S, Schwartz LM. Distribution of C-reactive protein values in the United States. N Engl J Med 2005; 352: 1611–13.

61. Ferrucci L, Penninx BW, Volpato S, et al. Change in muscle strength explains accelerated decline of physical function in older women with high interleukin-6 serum levels. J Am Geriatr Soc 2002; 50: 1947–54.

62. Payette H, Roubenoff R, Jacques PF, et al. Insulin-like growth factor-1 and interleukin 6 predict sarcopenia in very old community living men and women: the Framingham Heart Study. J Am Geriatr Soc 2003; 51: 1237–43.

63. Reuben DB, Judd-Hamilton L, Harris TB, Seeman TE. The associations between physical activity and inflammatory markers in high functioning older persons: MacArthur Studies of Successful Aging. J Am Geriatr Soc 2003; 51: 1125–30.

Medication and prescribing 9

Hilary A Wynne

INTRODUCTION

The use and misuse of medication increases markedly with advancing age, as a response to the greater prevalence of acute and chronic conditions requiring medicinal therapy.[1] Of equal importance, age-related changes in hepatic and renal function lead to alterations in drug clearance. Liver blood flow falls by about 35% between young adulthood and old age, and liver size diminishes by about 24–35%. Glomerular filtration, effective renal plasma flow, and renal tubular function fall, on average, with age, although there is a wide interindividual variability in the extent to which this occurs. The contribution of age to altered drug clearance in an individual older patient is difficult to predict. This is because interindividual variability, drug interactions (particularly in the form of induction or inhibition of metabolism), numbers and types of co-prescribed drugs, and underlying disease are superimposed on the aging process. As older patients are often excluded from clinical trials, only generalizations such as 'when prescribing for the older patient, it is wise to start low and increase dose slowly, starting with a dose some 30–40% smaller than the average dose for young or middle-aged adults' can be made. This chapter examines common problems in prescribing for elderly women: adverse drug reactions, drug adherence, drug interactions, pharmacokinetics, and pharmacodynamics. Awareness of these issues, hopefully, will lead to safer prescribing.

PRESCRIBING FOR ELDERLY WOMEN

Whereas those aged 65 years and older only account for 15% of the entire UK population, they receive 45% of the total prescriptions dispensed. Of great importance, the number of medications used per person has increased substantially over the past two decades, particularly among those aged 85 years or over, and especially in women.[2] This is because of a number of distinct factors, not the least of which is the introduction of new drugs and adoption of different uses for existing drugs, including for prophylaxis of disease, even in the very old. The widespread belief that the absolute benefit of drug treatment is likely to be at least as large in older as in younger patients has contributed to the increase in prescribing, as has the concept that no reasonable therapy should be withheld from elderly individuals on the basis of their age alone. Despite the presence of these 'positive forces', as it were, a conflict may present itself between recommendations for multiple drug interventions as treatment or prophylaxis and using the lowest effective dose of the least number of drugs per day for the shortest duration to reduce the incidence of adverse drug reactions, which are a risk from any drug. This conflict is particularly acute in the older elderly, especially when there are defects in mentation, and adherence with any prescribed medication is problematic.

Where life expectancy allows, it is appropriate to prescribe drugs which improve well-being as well as prognosis, although judgment on this point is often of necessity made without being able to apply randomized controlled trial evidence directly to older people, who most often have been excluded from clinical trials. Furthermore, women represent a special subset of older people which traditionally has been under-represented in drug studies and, even when included, are reported by gender in fewer than 20% of publications. Real-life trials with clinically relevant endpoints to improve the evidence base are obviously urgently required. Clinical trials in older women with multiple comorbidities can achieve high levels of adherence, although study medication discontinuation is predicted by fair to poor self-rated health or having four or more depressive symptoms.

Women account for two-thirds of those individuals who have survived to 65 years of age and, at each age, have more non-fatal diagnoses than men: they also receive more prescriptions. Age, income, and educational level account for 9% of the variation, with education level accounting for most variation in polypharmacy, at least in North America, where older more educated women are most likely to take multiple medicines.[3] Various explanations as to why women are more likely than men to consult their doctors and receive prescription medication have been proposed. These include the fact that it may be culturally more acceptable for women to report and medically treat their symptoms, with easier access to physicians, pharmacists, and the medicine cabinet as they spend more time at home than men. Also, their social roles may be less satisfying or more stressful than those of men, and health professionals may perceive them as being more ill than men; finally, they may have a greater range of morbidities amenable to drug therapy than do men.[4] The validity of all these points of view is open to question, however.

ADVERSE DRUG REACTIONS

Definition and scale of the problem

The World Health Organization's definition of an adverse drug reaction (ADR) is that of a noxious, unintended and undesired effect, which occurs at doses used in humans for prophylaxis, diagnosis or therapy.[5] This definition excludes adverse drug events (ADEs), which are due to errors in administration, intentional and accidental overdose, and omission or non-compliance of a degree that contributes to therapeutic failure. Adverse drug events are preventable, frequently severe and often result in hospital admission, especially in the elderly. In an Australian cohort of patients aged 75 years and over, ADEs explained 30% of emergency medical admissions for which non-compliance, omission or cessation of indicated treatment accounted collectively for 26%.[6] Further, in an American survey of 6365 patients, such events in women were more likely to be the result of therapeutic error, adverse drug reactions, inadvertent ingestions and acute-on-chronic adverse drug effects than was the case in men.[7] Older age was inversely associated with acute events, suspected suicide, food poisoning, and inhalation and derma exposures. Older women may be at especially high risk because of high medication use, both over-the-counter and prescribed as well as the effects of biological changes which affect drug metabolism.

A meta-analysis of 39 prospective US studie of ADRs as a cause of admission and during hospital stay reported an overall incidence of ADR requiring hospitalization, prolonging hospitalization, or causing permanent disability, or death as 6.7% and of fatal ADRs as 0.32% of hospitalized patients (Table 9.1).[8]

The number of drug exposures per patient length of hospital stay, and older age all affec ADR rates. Furthermore, the risk ratio for wome vs men may be as high as 1.5. Although th

Table 9.1 Adverse drug reactions (ADRs)

	Total no. patients studied	Incidence of ADRs (%)	95% CI	No. of studies
ADRs in patients while in hospital:				
All severities	34463	10.9	7.9–13.9	18
Serious	22505	2.1	1.9–2.3	12
Fatal	28872	0.19	0.13–0.26	10
Patients admitted to hospital due to an ADR:				
Serious	28017	4.7	3.1–6.2	21
Fatal	17753	0.13	0.04–0.21	6
Overall ADR incidence, while in hospital + causing admission to hospital:				
All severities	62480	15.1	12.0–18.1	39
Serious	50519	6.7	5.2–8.2	33
Fatal	46625	0.32	0.23–0.41	16

Patients had an average age of 54 years, proportion female 0.5, average drug exposure 8. Adapted from Lazarou et al.[8]

heterogeneity among the studies leads to uncertainty about the accuracy of their estimation that ADRs are between the fourth and sixth leading cause of death in the US, the burden from ADRs is clearly great.

Thus, a large study on ADR-related hospitalization in older people that paid special attention to measuring avoidability is particularly noteworthy. Pirmohamed et al,[9] in their prospective observational study of 18 820 patients admitted to two general hospitals in Merseyside, UK, between November 2001 and April 2002, noted 1225 admissions related to an ADR, giving a prevalence of 6.5%, with the ADR directly leading to admission in 80% of cases and accounting for 4% of hospital bed days used. Drug interactions accounted for one in six ADRs. Patients admitted with an ADR were significantly older than those without, being 76 and 66 years, respectively. The proportion of women in the ADR group (59%) was also significantly higher than in the non-ADR group (52%), p <0.0001.

Aspirin accounted for 18% of ADR admissions, other non-steroidal anti-inflammatory drugs (NSAIDs) 12%, and warfarin 11%, most commonly because of gastrointestinal bleeding. Self-medication with aspirin plays a substantial role in drug-related harm, being characterized by poor indication, uncontrolled use, polypharmacy, use for treatment of epigastric pain, and the patient's unawareness of potential adverse effects. This suggests the need for intensified information to the public concerning potential adverse effects of all drugs, not the least of which are the common over-the-counter medications.

The totality of ADEs represents a considerable public health and economic burden. Mean length of stay increases in patients who experience an ADR during hospitalization compared with those who do not, as do total hospitalization costs. The projected annual cost of ADR-related admissions to the NHS in the UK has been estimated to be £466 million (€706 million, $847 million). Estimates of ADR-related costs other than caused by hospitalization are scant and must be approached with caution, as they are based on uncertain assumptions and include issues such as cost of reduced quality of life, untreated indications, inappropriate drug costs, overdosages, and non-compliance.

Determinants of adverse drug reactions

The most important determinant of an ADR is the absolute number of concurrently used medications. A multicenter pharmacoepidemiological survey of 28 411 patients conducted between 1988 and 1997 in 81 hospitals in Italy reported that the number of drugs (odds ratio [OR] = 1.24, 95% confidence interval [CI] 1.20–1.27 for each drug increase) was an independent predictor of ADR-related hospital admissions, as were female gender (OR = 1.30, 95% CI 1.10–1.54), and alcohol use (OR = 1.39, 95% CI 1.20–1.60). For severe ADRs, age

(OR = 1.50, 95% CI 1.01–2.23 for age 65–79 and OR = 1.53, 95% CI 1.00–2.33 for age 80 and above), comorbidity (OR = 1.12, 95% CI 1.05–1.20 for each point in the Charlson Comorbidity Index), and number of drugs (OR = 1.18, 85% CI 1.11–1.25 for each drug increase) were the only predisposing factors.[10] Of 2.3 million case reports of adverse events reported to the US Food and Drug Administration's (FDA's) International Adverse Events Reporting System between 1969 and 2002, more reports referred to women (53%) than men (35%), with 12% not specifying gender.[11]

Four predictors are characteristic of older people in the community at high risk of an ADE:

- 12 or more doses of medication per day
- more than one prescriber
- having no caregiver to prompt medication-taking
- occasionally forgetting to take medication.

These circumstances are accentuated with multiple prescribers, as there often is a drug, dose and frequency disparity between the respective physicians' and patients' perceptions of the exact nature of the medication regimens.

COMPLIANCE AND ADHERENCE

Compliance is an older term that was defined as the extent to which a person's behavior (in terms of taking medication, following diets, or executing lifestyle changes) coincides with medical or health advice. Adherence is a newer and perhaps more politically correct term that has been suggested as being more neutral and more compatible of a partnership approach between the clinician and the patient. Concordance is an alternative descriptive term in which the patient and doctor exchange their differently informed health beliefs to form a therapeutic alliance whereby the patient makes as informed a choice as possible about the diagnosis and treatment. Because the term adherence is now widely used and accepted, it will be used here.

Poor adherence is an obstacle to patients experiencing optimal benefit from medical care. For example, good adherence to treatment advice following myocardial infarction is independently associated with improved survival. The importance of adherence was recognized by the World Health Organization in their report which commended training and reward of healthcare professionals for recognizing and overcoming the barriers faced by patients and their families in moving towards optimal health.[12]

Studies of the elderly report an adherence range from 40 to 75%, and the actual number is influenced by population demographics and regimen type. Variation is broad within and between individuals. Some drugs are better able to maintain a steady state of therapeutic coverage than others, with long-acting slow-release drugs, for example, compensating for imperfect adherence, albeit at a lower plasma level. In contrast, other drugs such as warfarin are less forgiving if adherence is imperfect. One of the major challenges in adherence research is finding a reliable measurement. As direct patient questioning tends to overestimate adherence, additional methods such as pharmacist questioning and/or review of computerized patient medication records should be used to increase reliability. In some instances, trials have utilized special medication containers which contain imbedded computer chips that assist in counting out the medication as it is being used.

Intentional and unintentional poor adherence

Patients' perceptions of their medication range from 'enabling and essential' to 'standby' or even 'little use or constraining, and therefore not worth taking at all'. Studies in elderly patients have described 70% of non-compliance episodes as intentional. Most commonly, patients felt that they did not need the medication in the dose prescribed and/or they expressed concern about negative consequences and side effects. Fortunately or unfortunately, attitudes to drug therapy are influenced by the presence of medical conditions. Thus, women admitted to hospital with a fracture are more receptive to education about osteoporosis and to the offer of further investigation and treatment than a control group with similar demographics but without recent fracture.[13] Of interest, intentionally non-adherent patients tend to consult more health professionals (doctors and/or pharmacists), and they tend to rely less on particular individuals to make decisions, and be less likely to follow a doctor's advice. In contrast, unintentional poor adherence occurs when the demands of the regimen exceed the patient's capacity to carry them out. Problems with understanding can occur if the healthcare professional has not communicated instructions or if the patient has cognitive problems and has forgotten them.

Hospital medical admissions of elderly patients due to non-adherence most commonly result from under-use, mainly intentional, through perceiving medication as unnecessary, forgetfulness, or in response to adverse effects.[14] Factors identified as being associated with a higher rate of hospitalization because of non-adherence in an Indian study included poor recall of medication regimen, treatment by numerous physicians, female gender, polypharmacy, drug costs, and switching to non-conventional forms of treatment.[15]

Whereas there is little evidence to indicate that the elderly are more likely to exhibit non-adherent behavior than younger patients, non-adherence represents a greater risk of poor disease control in the elderly, which may be compounded by comorbidities and polypharmacy.

Younger people are less regular in their timing of taking medicines owing to their more varied daily activities, whereas elders are more likely to forget, the very old having a lower rate of adherence than less elderly people. Although elderly individuals might admit to general memory problems, they are less likely to admit to specific medication-related memory problems: depression is a predictor of patients' overall self-rating of medication memory, whereas age is the best predictor of actual memory-related problems.

Improving adherence

Adherence improves with greater knowledge of the purpose for which the drug has been prescribed. Patients need clearly understandable written and oral information about both prescribed drugs and over-the-counter preparations. However, if contradictory information is obtained from different professionals, the likelihood of non-adherence increases. With non-adherent patients, expending resources on reviewing therapy, linking drug administration to daily events, counseling and providing drug reminder cards or facilitators which enable the physical administration of drugs, all help improve adherence. Having a caregiver assistant also improves adherence, as does the use of one pharmacy, which improves continuity of care and identification of potential adverse drug interactions as new prescriptions are received.

Adherence and access to medications

Adherence to medication is influenced by access to such medications. This is particularly important in healthcare systems that do not offer prescription benefits to older people. The inability to pay for medication or reduced access through government programs often result in 'enforced non-adherence'. For example, restricting the limit to three paid prescriptions per month under Medicaid in the US in the early 1990s resulted in a sustained drop of 30% in the number of prescriptions filled. Unfortunately, women, the elderly, and the disabled were most severely affected. The decrease was greatest for 'prophylactic drugs', but large drops were also observed for essential drugs such as insulin, thiazide diuretics, and furosemide. Further analysis revealed that this three-drug limit was associated with an increase in rates of admission to nursing homes. An increased use of emergency mental health services by patients with schizophrenia was also noted.[16] This was attributed to the restriction on payment for psychoactive drugs, which led to immediate and sustained reductions in the use of antipsychotics, antidepressants, and lithium. After the cap was discontinued, the use of medications and most mental health services reverted to baseline levels.

DRUG INTERACTIONS

Drug–drug interactions (DDIs) are a risk factor for adverse drug reactions and are common. Interaction between prescribed drugs and alternative and complementary therapies are covered in Chapter 10. Table 9.2 lists some common DDIs and their consequences.

Although many patients take drug combinations with the potential to induce dangerous DDIs, the proportion associated with relevant clinical consequences is relatively low.[17] A Swiss study of 500 medical patients found that whereas 60% were discharged from hospital with at least two prescriptions that could be expected to have at least one potentially interacting drug combination (70% of moderate and 12% major severity), only one patient was re-hospitalized within the next 2 months due to a problem associated with the potential DDI. Despite this seeming

Table 9.2   Some drug–drug interactions and their consequences

Drug group	Drug	Interacting drugs	Adverse effect
Antiarrhythmic agents	Beta-adrenergic antagonists	Verapamil	Bradycardia and asystole
Cardiac glycosides	Digoxin	Diuretics	Hypokalemia increases risk of ventricular arrhythmias
Anticoagulants (oral)	Warfarin	NSAIDs	Bleeding increased
Anticoagulants (oral)	Warfarin	Ciprofloxacin	Enzyme inhibition increases anticoagulant effect
Antihypertensives	ACE inhibitors	Potassium-sparing diuretics	Hyperkalemia
Hypnotics	Benzodiazepines	Alcohol	Sedation
Bisphosphonates	e.g. Etidronate	Calcium supplements	Concomitant ingestion decreases bioavailability and results in therapeutic failure
Dopaminergic agents	Levodopa	Anticholinergic drugs	Reduce bioavailability by delaying gastric emptying

ACE, angiotensin-converting enzyme; NSAIDs, non-steroidal anti-inflammatory drugs.

reassurance, the absolute numbers of patients harmed by DDIs per year is high given the widespread use of drugs. For example, warfarin, used commonly in those >65 years old to reduce the risk of thromboembolism associated with atrial fibrillation, has a narrow therapeutic index, high interindividual variability in dose requirements, and is much subject to influence by interacting drugs, both through pharmacokinetic and pharmacodynamic means. In patients ≥66 years old, concomitant use of a non-selective NSAID or a selective cyclooxygenase-2 (COX-2) inhibitor with warfarin doubles the risk of hospitalization for upper gastrointestinal hemorrhage compared with taking warfarin alone. Co-prescription should be avoided. Similarly, the concurrent use of anticholinergics such as antihistamines, tricyclic antidepressants and bladder antispasmodics with acetylcholinesterase inhibitors is common in patients with Alzheimer's disease, although rarely appropriate as they are likely to negate the latter's potential cognition enhancing effect. Although when initiating cholinesterase inhibitor treatments prescribers should attempt to eliminate concurrent anticholinergic agents, in an American study of 557 patients, 197 (35%) received anticholinergics concurrently, with prescribing actually increasing to counteract their adverse effects of urge incontinenece or gastrointestinal upset.[18]

Three population-based, nested case-control studies of all Ontario, Canada residents aged ≥66 years old treated with glyburide, digoxin, or an angiotensin-converting enzyme (ACE) inhibitor demonstrated that 909 elderly patients receiving glyburide were admitted with a diagnosis of hypoglycemia during the 7-year study period. In the primary analysis, those patients admitted for hypoglycemia were more than 6 times as likely to have been treated with co-trimoxazole in the previous week (adjusted OR = 6.6; 95% CI 4.5–9.7). Patients admitted with digoxin toxicity ($n = 1051$) were about 12 times more likely to have been treated with clarithromycin (adjusted OR = 11.7; 95% CI 7.5–18.2) in the previous week, and patients treated with ACE inhibitors admitted with a diagnosis of hyperkalemia ($n = 523$) were about 20 times more likely to have been treated with a potassium-sparing diuretic (adjusted OR = 20.3; 95% CI 13.4–30.7) in the previous week. No increased risk of drug toxicity was found for drugs with similar indications but no known interactions (amoxicillin, cefuroxime, and indapamide, respectively).[19] This study clearly demonstrates that many hospital admissions of elderly patients for drug toxicity occur after administration of two drugs known to be associated with DDIs. Many such interactions could have been avoided by better prescribing practice, by educating clinicians and patients about potential interactions and contraindications, and by greater controls applied at the level of the dispensing pharmacy. Although patient information leaflets about commonly prescribed medicines are generally well comprehended, information on risk of interactions and contraindications are poorly comprehended by older patients, particularly those aiming to deliver more complex messages.[20]

PHARMACOKINETICS AND PHARMACODYNAMICS

Pharmacokinetics is the area of science concerned with the fate of a drug once it arrives in the body, including protein binding, absorption, distribution, metabolism, and excretion. Although one can generalize about the effect of age upon drug disposition, factors including gender, race, diet and nutrition, frailty, disease states, and environmental factors such as smoking and other drug use all influence this phenomenon. Table 9.3 details the changes in pharmacokinetics with age. Furthermore, pharmacodynamics, i.e. the

Table 9.3 Changes of pharmacokinetics with age

Process	Changes with age	Drugs affected	Adverse effect
Absorption	No significant effect of aging on drug absorption		
Presystemic elimination	Reduced for drugs with extensive first-pass metabolism	Propranolol Nifedipine Triazolam	Hypotension Sedation
Distribution: non-polar drugs	Increased volume of distribution	Barbiturates	Not of clinical significance
Distribution: polar drugs	Smaller volume of distribution, higher serum levels	Alcohol Morphine	Sedation Respiratory depression
Protein binding	Decreased albumin	Propranolol Tolbutamide Warfarin Phenytoin Acetylsalicylic acid	Potentiating effect, e.g. between salicylates and warfarin
Renal clearance	Reduced renal excretion	Aminoglycosides Digoxin Lithium Atenolol	Increased risk of overdose effects
Hepatic clearance	Reduced hepatic metabolism	Benzodiazepines Phenytoin Theophylline	Sedation Ataxia Nausea, arrhythmias
Response to induction	Reduced induction of some enzymes in response to drugs and smoking	Propranolol	Bradycardia

body's response to a given concentration of a drug, will also determine the individual's overall response.

Pharmacokinetics

Absorption

Although some older individuals have reduced gastric acid secretion, gastric emptying, and blood flow, the gastrointestinal structure and function retain sufficient capacity so that age does not significantly alter drug absorption.

Presystemic elimination

After absorption from the gut, drugs are transported to the liver. Although drugs not metabolized in the liver, e.g. polar (water-soluble) drugs, pass into the systemic circulation unchanged, those with high hepatic extraction ratios, i.e. the non-polar (lipid-soluble) compounds, are avidly taken up. Liver volume and function fall with age, reducing the capacity for first-pass metabolism.[21] When a fall in first-pass clearance occurs, for example from 95% to 90%, this results in a significant doubling of systemic availability. In practical terms, this is something which should be anticipated for those drugs where the administered intravenous dose is significantly lower than the oral dose. This has been demonstrated, for example, for nifedipine, where response in terms of fall in blood pressure can be greater in older individuals.[22] Clomethiazole is subject to high first-pass metabolism, with around one-third of the oral dose becoming available systemically. As the extent of first-pass metabolism falls with age, plasma levels are higher in elderly than in young patients[23] although half-life after oral dose and pharmacodynamic sensitivity do not change.

Distribution and protein binding

The apparent volume of distribution of non-polar and polar drugs alter differentially with age due to the relative increase in body fat and decrease in total body water. That of most of the non-polar drugs, which include sedatives, hypnotics, and tranquillizers, rises in contrast to that of polar drugs, which include digoxin and alcohol, which falls. Thus, for example, a 15–30% higher plasma level of ethanol could be expected in an older compared with a younger woman after ingestion of a unit of alcohol due to a fall in volume of distribution and lean body mass. Also, ethanol is principally oxidized in the liver, primarily by the cytosolic enzyme alcohol dehydrogenase (ADH), first to acetaldehyde, and then to acetate. ADH activity in the gastric mucosa, which contributes substantially to the first-pass metabolism of ethanol, is lower in women than in men, who therefore have increased bioavailability and greater susceptibility to ethanol-induced impairment of muscle and neurological function.[24] Gastric ADH activity falls with age in men, but not in women,[25] whereas age has no effect on activity of ADH in the liver.[26]

The extent of protein binding of a drug is a function of its chemical properties, protein concentration and the number of protein-binding sites available as well as the affinity constant for the drug–protein interaction. Acid glycoprotein concentrations tend not to change with age, whereas albumin concentrations are generally reduced with age, and even more with frailty.[27] Age-related changes in protein binding are not generally clinically important in chronic therapy, although in acute drug administration these influence drug effect. With chronic administration of a drug, clearance acts as a homeostatic mechanism, increasing in response to any increase in free drug concentration as a result of reduced protein binding.

Drug clearance

Clearance (defined as the volume of blood from which the drug is cleared per unit time) is influenced by the physicochemical properties of the drug. Polar compounds can be excreted unchanged by the kidneys. Glomerular filtration, effective renal plasma flow, and renal tubular function fall, on average, with age, although there is a wide interindividual variability in the extent to which this occurs. For example, serum creatinine levels can remain stable with age in spite of a decline in creatinine clearance, as the decline in muscle bulk with age reduces creatinine production (see Chapter 8). Whereas a fall in renal function is unimportant for some drugs, this is not the case with renally excreted drugs with a narrow therapeutic index and serious side effects. Both concealed renal insufficiency, which is reduction in estimated glomerular filtration rate (GFR) in people with normal serum creatinine levels, and overt renal failure are associated with ADRs to polar drugs such as aminoglycoside antibiotics, digoxin, and lithium in the elderly. These agents should be prescribed with care.

Non-polar compounds, on the other hand, must undergo a chemical change in the liver, usually through a phase I (oxidative) reaction followed by a phase II (conjugative) reaction, although some drugs bypass the former step.

Hepatic drug clearance is influenced by the rate at which blood flow can deliver the drug to the liver for uptake as well as by activity of drug-metabolizing enzymes. Liver blood flow falls by about 35% between young adulthood and old age, with clearance falling in parallel. Liver size diminishes also by about 24–35%, resulting in a similar reduction in clearance.[21]

Drug clearance of beta-adrenergic antagonists and opioids

The effect of these changes is illustrated using beta-adrenergic antagonists and opioids as examples. Pharmacokinetic properties differ between beta-adrenergic antagonists. Thus, the polar compound atenolol is renally excreted and clearance falls with age.[28] Propranolol and metoprolol, both hepatically metabolized drugs, undergo significant age-related falls in first-pass metabolism and hepatic oxidation.[29] Although the decline in beta-adrenoceptor function which contributes to an age-related resistance to beta blockade counteracts the increase in plasma concentrations per unit dose, elderly people can be as, or even more, sensitive than younger individuals to the negative chronotropic effects of beta blockers.[27] Consequently, it is wise to start with a low dose and titrate upwards while, at the same time, monitoring cardiovascular and clinical responses.

Opioids are well absorbed from the gastrointestinal tract. Most are subject to high first-pass metabolism, and increased with age. Morphine is directly conjugated in the liver by glucuronidation, most importantly to its active metabolite morphine-6-glucuronide. The reduced liver clearance of morphine and this metabolite contributes to its age-related increase in analgesic effect and respiratory depression.[30] Furthermore, the relatively lower dose of intravenous fentanyl required to produce similar sedation provides evidence that pharmacodynamic

changes at the level of the opioid receptor also occur.[31]

Cytochrome P450 enzymes

The cytochrome P450 (CYP or P450) family of enzymes is the most important contributor to oxidative drug metabolism. There are 18 families in humans, of which CYP 1, 2, and 3 are involved in drug metabolism. The activity of these enzymes may differ between the genders and, furthermore, changes with age. Clearance of non-polar drugs metabolized by the cytochrome P450 enzymes is decreased in the elderly, probably as a result of reduced liver function.[32] Age, per se, generally does not impair cytochrome P450 function,[33] although an age-related fall in activity of a few enzymes has been described.[34] The most notable characteristic of liver function in the elderly is the increase in interindividual variability, a feature that may obscure age-related differences.

With regard to gender, the CYP3A4 isoenzyme, responsible for the metabolism of over 5% of therapeutic drugs, including diazepam, erythromycin, and prednisolone, and exhibits higher activity in women than in men.[35] Furthermore, in parallel with the higher content of CYP3A4, liver microsomes from females show faster *N*-dechloroethylation of the anticancer alkylating agent ifosfamide, which could result in a higher risk of neurotoxic side effects in women.[36] In contrast, the activity of CYP1A-dependent (CYP1C19, CYP2D6, and CYP2E1) isoenzymes and glucuronidation activity may be higher in men than in women.[35] No clear gender differences in individual contents and metabolizing activities have been detected in other cytochrome P450 enzymes.[35]

Few studies have evaluated age as well as gender changes in activities of specific cytochrome P450 enzymes. One found that both women and men were equivalent with respect to activity of most enzymes studied; although the activities of most did not change with age, one enzyme showed an age-related fall and one an increase in activity.[37] The clearance of drugs metabolized by the isoform CYP3A (quinidine, midazolam, triazolam, erythromycin, lidocaine) declines with age. However, the liver activity of CYP3A from patients aged 27–83 with normal liver function[38] does not correlate with age but varies fivefold between individuals.

Gender may affect the activity response of CYP isoenzymes in response to inducers, and this may vary with individual drugs.[39] With regard to age, elderly patients retain their sensitivity to dose-dependent autoinduction and induction by other enzyme inducers of CYP3A4 activity. However, as their CYP3A4-mediated drug metabolic rates remain considerably lower than in younger people, patients in old age require lower carbamazepine dosages to achieve serum concentrations comparable with those found in young adults.[40]

Frailty

Although activities of oxidative and conjugative enzymes can be well maintained into old age, falls in drug clearance noted in frail older people are explained by reductions in activity of some enzymes. Plasma aspirin esterase activity is similar in healthy young and older adults, but is significantly lower in the frail elderly,[27] owing to a reduction in quantity of esterase. This pharmacokinetic change is not regarded great enough to justify aspirin dosage adjustment, however. Paracetamol is a useful model substrate for the study of hepatic conjugation, being extensively metabolized, primarily to the glucuronide and sulfate conjugates, prior to excretion in the urine. Systemic availability is variable. Clearance, expressed per unit body weight, is reduced by 21% in the fit elderly compared with young individuals, but clearance per unit volume of liver is preserved.[41] In the frail elderly clearance is further reduced, not only by 47% per unit body weight but also by 37% per unit liver volume. This underlines the importance of adding chronic but stable diseases to the list of influences upon drug metabolism in the elderly. In routine practice, however, a significant hepatic and renal toxicity is only noted after acute overdose. Dosage reduction of paracetamol in old age is not required.

Disease

Drug metabolism is also affected by ill health. Liver disease, both acute hepatitis and chronic cirrhosis, with or without cholestasis, can impair hepatic function, with variation according to enzyme studied and disease state. Reduced activities of some enzymes have also been noted in cancer, trauma, sepsis, and critical illness. Renal failure also affects hepatic metabolism, the degree of impairment differing between drugs.

Pharmacodynamics

Pharmacodynamics, i.e. the body's response to a given concentration of a drug, changes with age. The examples given below are warfarin and antipsychotropic drugs, which are commonly used in the elderly.

Warfarin

Warfarin is metabolized by cytochrome P450 enzymes. Clearance falls with age and, as sensitivity to warfarin also increases with age, there is a 21% fall in dose requirements in the elderly over a 15-year period to achieve the same level of anticoagulation.[42] The increased target organ sensitivity may be because the fall in functional hepatic mass leads to a fall in total content of the warfarin receptor, vitamin K epoxide reductase, with age. The age-related fall in racemic warfarin clearance also contributes to lower warfarin maintenance dose requirements.

Antipsychotropic drugs

The antipsychotropics discussed are tricyclic antidepressants, selective serotonin reuptake inhibitors (SSRIs), and benzodiazepines. The National Service Framework in the UK recommends that tricyclic antidepressants should not be prescribed for patients over 70 years old because of the increased likelihood of anticholinergic adverse effects. The fall in the rate of hepatic oxidative metabolism with age, which results in reduced clearance and higher plasma levels, is partly responsible.[43] The noted increase in binding of imipramine in several brain regions suggests that pharmacodynamic changes also contribute.[44]

Clinical evidence supports the use of SSRIs as first-choice agents for treatment of late-life depression. There are few data and no clear evidence about differences in efficacy between antidepressants, although younger women may be more responsive to serotonergic antidepressants than older women.[45] Marked differences in the effects of SSRIs on specific cytochrome P450 isoenzymes influence their potential for pharmacokinetic interactions at this level. The half-life of fluoxetine is long, at 1–3 days; that of norfluoxetine, its active metabolite is even longer, at 5–7 days; and clearance falls with age. Dose in elderly patients should therefore be around half the dose of younger patients. Sertraline and paroxetine have half-lives of around 24 hours. Although metabolism of sertraline falls in old age, dose reduction is not normally required. Fluoxetine, norfluoxetine, and paroxetine are inhibitors of CYP2D6 and, as they are themselves metabolized by this isoenzyme, can accumulate in the elderly. Selection of an SSRI requires consideration of safety and

pharmacokinetic issues as well as comorbid conditions and concurrent drug therapy (see Chapter 6).

Benzodiazepines are non-polar drugs and the half-lives of those metabolized by hepatic oxidation (e.g. diazepam, desmethyldiazepam, chlordiazepoxide) increase with age.[46] However oxazepam and lorazepam undergo glucuronidation and their half-lives do not increase with age.[47] As well as pharmacokinetic changes, increased sensitivity to sedative effects are noted with age.[48]

CONCLUSION

Older people are major consumers of drugs and, because of this, comorbidity and age-related changes in pharmacokinetics and pharmacodynamics, are at risk in terms of associated ADRs. Practice points are listed in Table 9.4. Unfortunately, older patients are often excluded from clinical trials. Inclusion of older people with comorbidity, with clinically relevant endpoints, would improve knowledge about real-life treatment of the elderly. Information is currently largely derived from laboratory studies and investigations of carefully selected normal, healthy individuals. Trials which investigate geriatric pharmacotherapy in both men and women are needed to enhance the safety and efficacy of drug therapy in this pharmacologically sensitive subpopulation.

Table 9.4 Practice points

- Older people are major consumers of drugs
- Adverse drug events are a considerable health burden
- Poor adherence reduces optimal benefit of therapy
- Pharmacokinetics and pharmacodynamics alter with age
- Most clinical trials have not been undertaken in the elderly

REFERENCES

1. Department of Health. Prescriptions Dispensed in the Community: Statistics for 1993 to 2003. London: Department of Health; 2004.

2. Linjakumpu T, Hartikainen S, Klaukka T, et al. Use of medications and polypharmacy are increasing among the elderly. J Clin Epidemiol 2002; 55: 809–17.

3. Perry BA, Turner LW. A prediction model for polypharmacy: are older, educated women more susceptible to an adverse drug event? J Women Aging 2001; 13: 39–51.

4. Lipton H, Lee P. Drugs and the Elderly: Clinical, Social and Policy Perspectives. Stanford: Stanford University Press; 1988.

5. World Health Organization (WHO). International Drug Monitoring: The Role of the Hospital. Technical Report Series No 425. Geneva: WHO; 1996.

6. Chan M, Nicklason F, Vial JH. Adverse drug events as a cause of hospital admission in the elderly. Int Med J 2001; 31: 199–205.

7. Skarupski KA, Mrvos R, Krenzelol EP. A profile of calls to a poison information service regarding older adults. J Aging Health 2004; 16: 228–47.

8. Lazarou J, Pomeranz BH, Covey PW. Incidence of adverse drug reactions in hospitalized patients. A meta-analysis of prospective studies. JAMA 1998; 279: 1200–5.

9. Pirmohamed M, James S, Meakin S, et al. Adverse drug reactions as a cause of admission to hospital: prospective analysis of 18820 patients. BMJ 2004; 329: 15–19.

10. Onder G, Pedone C, Landi F, et al. Adverse drug reactions as a cause of hospital admissions: results from the Italian Group of Pharmacoepidemiology in the Elderly (GIFA). J Am Geriatr Soc 2002; 50: 1962–8.

11. Wysowski DK, Swartz L. Adverse drug event surveillance and drug withdrawals in the United States, 1969–2002: the importance of reported suspected reaction. Arch Intern Med 2005; 165: 1363–9.

12. World Health Organization (WHO). Adherence to Long-Term Therapies: Evidence for Action. Geneva: WHO; 2003.

13. Brennan NJ, Caplan GA. Attitudes to osteoporosis and hormone replacement therapy among elderly women. Osteoporosis Int 1999; 9: 139–43.

14. Levy M, Mermelstein L, Hemo D. Medical admissions due to non-compliance with drug therapy. Int J Clin Pharmacol Ther Toxicol 1982; 20: 600–4.

15. Malhotra S, Karan RS, Pandti P, Jain S. Drug related medical emergencies in the elderly: role of adverse drug reactions and non-compliance. Postgrad Med J 2001; 77: 703–7.

16. Soumerai SB, McLaughlin TJ, Ross-Degnan D, et al. Effects of a limit on Medicaid drug-reimbursement benefits on the use of psychotrophic agents and acute mental health services by patients with schizophrenia. N Engl J Med 1994; 331: 650–5.

17. Egger SS, Drewe J, Schlienfer RG. Potential drug–drug interactions in the medication of medical patients at hospital discharge. Eur J Clin Pharmacol 2003; 58: 773–8.

18. Carnahan RM, Lund BC, Perry PJ, Chrischilies EA. The concurrent use of anticholinergics and cholinesterase inhibitors: rare event or common practice. J Am Geriatr Soc 2004; 52: 2982–7.

19. Juurlink DN, Mamdani M, Kopp A, Laupacis A, Redelmeier DA. Drug–drug interactions among elderly patients hospitalized for drug toxicity. JAMA 2003; 289: 1652–8.

20. Gustafsson J, Kalvemark S, Nilsson G, Nilsson JL. Patient information leaflets – patients' comprehension of information about interactions and contraindications. Pharm World Sci 2005; 27: 35–40.

21. Wynne HA, Cope E, Mutch E, et al. The effect of age upon liver volume and apparent liver blood flow in healthy man. Hepatology 1989; 9: 297–301.

22. Robertson DR, Waller DG, Renwick AG, George CF. Age-related changes in the pharmacokinetics and pharmacodynamics of nifedipine. Br J Clin Pharmacol 1988; 25: 297–305.

23. Jostell KG, Fagan D, Bjork M, et al. The bioavailability and pharmacodynamics of chlormethiazole in healthy young and elderly volunteers: preliminary findings. Acta Psychiatr Scand Suppl 1986; 329: 32–3.

24. Frezza M, di Padova C, Pozzato G, et al. High blood alcohol levels in women. The role of decreased gastric alcohol dehydrogenase and first-pass metabolism. N Engl J Med 1990; 322: 95–9.

25. Seitz HK, Egerer G, Oertel UK, et al. Biochemical and immunohistological studies of alcohol dehydrogenase in human stomach: effect of age, sex, alcoholism and cimetidine. Gastroenterology 1998; 98: A629.

26. Wynne HA, Wood P, Herd B, et al. The association of age with the activity of alcohol dehydrogenase in human liver. Age Ageing 1992; 21: 417–20.

27. Williams FM, Wynne H, Woodhouse KW, Rawlins MD. Plasma aspirin esterase: the influence of old age and frailty. Age Ageing 1989; 18: 39.

28. Sowinski KM, Forrest A, Wilton JH, et al. Effect of ageing on atenolol pharmacokinetics and pharmacodynamics. J Clin Pharmacol 1995; 35: 807–14.

29. Tateishi T, Fujimura A, Shiga T, Ohashi K, Ebihara A. Influence of aging on the oxidative and conjugative metabolism of propranolol. Int J Clin Pharmacol Res 1995; 15: 95–101.

30. Sear JW, Hand CW, Moore RA. Studies on morphine disposition: plasma concentrations of morphine and its metabolites in anaesthetized middle-aged and elderly surgical patients. J Clin Anesth 1989; 1: 164–9.

31. Scott JC, Stanski DR. Decreased fentanyl and alfentanil dose requirements with age. A simultaneous pharmacokinetic and pharmacodynamic evaluation. J Pharmacol Exp Ther 1987; 240: 159–66.

32. Woodhouse KW, James OFW. Hepatic drug metabolism and ageing. Br Med Bull 1990; 46: 22–35.

33. Schmucker DL, Woodhouse KW, Wang RK, et al. Effects of age and gender on in vitro properties of human liver microsomal monooxygenases. Clin Pharmacol Ther 1990; 48: 365–74.

34. Tanaka E. In vivo age-related changes in hepatic drug-oxidizing capacity in humans. J Clin Pharm Ther 1998; 23: 247–55.

35. Tanaka E. Gender-related differences in pharmacokinetics and their clinical significance. J Clin Pharm Ther 1999; 24: 339–46.

36. Schmidt R, Baumann F, Hanschmann H, Geissler F, Preiss R. Gender differences in ifosfamide metabolism by human liver microsomes. Eur J Drug Metabol Pharmacokinet 2001; 26:93–200.

37. Bebia Z, Buch SC, Wilson JW, et al. Bioequivalence revisited: influence of age and sex on CYP enzymes. Clin Pharmacol Ther 2004; 76: 618–27.

38. Hunt CM, Westerkam WR, Stave GM. Effect of age and gender on the activity of human hepatic CYP3A. Biochem Pharmacol 1992: 44: 275–83.

39. Gorski JC, Vannaprasaht S, Hamman MA, et al. The effect of age, sex and rifampicin administration on intestinal and hepatic cytochrome P4503A activity. Clin Pharmacol Ther 2003; 74: 275–87.

40. Battino D, Croci D, Rossini A, et al. Serum carbamazepine concentrations in elderly patients: a case-matched pharmacokinetic evaluation based on therapeutic drug monitoring data. Epilepsia 2003; 44: 923–9.

41. Wynne HA, Cope LH, Herd B, et al. The effect of age and frailty upon paracetamol clearance in man. Age Ageing 1990; 19: 419–24.

42. Loebstein R, Yonath H, Peleg D, et al. Intraindividual variability in sensitivity to warfarin – Nature or nurture? Clin Pharmacol Ther 2001; 70: 159–64.

43. Ereshefsky L, Tran-Johnson T, Davis CM, LeRoy A. Pharmacokinetic factors affecting antidepressant drug clearance and clinical effect: evaluation of doxepin and imipramine – new data and review. Clin Chem 1988; 34: 863–80.

44. Gross-Isseroff R, Biegon A. Autoradiographic analysis of [^{3}H] imipramine binding in the human brain postmortem: effects of age and alcohol. J Neurochem 1988; 51: 528–34.

45. Gridgoriadis S, Kennedy SH, Bagby RM. A comparison of antidepressant response in younger and older women. J Clin Psychopharmacol 2003; 23: 405–7.

46. Klotz U, Avant GR, Hoyampa A, et al. The effects of age and liver disease on the disposition and elimination of diazepam in adult man. J Clin Invest 1975; 55: 347–59.

47. Kraus JW, Desmond PV, Marshall JP, et al. Effects of aging and liver disease on disposition of lorazepam. Clin Pharmacol Ther 1978; 24: 411–19.

48. Reidenberg MM, Levy M, Warner H, et al. Relationship between diazepam dose, plasma level, age and central neurosystem depression. Clin Pharmacol Ther 1978; 23: 371–4.

Complementary and alternative medicine

10

Alyson L Huntley

INTRODUCTION

Among the most frequently cited reasons for use of complementary and alternative medicine (CAM) are quality of life issues, prevention of illness, coping with a chronic illness, and boosting the immune system. Getting older is associated with an increase in all these concerns, and the use of CAM is pertinent to any discussion of older women. Indeed, the prevalence of chronic conditions is a reliable predictor of CAM utilization. In addition, the most common reason for CAM use is dissatisfaction and failure of conventional medical care.

The frequency of CAM use by elderly individuals is unclear. Studies undertaken in individuals aged 65 or over give a wide range of use throughout the world. One study by Foster et al found that 30% of the general older American population had used at least one modality of CAM in the previous year.[1] Another American study suggested 58% of older people in an urban population used some form of CAM.[2] Ernst and White found an 11% use of CAM in the UK.[3] A survey in an Italian urban center reported the use of at least one CAM therapy was 29.5% amongst the elderly population.[4]

How does the woman over 70 fit into all of this? One of the major features of use of CAM is gender bias in favor of women. Although the user profile is that of white middle-aged women, it is also important to consider the future use of CAM by older people in general.

Wellman et al have suggested that many CAM users (50–60 years old) are likely to mature into older users.[5]

Table 10.1 shows which CAM therapies are popular with the aging population from survey data. Of the CAM therapies cited, herbal medicine, chiropractic, massage, and acupuncture appear to be the most popular. This chapter describes clinical trial research in those areas of CAM that are pertinent to women over 70. All studies described in this chapter involve both men and women unless stated.

HERBAL MEDICINES

Over-the-counter (OTC) herbal medicines can contain either one herb alone or a mixture of herbs. Until recently, UK regulation meant that the vast majority of herbal medicines were sold as food supplements with little control over their contents. New European Union (EU) regulations, brought into force in October 2005, provide better control over what is sold, the quality of its content, and the claims made for medicinal value.[9] However, this change does not prevent older women from using herbal medicines in addition to medications prescribed by their health practitioners with or without consultation.

In general, communication about CAM therapies between patients and health providers is often unsatisfactory.[10,11] The focus of healthcare in older patients is control of chronic diseases,

Table 10.1 Data from surveys of types of complementary and alternative medicine (CAM) used by older people

	Williamson[6]	Dello Buono[4]	Flaherty[7]	Andrews[8]	Foster[1]
Country	Canada	Italy	Japan and US	UK	US
Number	42	655	307	144	311
Percent women	71.4	63	64.2	76.3	52
Ages (years)	66–100	<65	>59	68% >70	65+
Top 4 CAM modalities					
1	Chiropractic	Herbal medicine	Lifestyle diet	Reflexology	Chiropractic
2	Herbal medicine	Acupuncture	Herbal medicine	Massage	Herbal medicine
3	Massage	Relaxation therapies	Massage	Acupuncture	Relaxation therapies
4	Acupuncture	Homeopathy	Acupressure	Chiropractic	High-dose vitamins

and most are treated with multiple drug therapy. The average older adult takes five prescription drugs every day.[12] The addition of herbal medicines, mostly self-prescribed, to multiple drug therapy holds the potential for adverse drug–herb interactions.

A national survey of herbal use amongst the US elderly (31 044, of whom 57.2% were females and 5860 were ≥65 years old) concluded that use of herbal medicines was correlated with being female, greater income, higher educational level, and a more positive self-reported health status.[13] Some of the most popular herbal medicines reported in this study, as well as an academic review on herbal use by women, were Echinacea (E. angustifolia, E. purpurea, E. pallida) garlic (Allium sativum), ginkgo (Ginkgo biloba), ginseng (Panax ginseng), St John's wort (Hypericum perforatum), and valerian (Valeriana officinalis).[14] All six of these herbals have indications relevant to the health of women over 70, and thus their efficacy and safety will be discussed.

Echinacea spp.

Echinacea spp. are native to North America and were traditionally used by Indian tribes for a variety of ailments, including mouth sores and colds. The three most commonly used Echinacea spp. are E. angustifolia, E. pallida, and E. purpurea. The most common present-day applications of Echinacea spp. are prevention and treatment of respiratory tract infections. In appropriate cases, CAM or relevant substances may be administered in addition to conventional medicine as supportive measures in preventing infection and preserving health.

A Cochrane review of the effects of Echinacea in preventing or treating the common cold summarized 16 randomized controlled trials (RCTs), including a total of 22 comparisons of an Echinacea preparation and a control group (19 with placebo, 2 with no treatment, 1 with another herbal preparation).[15] Although most trials reported results in favor of Echinacea preparations, variations in the products used, methodological weakness, and suspected publication bias prevented the authors from making many clinical recommendations. A double-blind, placebo-controlled, seven-arm RCT study investigated various preparations of E. angustifolia for preventing and treating experimental Rhinovirus infections in 399 healthy young adult students. The results concluded that none of the Echinacea preparations, either alone or in combination, had any clinically significant effect on Rhinovirus or treatment of its symptoms.[16]

That being said, no serious risks have been reported with *Echinacea* spp. and adverse events in adults seem to be rare (allergic reactions, gastrointestinal complaints).[17] *Echinacea* spp. could theoretically decrease effects of immunosupression.[17]

Garlic

Garlic (*Allium sativum*) has been used as a food and spice as well as medically for various ailments for centuries. In recent years, however, garlic has been the focus of serious medical and clinical attention, with research focusing on its role in cardiovascular-related factors. Coronary heart disease is a leading cause of death in women over 60 years and yet few women appear to be aware of this (see Chapter 4).

A comprehensive review of the literature based on 45 RCTs concluded that, compared with placebo, garlic may lead to small reductions in total cholesterol level at 1 month (0.03–0.45 mmol/L) and at 3 months (0.32–0.66 mmol/L) but not at 6 months.[18] Changes in low-density lipoprotein (LDL) and triglyceride levels paralleled total cholesterol levels. Trials also reported significant reductions in platelet aggregation and mixed effects on blood pressure outcomes. No effects on glycemic-related outcomes were found.

Garlic is worth considering as an adjunct to other dietary and lifestyle measures. The most frequent adverse events are breath and body odors; other effects are rare. Garlic can increase the effects of anticoagulants and could theoretically enhance hypoglycemic effects of antidiabetic medications.[19]

Ginkgo

The ginkgo tree (*Ginkgo biloba*) is native to China, Korea, and Japan, although it is commercially cultivated in the South of France and parts of the US. It is one of the most extensively researched medicinal plants. Its main indications are cognitive impairment, dementia, intermittent claudication, and tinnitus. The annual incidence of intermittent claudication in women in the 65–74 age range is 54 per 10 000 at risk.[20] A meta-analysis of double-blind RCTs of ginkgo for treating intermittent claudication suggested a modest increase of pain-free walking distance compared with placebo (weighted mean difference=34 meters; 95% CI 26–43 meters) (Figure 10.1).[21] This conclusion is confirmed by another meta-analysis of all double-blind, placebo-controlled RCTs of an extract of *Ginkgo biloba*.[22]

In terms of cognitive impairment and dementia, a Cochrane review cautiously concludes that, overall, there is promising evidence of improvement in cognition and function associated with ginkgo.[23] A delay in the loss of capacities needed to cope with the demands of daily living may also be achieved.

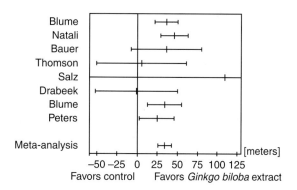

Figure 10.1 Effects of *Ginkgo biloba* extract in patients with intermittent claudication. The weighted mean differences in the change in pain-free walking distance from baseline are given with 95% confidence intervals. The vertical line represents no difference between *Ginkgo biloba* extract and placebo. (Reproduced with permission from Pittler et al.[21])

Another Cochrane review concluded that the limited evidence did not demonstrate that gingko was effective for treating tinnitus.[24] However, no reliable evidence as yet addresses the question of ginkgo for tinnitus associated with cerebral insufficiency. Beneficial effects were reported in double-blind RCTs for treating sudden hearing loss.[25] Regarding treating age-related macular degeneration, a Cochrane review identified one published trial and concluded that the question as to whether people with age-related macular degeneration should take ginkgo extract to prevent progression of the disease has not been answered to date.[26] For pre-existing visual field damage in normal tension glaucoma, some positive effects have been reported.[27]

Adverse effects of ginkgo can include gastrointestinal disturbances, diarrhea, vomiting, allergic reactions, pruritus, headache, dizziness, epileptic seizures, and Stevens–Johnson syndrome.[21] Drug–herb interactions with Ginkgo are reported in Table 10.2.

Ginseng

Asian ginseng (*Panax ginseng*) is a perennial herb native to the mountain forests of China and Korea. Today, however, it is rarely found in the wild. It is thought of as a 'cure-all' and is widely available as an OTC supplement. Conditions that are frequently treated with Asian ginseng are cancer, cardiovascular diseases, diabetes, immune function, sexual disfunction, and general level of vitality.

A systematic review assessed the clinical evidence from all double-blind RCTs of Asian ginseng for any indication.[29] The limited number of rigorous clinical trials relate to physical performance, psychomotor performance, cognitive function, immunomodulation, type II diabetes, cancer, and herpes simplex type II infections. This review, as well as a more recent systematic review, concluded that the effectiveness of Asian ginseng is not established beyond reasonable doubt for any indication.[29,30] Asian ginseng might improve pulmonary function, health-related

Table 10.2 Drug interactions with ginkgo (*Ginkgo biloba*)

Drug group	Interaction effect
Analgesics/NSAIDs	Aspirin, ibuprofen: increased risk of bleeding
Anticoagulants	Increased risk of bleeding
CNS agents	Alprazolam: AUC may be decreased slightly
	Haloperidol: increases effectiveness, reduces extrapyramidal side effects
	Trazodone: increased risk of sedation
Insulin/oral hypoglycemic agents	Increases fasting insulin in healthy subjects
	Effects in diabetics unknown
Cardiovascular agents	Plasma concentrations of nifedipine elevated in healthy human subjects
Proton pump inhibitors/antacids	Omeprazole and possibly other drugs in this class
	Reduction in plasma concentrations; therefore decreased therapeutic effect
Surgery	Risk of increased postoperative bleeding
	Animal studies show decreased sleep time induced by anesthetics
	Theoretically may alter heart rate or blood pressure
Thiazide diuretics	Potential increase in blood pressure

Created by A Huntley, based on information from references 19 and 28.

NSAIDs, non-steroidal anti-inflammatory drugs; AUC, area under concentration-time curve.

quality of life, and memory, but has shown no effect on psychological well-being in healthy young adults, on glycemic control, and on memory and concentration in postmenopausal women. A systematic review of potential cancer-preventive effects found that the evidence is inconclusive in terms of its effects in humans.[31]

Siberian ginseng (*Eleutherococcus senticosus*) is a shrub native to Siberia and northern China. It is in the same family, but is a different genus than Asian ginseng, and is therefore not considered a true ginseng despite pharmacologically exerting similar effects to *Panax ginseng*. Siberian ginseng has similar indications to its Asian counterpart. A systematic review assessed all available double-blind RCTs of Siberian ginseng root extract for any indication.[29] This study identified three trials that reported positive effects on psychomotor performance, cognitive function, and herpes simplex type II infections. The overall conclusion was that the effectiveness of Siberian ginseng is

not established beyond reasonable doubt for any indication.

Adverse events with *Panax ginseng* and Siberian ginseng include insomnia, anxiety, and manic symptoms.[32] Thus, recommendations cannot be given at present for either ginseng preparation as a therapeutic intervention. Drug–herb interactions with ginseng are given in Table 10.3.

St John's wort

St John's wort (SJW; *Hypericum perforatum*) is an herbaceous perennial native to most of Europe, Asia, and northern Africa that now also grows in the US and Australia. SJW has been used for medicinal purposes since antiquity, is one of the most well-known OTC herbals, and is used to treat mild to moderate depression and low mood. Depression may affect up to 50% of people in older groups, with women being more susceptible (see Chapter 6) . These figures are set to increase with an aging population.

Table 10.3 Drug interactions with ginseng (*Panax ginseng*)

Drug group	Interaction effect
Anticoagulants	Theoretical, based on animal studies
Antihypertensives	Possible additive effects
Anxiolytics	Theoretical additive effects based on animal studies
Cardiovascular agents	Increased plasma concentrations of nifedipine plus increased pharmacological and adverse effects
CNS agents	With isocarboxazid, tranylcypromine, increased risk of occurrence of CNS effect, e.g. manic symptoms, headache, insomnia. Aprazolam no interaction, but interaction with Siberian ginseng
Digoxin/cardiac glycosides	Concurrent use: enhanced effect of drug in chronic heart failure patients
Immunosuppressants	Not advised, as ginseng has immunostimulant activity
Insulin/oral hypoglycemic drugs	Theoretical effect on blood glucose levels based on animal studies
Monoamine oxidase inhibitors	Potentiates phenelzine, causing manic symptoms
Renal and genitourinary agents	Decreased diuretic effect
Surgery	Recommended to discontinue 7 days before surgery, owing to risk of hypoglycemia and bleeding

Created by A Huntley based on information from references 19 and 32.
CNS, central nervous system.

Numerous double-blind, placebo-controlled RCTs demonstrate the efficacy of SJW in treating mild to moderate depressive disorders and are confirmed by meta-analysis.[33] At the same time, comparative RCTs indicate that SWJ may be as effective as conventional antidepressants, including trials with severely depressed patients. However, recent RCT data were mixed: two placebo-controlled RCTs generated ambiguous or negative results, whereas others produced positive findings. When these new data were included in a meta-analysis, the risk ratio decreased from 1.97 to 1.73 but was still positive.[33] Further studies suggest that SJW may be effective for seasonal affective disorder and somatoform disorders (psychiatric disorders characterized by physical symptoms), but ineffective for social phobia.[34,35]

Most commonly reported side effects include gastrointestinal symptoms, allergic reactions, fatigue, and anxiety.[36] RCT data suggest that adverse events of SJW are similar to placebo. Several cases of mania and one of subacute toxic neuropathy have been reported. Unquestionably, SJW interacts with a wide range of other drugs (Table 10.4). Nonetheless, it can be recommended for mildly or moderately depressed patients as a monotherapy.

Valerian

Valeriana officinalis is an herbaceous perennial native to most of Europe and Asia. *Valeriana edulis* is widely used in South America. Both species are used for insomnia and anxiety. A recent meta-analysis on insomnia confirms the epidemiological evidence of the female predisposition for insomnia.[37] The trend of female predisposition was consistent and progressive across age, and more significant in the elderly.

A systematic review of the hypnotic effects of valerian concluded that the evidence was promising but not conclusive, owing to inconsistent results and methodological limitations.[38] RCTs published subsequently found valerian to

Table 10.4   Drug interactions with St Johns wort (*Hypericum perforatum*)

Drug group	Drug/interaction effect
Antiarrhythmic agents	Digoxin: blood levels reduced
Anticoagulants	Warfarin: decreased plasma levels and anticoagulant effect
Antihistamines	Fexofenadine: plasma levels and activity reduced
Cardiovascular agents	Nifedipine, simvastatin: plasma levels and activity reduced
CNS agents	Amitriptyline: blood level reduced
	Midazolam: reduced plasma levels
	Nortriptyline: reduced plasma levels
	Paroxetine: increased sedative–hypnotic effect
	Quazepam: decreased plasma levels but no clinical effect
	Sertraline: serotonin syndrome
Immunosuppressants	Cyclosporine: reduced blood levels, caused transplant rejections
	Tacrolimus: reduced plasma concentrations, risk of transplant rejection
Respiratory agents	Theophylline: reduced plasma levels
Surgery	Recommendation to discontinue use 5 days prior to surgery

Created by A Huntley based on information from references 19 and 36.

CNS, central nervous system.

be as effective as oxazepam in enhancing the sleep quality of insomniacs after 4 weeks. A sizable ($n = 202$) RCT with patients suffering from insomnia confirmed that valerian extract (600 mg/day) is at least as effective as oxazepam (10 mg/day) in increasing sleep quality when taken for 6 weeks.[39] Recent placebo-controlled RCTs generated mixed results: two small studies suggested efficacy in enhancing sleep, while a series of 42 n-of-1 trials failed to show such effects in any individual patient with insomnia or for the group a whole.[40–42] One comparison between *V. officinalis* and *V. edulis* concluded that both have equal hypnotic activity.[43] A further crossover RCT ($n = 16$) conducted under sleep laboratory conditions tested 300 mg vs 600 mg valerian extract vs placebo.[44] No electroencephalographic or psychometric changes were noted suggestive of sleep promotion actions.

In addition to single herb preparations, several combinations are available for which promising data have emerged; these include valerian/hops, valerian/lemon balm, and valerian/kava.[45–47]

Encouraging data from RCTs or controlled clinical trials (CCTs) are available as a treatment for situational anxiety, generalized anxiety disorder, reducing mental stress under experimental conditions, and as an aid during benzodiazepine withdrawal.[48]

Headache and gastrointestinal symptoms are occasionally reported with valerian preparations.[19] Potentiation of the effects of sedatives, hypnotics, or other CNS depressants is possible at high doses.

CHIROPRACTIC

Decreases in musculoskeletal functioning, endurance, lean body mass, strength, and flexibility can result from disuse. Older individuals are susceptible to disuse, particularly if they have one or more chronic conditions that hinder or prevent them from being active.

Chiropractic is a health profession concerned with the diagnosis, treatment, and prevention of mechanical disorders of the musculoskeletal system, and the effects of these disorders on the function of the nervous system and general health. There is an emphasis on manual treatment, including spinal manipulation or adjustment. Related techniques include osteopathy, manual therapy, and spinal mobilization/manipulation.

Conditions frequently treated include headache, migraine, musculoskeletal problems, and other pain syndromes.

A systematic review of spinal manipulative therapies for back pain included 39 RCTs: of which 29 assessed acute pain, 29 chronic pain, and 14 studies mixed or indeterminate durations of pain.[49] For patients with acute low-back pain, spinal manipulative therapy was superior only to sham therapy or therapies judged to be ineffective or even harmful. Spinal manipulative therapy had no statistically or clinically significant advantage over general practitioner care, analgesics, physical therapy, or exercises. Results for patients with chronic low-back pain were similar. The reviewers concluded that there is no evidence that spinal manipulative therapy is superior to other standard treatments for patients with acute or chronic low-back pain.

A Cochrane review of spinal manipulation and mobilization for neck pain included 33 trials and found that, administered alone, these treatments were not beneficial.[50]

Eight RCTs were included in a systematic review of spinal manipulation for headache disorders.[51] These results were inconclusive and no definitive conclusion about the effectiveness of this approach was drawn.

With regard to risks, prospective studies suggest that minor, transient adverse events occur in approximately half of all patients receiving spinal manipulation.[52] The most common serious adverse events are vertebrobasilar accidents, disk herniation, and cauda equina syndrome. Estimates of the incidence of serious complications range from 1 per 2 million manipulations to 1 per 400 000. Patients on anticoagulants may be at risk of cerebrovascular accidents after manipulations of the upper spine.

It is important to consider the implications for these therapies, specifically for the older individual. Obviously, too much manual therapy can be dangerous. It is reasonable that older individuals should consider manual therapies for short durations, but the primary care provider should be involved to ascertain safety.

MASSAGE

Massage is defined as manipulation of the soft tissue of whole body areas using pressure and traction. The most popular version is Swedish massage. Related therapies are aromatherapy, reflexology, and shiatsu.

Use of massage therapy increases with the number of chronic illnesses in individuals aged 50 and over.[53] Massage is thought to help individuals deal with their chronic illness and potentially help older people maintain a more independent life within their home or community.

A Cochrane review of massage therapy for low-back pain concluded that massage might be beneficial for patients with subacute and chronic non-specific low-back pain, especially when combined with exercises and education.[54] Another systematic review concluded that vibratory massage might be of benefit for muscloskeletal pain.[55] For treating constipation, a systematic review assessed the evidence on abdominal massage and cautiously concluded that abdominal massage could be a promising treatment option.[56]

In 102 elderly stroke patients (50% female, mean age 73.2 years), an RCT reported reduced levels of pain and anxiety with an intervention consisting of 10 minutes of slow stroke massage for seven consecutive evenings.[57] A meta-analysis of RCTs suggested that the largest effects of massage therapy are on trait anxiety and depression.[58] Single applications of massage therapy reduced state anxiety, blood pressure, and heart rate, but not negative mood, immediate assessment of pain, and cortisol level. Multiple applications reduced delayed assessment of pain. Reductions of trait anxiety and depression were the largest effects, with a course of treatment providing benefits similar in magnitude to those of psychotherapy.

There are some trials on massage and or aromatherapy for agitated behaviour associated with dementia (Table 10.5). These trials are generally small and differing in their approaches but the results seem to suggest that physical touch is more important than the olfactory experience. This fits with the significant evidence in the neurologic and neuropsychologic literature that persons with dementia have impaired olfactory abilities. Massage is generally considered to be a safe therapy as an adjunctive treatment to conventional care. Contraindications are cancer, myocardial infarction, osteoporosis, and individuals who feel uncomfortable with close contact.

ACUPUNCTURE

Acupuncture originated in China and is an integral part of traditional oriental medicine. In the West, its popularity has grown rapidly in the last few decades, particularly as a treatment for pain. Numerous systematic reviews of acupuncture trials have been published. Included in these data is documented effectiveness for various painful conditions, including back pain, dental pain, headache, and osteoarthritis (OA) of the knee. The prevalence of OA is about 70% in women after the age of 65 years. A systematic

Table 10.5 Massage and/or aromatherapy for dementia

Study and design	Patient details as available	Interventions	Results
Smallwood 2001[59] RCT	21 (12 female) patients, inpatients with dementia; mean age 69 years	Aromatherapy and massage, conversation and aromatherapy, or massage (lavender oil was used)	All groups improved in terms of frequency of excessive motor behavior, with aromatherapy massage having the greatest effect
Holmes 2002[60] CCT	15 patients with severe dementia	2% lavender oil aromatherapy stream in the ward for 2 hours alternated with placebo (water) every other day for 10 sessions	Lavender oil in aromastream had modest efficacy in agitated behavior in severe dementia
Ballard 2002[61] RCT	72 patients (43 female) with clinically significant agitation with severe dementia; mean age 78.5 ± 8.1 years	Aromatherapy with Melissa essential oil or placebo (sunflower oil); faces and arms twice daily	Significant overall improvement in agitation scores and quality of life with Melissa oil compared with placebo
Remington 2002[62] RCT	68 nursing home residents with dementia with agitated behaviors	10 min/day of either calming music, hand massage, or calming music and hand massage simultaneously or no intervention	Each of the interventions reduced agitation more than the control for up to 1 hour, significantly reducing physically non-aggressive behaviors but not aggressive behaviors
Gray 2002[63] RCT	13 (6 women) in residential care with confusion due to dementia and agitated behaviors during medication administration	Subjects were exposed to 4 aroma interventions during medication procedures: *Lavandula officinalis, Citrus aurantium, Melaleuca alternifolia*, or no aroma (control)	No statistically significant differences across all interventions
Snow 2004[64] CCT	7 nursing home residents with dementia with marked agitation	Study design was within subjects ABCBA (A = lavender oil, B = thyme oil, C = unscented grapeseed oil) each for 2 weeks, with oil being placed every 3 hours on the participant's shirt	None of the interventions decreased agitation
Woods 2005[65] RCT	57 residents (46 female) 67–93 years with behavioral symptoms of dementia	Participants received either therapeutic touch, placebo therapeutic touch, or usual care	Significant difference in overall behavioral symptoms of dementia with therapeutic touch compared with the other groups

RCT = randomized controlled trial, CCT = controlled clinical trial.

review identified seven trials, representing 393 patients with knee OA.[66] The authors concluded that for pain, there was strong evidence that real acupuncture is more effective than sham acupuncture, in contrast to the results for function, where no benefit was seen. Overall, there was insufficient evidence to determine whether the efficacy of acupuncture is similar to other treatments.

Acupuncture has been used for stroke in China and Korea for centuries, but scientific studies on this topic have only recently started to emerge. A Cochrane review assessing the effectiveness and safety of acupuncture in patients with acute stroke showed it to be safe, albeit without clear evidence of benefit.[67] Fourteen trials, involving 1208 patients, were included, with 10 consisting of ischemic stroke patients only. Comparison of acupuncture with sham acupuncture only showed a significant difference on death or requiring institutional care, but not death or dependency or change of global neurological deficit score. Severe adverse events with acupuncture were rare: dizziness, intolerable pain, and infection of acupoints (1.55%).[67]

CONCLUSION

In summary, little or no research on CAM therapies specifically addresses women over 70.

However, many of the major CAM therapies have applications for this group of women. In view of the aging population and the popularity of CAM with women, more clinical trials in elderly women are required. Overall, CAM interventions can add to the health and well-being of women over 70. It is important, however, that the relevant safety issues be taken into consideration. The most significant of these are drug–herb interactions, but also the adaptation of the physical therapies for the more fragile older body.

The use of CAM approaches by women over 70 is a question of choice. If chosen properly, this can lead to a sense of empowerment and control over an individual's health care. As with other medical decisions, good communication between patient and health provider is essential to ensure a safe approach and maximum benefit from these therapies.

EDITORS NOTE

As the author so carefully noted, most of these therapies are patient chosen, not physician prescribed. Patients do not make choices based on evidence in Cochrane Reviews. These therapies would not be popular if patients did not *perceive* their value.

REFERENCES

1. Foster DF, Phillips RS, Hamel MB, et al. Alternative medicine use amongst older Americans. J Am Geriatr Assoc 2000; 48: 1560–5.
2. Cherniack EP, Senzel, Pan CX. Correlates of use of alternative medicine by the elderly in an urban population. J Altern Complement Med 2001; 7: 277–80.
3. Ernst E, White A. The BBC survey of complementary medicine use in the UK. Complement Ther Med 2000; 8: 32–6.
4. Dello Buono M, Uriciuoli O, Marietta P, et al. Alternative medicine in a sample of 65 community-dwelling elderly. J Psychosom Res 2001:50: 147–54.
5. Wellman B, Kelner M, Wigdor B. Older adults use of medical and alternative care. Appl Gerontol 2001; 20(1): 3–23.
6. Williamson AT, Fletcher PC, Dawson KA. Complementary and alternative medicine. Use in an older population. J Gerontol Nurs 2003 29: 20–8.

7. Flaherty JH, Takahashi R, Teoh J, et al. Use of alternative therapies in older outpatients in the United States and Japan: prevalence, reporting patterns, and perceived effectiveness. J Gerontol A Biol Sci Med Sci 2001; 56: M650–5.

8. Andrews GJ. Private complementary medicine and older people: service use and user empowerment. Ageing and Society 2002; 22: 343–8.

9. The Traditional Herbal Medicines Registration Scheme at http://www.mhra.gov.uk/home. Accessed February 22, 2006.

0. Suchard JR, Suchard MA, Steinfeldt JL. Physician knowledge of herbal toxicities and adverse herb–drug interactions. Eur J Emerg Med 2004; 11: 193–7.

1. Giveon SM, Liberman N, Klang S, et al. A survey of primary care physicians' perceptions of their patients' use of complementary medicine. Complement Ther Med 2003; 11: 254–60.

2. Bressler R, Bahl JJ. Principles of drug therapy for the elderly patients. Mayo Clin Proc 2003; 78: 1564–77.

3. Bruno JJ, Ellis JJ. Herbal use among US elderly: 2002 National Health Interview Survey. Ann Pharmacother 2005; 39: 643–8.

4. Tesch BJ. Herbs commonly used by women: an evidence based review. Clin J Women's Health 2001; 1: 89–102.

5. Linde K, Barrett B, Wolkart K, Bauer R, Melchart D. Echinacea for preventing and treating the common cold. Cochrane Database Syst Rev 2006; (1): CD000530.

6. Turner RB, Bauer R, Woelkart K, Hulsey TC, Gangemi JD. An evaluation of Echinacea angustifolia in experimental rhinovirus infections. N Engl J Med 2005; 353: 341–8.

7. Huntley AL, Thompson Coon J, Ernst E. The safety of herbal medicinal products derived from Echinacea species a systematic review. Drug Saf 2005; 28: 387–400.

8. Ackermann RT, Mulrow CD, Ramirez G, et al. Garlic shows promise for improving some cardiovascular risk factors. Arch Intern Med 2001; 161: 813–24.

9. Herr SM. Herb–Drug Interaction Handbook, 2nd edn. Nassau, NY: Church Street Books; 2002.

20. Kannel WB, Skinner JJ Jr, Schwartz MJ, et al. Intermittent claudication. Incidence in the Framingham Study. Circulation 1970; 41: 875–83.

21. Pittler KH, Ernst E. The efficacy of Ginkgo biloba for the treatment of intermittent claudication. A meta-analysis of randomized clinical trials. Am J Med 2000; 108: 276–81.

22. Horsch S, Walther C. Ginkgo biloba special extract EGb 761 in the treatment of peripheral arterial occlusive disease (PAOD) – a review based on randomized controlled studies. Int J Clin Pharmacol Ther 2004; 42: 63–72.

23. Birks J, Grimley Evans J. Ginkgo biloba for cognitive impairment and dementia. Cochrane Database Syst Rev 2002; (2): CD003120.

24. Hilton M, Stuart E. Ginkgo biloba for tinnitus. Cochrane Database Syst Rev 2004; (2): CD003852.

25. Reisser CH, Weidauer H. Ginkgo biloba extract EGb 761 or pentoxifylline for the treatment of sudden deafness: a randomized, reference-controlled, double-blind study. Acta Otolaryngol 2001; 121: 579–84.

26. Evans JR. Ginkgo biloba extract for age-related macular degeneration. Cochrane Database Syst Rev 2000; (2): CD001775.

27. Quaranta L, Bettelli S, Uva MG, et al. Effect of Ginkgo biloba extract on preexisting visual field damage in normal tension glaucoma. Ophthalmology 2003; 110: 359–62.

28. Bressler R. Herb–drug interactions: interactions between Ginkgo biloba and prescription drugs. Geriatrics 2005; 60(4): 30–3.

29. Vogler BK, Pittler MH, Ernst E. The efficacy of ginseng. A systematic review of randomised clinical trials. Eur J Clin Pharmacol 1999; 55: 567–75.

30. Ernst E. The risk-benefit profile of commonly used herbal therapies: Ginkgo, St John's Wort, Ginseng, Echinacea, Saw Palmetto, and Kava. Ann Intern Med 2002; 136: 42–53.

31. Shin HR, Kim JY, Yun TK, Morgan G, Vainio H. The cancer-preventive potential of Panax ginseng: a review of human and experimental evidence. Cancer Causes Control 2000; 11: 565–76.

32. Bressler R. Herb–drug interactions: interactions between ginseng and prescription drugs. Geriatrics 2005; 60(8): 16–17.

33. Linde K, Milrow C, Berner M, et al. St John's wort for depression. Cochrane Database Syst Rev 2005; (2): CD000448.

34. Martinez B, Kasper S, Ruhrmann S, Moller HJ. Hypericum in the treatment of seasonal affective disorders. J Geriatr Psychiatry Neurol 1994; 7(Suppl 1): S29–33.

35. Kobak KA, Taylor LV, Warner G, Futterer R. St. John's wort versus placebo in social phobia: results from a placebo-controlled pilot study. J Clin Psychopharmacol 2005; 25(1): 51–8.

36. Bressler R. Herb–drug interactions: interactions between St John's wort and prescription drugs. Geriatrics 2005; 60(7): 21–3.

37. Zhang B, Wing YK. Sex differences in insomnia: a meta-analysis. Sleep 2006; 29: 85–93.

38. Stevinson C, Ernst E. Valerian for insomnia: systematic review of randomised placebo-controlled trials. Sleep Med 2000; 1: 91–9.

39. Ziegler G, Ploch M, Miettinen-Baumann A, Collet W. Efficacy and tolerability of valerian extract LI 156 compared with oxazepam in the treatment of non-organic insomnia – a randomized, double-blind, comparative clinical study. Eur J Med Res 2002; 7(11): 480–6.

40. Donath F, Quispe S, Diefenbach K, et al. Critical evaluation of the effect of valerian extract on sleep structure and sleep quality. Pharmacopsychiatry 2000; 33: 47–53.

41. Francis AJP, Dempster RJW. Effect of valerian, Valerian edulis, on sleep difficulties in children with intellectual deficits. Phytomedicine 2002; 9: 273–9.

42. Coxeter PD, Schluter PJ, Eastwood HL, Nikles CJ, Glasziou PP. Valerian does not appear to reduce symptoms for patients with chronic insomnia in general practice using a series of randomised n-of-1 trials. Complement Ther Med 2003; 11: 215–22.

43. Herrera Arellano A, Luna Villegas G, Cuevas Uriostegui ML. Polysomnographic evaluation of the hypnotic effect of Valeriana edulis standardized extract. PlantaMed 2001; 67: 695–9.

44. Diaper A, Hindmarch I. A double-blind placebo-controlled investigation of the effect of two doses of a valerian preparation on the sleep, cognitive and psychomotor function of sleep-disturbed older adults. Phytother Res 2004; 18: 831–6.

45. Vonderheid-Guth B, Todorova A, Brattström A, Dimpfel W. Pharmacodynamic effects of valerian and hops extract combination (Ze 91019) on the quantitative-topographical EEG in healthy volunteers. Eur J Med Res 2000; 5: 139–44.

46. Cerny A, Schmid K. Tolerability and efficacy of valerian/lemon balm in healthy volunteers (a double-blind, placebo-controlled, multicentre study). Fitoterapia 1999; 70: 221–8.

47. Wheatley D. Stress-induced insomnia treated with kava and valerian: singly and in combination. Hum Psychopharmacol 2001; 4: 353–6.

48. Ernst E. Herbal remedies for anxiety – a systematic review of controlled clinical trials. Phytomedicine 2006; 13: 205–8.

49. Assendelft WJJ, Morton SC, Yu EI, et al. Spinal manipulation therapy for low back pain. Cochrane Database Syst Rev 2004; (1) CD000447.

50. Gross AR, Hoving JL, Haines TA, et al. A Cochrane review of manipulation and mobilization for mechanical neck disorders. Spine 2004; 29: 141–8.

51. Astin JA, Ernst E. The effectiveness of spinal manipulation for the treatment of headache disorders: a systematic review of randomized clinical trials. Cephalagia 2002; 22: 617–23.

52. Stevinson C, Ernst E. Risks associated with spinal manipulation. Am J Med 2002; 112: 566–71.

53. Votova K. Complementary and alternative medicine use among older adults. The role of health beliefs. Unpublished Masters thesis, Simon Fraser University (B.C.). Lecture presented at the 32nd Annual Scientific and Educational Meeting, 'Bringing the pieces together,' Canadian Association on Gerontology, Toronto Canada, November 1, 2003.

54. Furlan AD, Brosseau L, Imamura M, Irvin E. Massage for low back pain: a systematic review

within the framework of the Cochrane Collaboration Back Review Group. Spine 2002; 27: 1896–910.

55. Gottschild S, Kröling P. Vibrationsmassage Eine Literaturübersicht zu physiologischen Wirkungen und therapeutischer Wirksamkeit. Phys Med Rehab Kuror 2003; 13: 85–95.

56. Ernst E. Abdominal massage therapy for chronic constipation: a systematic review of controlled clinical trials. Forsch Komplementärmed 1999; 6: 149–51.

57. Mok E, Woo CP. The effects of slow-stroke back massage on anxiety and shoulder pain in elderly stroke patients. Complement Ther Nurs Midwifery 2004; 10: 209–16.

58. Moyer CA, Rounds J, Hannum JW. A meta-analysis of massage therapy research. Psychol Bull 2004; 130: 3–18.

59. Smallwood J, Brown R, Coulter F, et al. Aromatherapy and behaviour disturbances in dementia. Int J Geriatr Psychiatry 2001; 16(10): 1010–13.

60. Holmes C, Hopkins V, Hensford C, et al. Lavender oil as a treatment for agitated behaviour in severe dementia: a placebo controlled study. Int J Geriatr Psychiatry 2002; 17(4): 305–8.

61. Ballard CG, O'Brien JT, Reichelt K, et al. Aromatherapy as a safe and effective treatment for the management of agitation in severe dementia: the results of a double-blind placebo controlled trial with Melissa. J Clin Psychiatry 2002; 63(7): 553–8.

62. Remington R. Calming music and hand massage with agitated elderly. Nurs Res 2002; 51(5): 317–23.

63. Gray SG, Clair AA. Influence of aromatherapy on medication administration to residential-care residents with dementia and behavioral changes. Am J Alzheimers Dis Other Demen 2002; 17(3): 169–74.

64. Snow AL, Hovanec L, Brandt J. A controlled trial of aromatherapy for agitation in nursing home patients with dementia. J Altern Complement Med 2004; 10(3): 431–7.

65. Woods DL, Craven RF, Whitney J. The effect of therapeutic touch on behavioural symptoms of persons with dementia. Altern Ther Health Med 2005; 11(1): 66–74.

66. Ezzo J, Hadhazy V, Birch S, et al. Acupuncture for osteoarthritis of the knee: a systematic review. Arthritis Rheum 2001; 44: 819–25.

67. Zhang SH, Liu M, Asplund K, et al. Acupuncture for acute stroke. Cochrane Database Syst Rev 2005; (2): CD0003317.

Section IV
Common gynecological problems

Prolapse

11

Themos Grigoriades and Andrew Hextall

INTRODUCTION

The vagina, bladder, and muscles of the pelvic floor are sensitive to estrogen deficiency and the effects of aging. It is therefore not surprising that a variety of urogenital problems, including prolapse, occur more commonly in the postmenopausal years and are a particular concern for older women. Although rarely the cause of mortality, pelvic organ prolapse (POP) and related urinary and fecal problems may lead to significant morbidity and impairment in quality of life. Women often withdraw from their normal daily activities, and this circumstance may have a negative impact on their physical as well as their psychological well-being. The economic burden on healthcare systems from pelvic floor disorders is also significant, and likely to rise as the number of elderly women increases. It is therefore imperative that clinicians be aware of both the implications of prolapse and the available management options, particularly in the elderly and frail.

DEFINITION

The American College of Obstetricians and Gynecologists (ACOG) in 1995 defined prolapse as the protrusion of the pelvic organs into or out of the vaginal canal.[1] The problem with this definition is that it includes a wide range of situations from a slight descent of the cervix (which occurs commonly in multiparous women) to a complete procidentia, making it difficult to determine the transition between normal and pathological POP. Part of this difficulty arises because the degree and stage of POP in the general female population has not been well described. Unfortunately, many investigators have used differing examination techniques and reporting systems, so that historical data are difficult to interpret. In 1996, the Pelvic Organ Prolapse Quantification (POPQ) staging system was introduced which, unlike previous systems, has since been validated with high intra- and interobserver reproducibility.[2,3] In this system, specific measurements are made at different vaginal sites, allowing an objective evaluation of prolapse and the assignment of an overall stage, without consideration for symptoms perceived by the woman.

The quantitative POPQ examination measures the position of midline vaginal structures (in centimeters) relative to the hymenal ring, which is a fixed and easily identified landmark. The examination is performed both at rest and during straining, with structures above the hymenal ring given negative measurements (in centimeters) and those which prolapse beyond positive values. Stages of prolapse range from 0 to 4, and are analogous to staging systems used for cancer, with stage 0 corresponding to normal support and stage 4 corresponding to complete uterine or vaginal vault prolapse (Table 11.1 and Figure 11.1a).

One aspect of this system is the avoidance of terms such as cystocele (prolapse of the bladder),

Table 11.1 Staging of pelvic prolapse[2]

Stage	Description
0	No descensus of pelvis structures during straining
I	The leading surface of the prolapse does not descend below 1 cm above the hymenal ring
II	The leading edge of the prolapse extends from 1 cm above the hymen to 1 cm through the hymenal ring
III	The prolapse extends more than 1 cm beyond the hymenal ring, but there is not complete vaginal eversion
IV	The vaginal is completely everted

rectocele (prolapse of the rectum), or enterocele (prolapse of small bowel) (Figure 11.1b). The underlying rationale is that these phrases may imply an unrealistic certainty as to the structures on the other side of the vaginal bulge, particularly in women who have had previous prolapse surgery. Regardless, these terms are still widely used in clinical practice along with a visual description of severity such as mild, moderate, or severe.

PREVALENCE

The exact prevalence of prolapse is unknown. A few studies,[4,5] using the POPQ system on general populations, suggest that no prolapse (stage 0) is found in about 20–25% of a general population, stage 1 in about 35%, stage 2 in about 30%, and stages 3 and 4 in about 10% of the women. Of these, only about one in five women with a prolapse on examination are symptomatic and require treatment.[6] In the UK, prolapse accounts for the 20% of women on the waiting list for major gynecological surgery, and up to 11% of women have surgery for POP or related conditions by age 80 years.[7]

PELVIC FLOOR ANATOMY

The *pelvic floor* consists of several components lying between the pelvic peritoneum and the vulvar skin. These are (from above downwards) the visceral pelvic peritoneum, the endopelvic fascia, the levator ani muscles, the perineal membrane, and external pelvic muscles. The pelvic floor closes the bony pelvic outlet and supports the pelvic organs. The urethra, vagina, and rectum pass through the pelvic floor and are surrounded by the pelvic floor muscles.

DeLancey describes three levels of vaginal support.[8,9] The cervix and upper third of the vagina are supported by the uterosacral and cardinal ligament complex, which form the level I support. Although these tissues are termed 'ligaments', their mixed composition of blood vessels, nerves, and fibrous connective tissue reflects their combined function as mesenteries (supplying the genital tract bilaterally) as well as supportive structures. Contiguous with the uterosacral/cardinal ligament complex is the level II support – the paravaginal attachments. The middle third of the vagina is attached by endopelvic fascia to the arcus tendinous fasciae pelvis (the so-called white line that runs between the symphysis pubis and ischial spine). Level III support is provided by the perineal membrane, the muscles of the deep perineal space, and the perineal body. These structures provide support and maintain the normal anatomical position of the urethra and the distal third of the vagina.

Normal pelvic organ support depends on a dynamic interaction between pelvic floor muscles and the endopelvic fascia. In a standing woman the endopelvic fascia suspends the upper vagina, the bladder, and the rectum over the levator ani plate, while the pelvic floor muscles close the urogenital hiatus and provide a stable platform on which the pelvic viscera rests. This theory was put forth almost a century ago by Paramone who described the uterus 'as a floating organ'

(a)

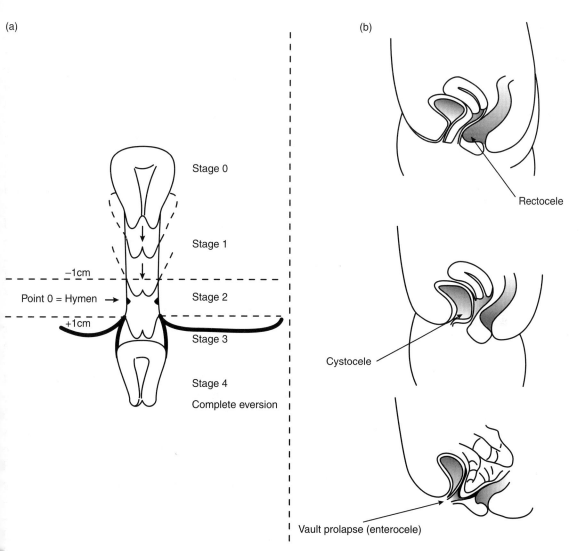

Stage 0

Stage 1

−1cm

Point 0 = Hymen →

Stage 2

+1cm

Stage 3

Stage 4

Complete eversion

(b)

Rectocele

Cystocele

Vault prolapse (enterocele)

Figure 11.1 (a) Classification of stages of prolapse. (b) Former dicriptive terminology.

akin to a ship held in place at dock by rope (ligaments) and water (pelvic floor muscles).[10]

The location of damage to these supports determines whether a woman has cystocele, rectocele, or vaginal vault prolapse. Disruption of the level I support may lead to prolapse of the vault or procidentia if the uterus is still in situ, whereas damage to level II and III supports predisposes to anterior and posterior vaginal prolapse. For the anterior vaginal wall prolapse, Nichols and Randall describe two types of prolapse – distention and displacement.[11] Distention is thought to occur as a result of overstretching and attenuation of the anterior vaginal wall (due to vaginal delivery or to postmenopausal atrophic changes). On examination, this type of prolapse is described as diminished or absent rugal folds of the anterior vaginal wall due to thinning or loss of midline vaginal fascia. The other type of anterior vaginal wall prolapse, displacement, is attributed to pathological detachment of the anterolateral vaginal supports to the arcus tendineus fascia pelvis (ATFP) unilaterally or bilaterally. In this type of prolapse, rugal folds may or may not be preserved. Richardson et al[12] attribute most cases of anterior prolapse to detachment of the lateral connective tissue from the ATFP, resulting in a paravaginal defect.

Damage to the pelvic floor muscles due to neuropathic or mechanical muscular damage can lead to a widening of the genital hiatus, resulting in a vagina further exposed to the effects of an abdominal pressure that is much greater than atmospheric pressure. This means that the endopelvic fascia becomes the primary mechanism of support. As long as the fascial layer is intact, the vagina may be adequately supported. However, over time, prolapse may result, after breaks, stretching, or attenuation occur in the endopelvic fascia.

PATHOPHYSIOLOGY OF PROLAPSE

Evolutionary changes and the development of a more upright posture placed greater strain on the supportive role of the pelvic floor. A multitude of physiological and lifestyle risk factors are independently linked to the development of the pelvic organ or vaginal prolapse. For most women the etiology of the POP appears to be a combination of various risk factors, with pathological processes occurring over time. However, some women may relate their initial detection of a prolapse to a strenuous event such as a vigorous cough or heavy lifting when they felt tissues give way.

The main pathophysiological factors associated with the development of prolapse are shown in Figure 11.2.

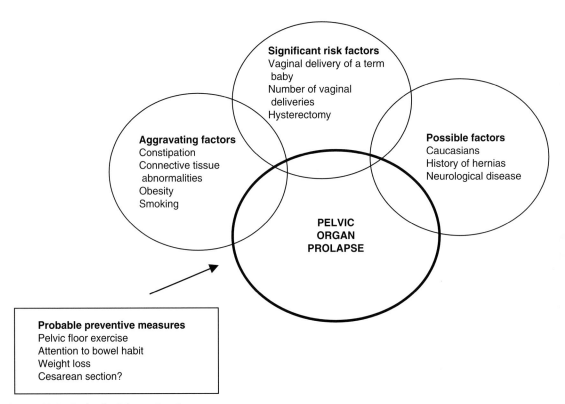

Figure 11.2 Pathophysiology of prolapse.

Obstetric factors

Several studies confirm an important association between the role of the past obstetric history and POP. Pregnancy itself, the number of vaginal deliveries, instrumental delivery, macrosomia, episiotomy, management of second stage, and type of anesthesia are all linked to the development of prolapse. There are sufficient grounds to assume that vaginal delivery (or even the attempt of a vaginal delivery) can cause damage to the pudendal nerve, the inferior aspects of the levator ani muscle, and fascial pelvic organ supports. Various studies show that increasing parity is associated with advancing prolapse. One vaginal delivery gives an odds ratio (OR) of 1.2–2.6, whereas a parity of ≥3 confers an OR of 3.0–5.4 compared with a nulliparous postmenopausal woman.[4,5,13]

Aging process

The Pelvic Organ Support Study (POSST) documented a 100% increased risk of prolapse for each decade of life.[4] Slieker-ten Hove et al used the POPQ system to examine 653 women randomly selected from the entire population of a small town of Holland.[14] Advancing age was a statistically significant cause of an increased POPQ score. Of those women >70 years old, 15% had a grade 4 POPQ score, compared with less than 1% of those <65 years old. Handa et al followed up 394 women who participated in the Women's Health Initiative (WHI) trial for a mean 5.7 years.[15] New cystocele, rectocele, and uterine prolapse occurred in 9%, 6%, and 2% of women per year, respectively. However, this study did not use an objective and quantitative classification system such as the POPQ.

Nerve injury

Some evidence shows that vaginal delivery and chronic excessive straining to achieve defecation is associated with pelvic muscle denervation. Also, pudendal neuropathy can play a role in the pathophysiology of prolapse.

Genetic predisposition

Some women develop uterine prolapse without presenting risk factors, whereas others do not develop this problem despite having had difficult obstetric deliveries. Thus, risk factors are only important when there is a predisposition to genital prolapse.

A few reports suggest that genetic or familial factors may increase a woman's risk of developing a prolapse, particularly if they are nulliparous. Rinne and Kirkinen[16] found that the familial incidence of genital prolapse was 30% in women aged ≤45 years old who underwent pelvic prolapse repair. Another study[17] found that familial clustering and transmission of pelvic prolapse occurs in a subset of patients and, within these families, there is a dominant pattern of inheritance, with high degree of penetrance and an increased relative risk to siblings.

Abnormalities of connective tissue and connective tissue repair may also predispose women to prolapse.[18] Women with joint hypermobility or connective tissue disorders such as Ehlers–Danlos syndrome or Marfan syndrome are more likely to develop pelvic prolapse.[18] In a small case series studying symptoms of prolapse in patients with connective tissue disorders, one-third of women with Marfan syndrome and three-fourths of women with Ehlers–Danlos syndrome reported a history of pelvic organ prolapse.[19]

Quantitative or qualitative deficiencies in collagen have been also associated with the development of pelvic organ prolapse, but it is unclear if the above findings are the cause or effect of prolapse. Prospective studies might help to identify patients at high risk of developing POP in the future, allowing them to be counseled regarding mode of delivery and prognosis for recurrent prolapse after reconstructive surgery.

Ethnic and racial variations in the incidence of prolapse are described. Women of European and Hispanic ancestry may be at greater risk for the development of prolapse and urinary incontinence compared with women of Asian, African, and Native American ethnicity.[20,21]

Chronic diseases

Conditions that lead to a chronically increased intra-abdominal pressure are thought to be predisposing factors for the development of prolapse, although there are few data in the literature to substantiate this. Obesity is an independent risk factor for urinary stress incontinence,[22,23] but the evidence of association between obesity and POP is conflicting.[24]

Chronic constipation, chronic cough, and chronic obstructive pulmonary disease (COPD) are also thought to increase the risk of POP. Whereas cigarette smoking may increase the risk of lung disease and coughing, surprisingly the WHI study suggested it is protective against the development of prolapse. However, in this study, prolapse was only assessed by inspection without any validated examination protocol (such as the POPQ). Recently, Wieslander et al assessed women taking part in the POSST, and showed that tobacco smoking was an independent risk factor for POP; the risk of POP in nulliparous smokers (OR = 1.95) was greater than that conferred by one vaginal delivery in non-smokers (OR = 1.34).[25]

Gynecological surgery

Nearly a third of women undergoing prolapse surgery require a further operation at some point in their lifetime.[26] Although this may be due to failure to re-establish adequate ligamentous or fascial support of the vagina, it is more likely secondary to generalized pelvic floor weakness, which leads to the initial development of a prolapse. Vaginal vault and posterior wall (rectocele and enterocele) prolapse are more common after hysterectomy.

PATIENT ASSESSMENT

Prolapse symptoms

Several studies find only weak to moderate correlations between the degree of vaginal prolapse and the presence of specific symptoms such as vaginal bulging, pelvic heaviness, and voiding dysfunction.[27–30] Swift et al evaluated symptoms and pelvic organ support in 477 women presenting for annual gynecological examination and found that the number of pelvic floor symptoms increased from an average of 0.5 symptom for patients with stage 1 pelvic support to 2.1 symptoms for women when the leading edge of the prolapse extended beyond the hymen.[31] Thus the hymen appears to be an important anatomical landmark for symptom development. Significantly increasing symptoms are present when the leading edge of the prolapse protrudes beyond the hymenal remnants compared with a low incidence of symptoms when the prolapse remains at or above the hymenal level.[31] In contrast, the prevalence of some symptoms, particularly urinary stress incontinence, appears to decline as prolapse extends beyond the hymen, probably because of increased resistance from the urethral kinking. Because interviewing a woman about her symptoms associated with urogenital prolapse may cause embarrassment, overall assessment may be difficult or inaccurate. Common symptoms secondary to prolapse are shown in Table 11.2.

During the last few years, quality of life questionnaires have been introduced as useful instruments to help the clinician to assess the severity of symptoms of POP and their impact on the quality of life in women with urogenital prolapse

Table 11.2 Symptoms of prolapse

Local symptoms

Sensation or awareness of lump/protrusion from the vagina

Feeling of pressure/heaviness/pain in the vagina

Lower abdominal dragging

Low-back pain, which is eased with lying down

Bloodstained and purulent discharge (sinister pathology must be excluded)

Urinary symptoms

Incontinence (stress and/or urge)

Frequency and nocturia

Difficulty empting (hesitancy, poor flow, incomplete evacuation)

Manual reduction of prolapse (digitation) or change of position required to start or complete emptying

Bowel symptoms

Incontinence (flatus, liquid, or solid stool)

Urgency of defecation

Constipation or difficulty evacuating completely

Digitation/splinting of vagina, perineum, or anus to complete defecation

Rectal protrusion during or after defecation (rectal prolapse)

Sexual symptoms

Dyspareunia

Lack of satisfaction or orgasm

Incontinence during sexual activity

Loss of libido

Questionnaires such as the Pelvic Floor Distress Inventory (PFDI) and the Pelvic Floor Impact Questionnaire (PFQI) have been introduced in the US, but with limited use in view of their size, with 46 and 93 items, respectively. Recently, the King's Prolapse Quality of Life (P-QOL) questionnaire has been introduced. This includes 20 questions representing nine quality of life domains that cover general health, prolapse impact, role, physical and social limitations,

personal relationships, emotional problems, and sleep/energy disturbance, as well as measurements of symptom severity. The P-QOL is reliable and valid, and provides an instrument to characterize symptom severity, impact on quality of life, and evaluation of treatment outcome.[32] Radley et al[33] devised a web-based, electronic pelvic floor symptoms assessment questionnaire (e-PAQ) that can be accessed online at www.epaq.co.uk.

Physical examination

Clinical examination is the main tool used for evaluating a patient with pelvic organ or vaginal prolapse. It is particularly important to consider the general well-being and mental state of an elderly patient, as this may influence the treatment options suitable for her. In addition to a general assessment, it is useful to palpate the abdomen so as to exclude causes of increased intra-abdominal pressure such as a pelvic mass or ascites. Marked striae gravidarum may suggest an underlying collagen disorder that may have also predisposed to the development of a prolapse.

Vaginal examination outside of a research setting will largely involve inspection and palpation in both the supine and erect positions, aided by the use of a good light and a speculum. In addition to a description of area(s) prolapsing, note should be made of atrophic changes secondary to estrogen deficiency or ulceration, especially if the prolapse has been extending beyond the introitus and rubbing on undergarments. Digital assessment should exclude significant uterine enlargement and adnexal masses. Occasionally, rectal examination can help to differentiate between a high rectocele and an enterocele.

Investigation

Women with prolapse and urinary symptoms should be investigated with cystometry prior to surgery, as they may have coexistent problems, such as bladder overactivity, urethral sphincter incompetence, or difficulty emptying, that may need to be addressed. Potential stress incontinence may be masked by prolapse; therefore, urodynamic studies with a ring pessary in situ may also be useful in predicting which women with a cystocele are likely to develop incontinence following anterior repair when any urethral kinking is corrected.[34]

If a pelvic mass or uterine enlargement is suspected, imaging with ultrasound may be necessary. Rarely, women with a large cystocele or procidentia may develop ureteric obstruction that requires estimation of urea and electrolytes and ultrasound of the renal tract. Anorectal imaging and manometry can be useful if there are concurrent bowel symptoms.

MANAGEMENT

A number of factors must be taken into consideration when advising a patient regarding treatment of prolapse. For asymptomatic patients, and those with only mild symptoms which are not bothersome, simple reassurance may be all that is required. However, women whose quality of life is impaired, as well as those who find their prolapse uncomfortable, will require treatment. The approach taken should depend upon the general health of the patient, severity of symptoms, the area of the vagina prolapsing, and the need to treat coexistent problems such as urinary incontinence. In general, conservative management should always be considered before undertaking any invasive or surgical therapy.

Simple measures

Simple measures could include lifestyle changes aimed towards providing symptom relief. A patient whose symptoms are related to posterior vaginal wall prolapse might benefit from attention to dietary fiber, with appropriate use of laxatives and suppositories, to improve defecatory habits. For women with symptoms due to vaginal atrophy, topical estrogen can be prescribed.

Pelvic floor exercises may limit the progression of mild prolapse and alleviate mild symptoms such as low backache and pelvic pressure.[35] However, they are not particularly useful if the prolapse extends to or beyond the vaginal introitus.[36]

Vaginal pessaries

A pessary is a device placed in the vagina in order to mechanically support prolapsed tissues. Detailed instructions of how to use pessaries can be found from as early as the 5th century BC in documents written by Hippocrates. He described the therapeutic effects of placing a pomegranate in the vagina for 40 days. In the late 1800s, there were over 100 different types of pessaries and, similarly, today many pessaries are available in a variety of shapes and sizes.

Pessaries are preferred for very elderly women who are unfit or decline surgery and can be used for the symptomatic relief of women on the waiting list for prolapse surgery. Limited evidence suggests that the degree of prolapse is unlikely to worsen during use of a supportive pessary after 1 year.[37] A recent prospective study showed that at 1 year, successful pessary treatment can be as effective as surgical treatment of POP. In this study, 12 months after treatment there was no statistical difference in general bladder, bowel, and sexual symptoms between women who had surgical treatment of their POP and women who had successful pessary treatment. This study provides important information that can be used during counselling for women who have symptomatic POP.[38] Pessaries are particularly useful for women with anterior vaginal wall or uterine descent and less successful for patients with a short vagina, significant posterior defect or those with a large genital hiatus secondary to perineal deficiency.

The selection of type and size of the pessary is usually made by trial and error, although during a bimanual examination the index finger can be used as a measure of the length of the vagina. Most pessaries can stay in situ and be changed only every 6–12 months by a health professional if there are no adverse symptoms. Careful inspection of the vagina and the cervix is performed, looking for signs of infection, erosions, or ulcerations. However, the cube pessary must be removed and then reinserted daily for cleansing, since this pessary has no area for drainage of vaginal secretions. This limits its use in women with limited manual dexterity, since a health professional may not be available on a daily basis to undertake this procedure (Figure 11.3).

Surgical treatment

Although elderly and frail women may be reluctant to consider surgery for their prolapse, particularly if they have multiple medical disorders,

this is the only definitive treatment. Although the absolute risk of death following surgery for POP is low, elderly women (>80 years old) have a significantly higher risk of mortality and perioperative complications compared with women of a younger age (<60 years old) undergoing the same type of operation.[39] However, advances in surgical techniques and anesthesia mean that it is increasingly rare for the very elderly to be considered truly unfit for surgery.

A number of factors influence the patient's and surgeon's choice of procedure for POP. These include the specific defects in pelvic organ support unique to each individual, associated urinary and rectal symptoms, the desire to maintain or restore vaginal anatomy to accommodate sexual intercourse, and the medical condition of the patient. Appropriate anesthetic techniques (including the use of regional and local blockade), careful perioperative pulmonary care, cautious intravenous hydration, thrombotic prophylaxis, perioperative antibiotics, and minimization of intraoperative blood loss all improve patient recovery from surgery.

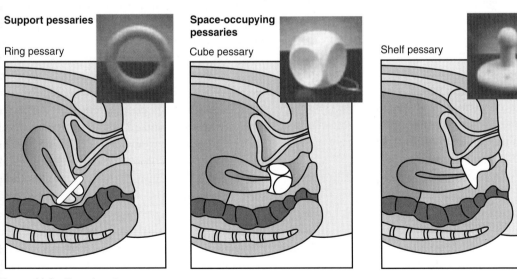

Figure 11.3 Pessaries.

Surgery for the anterior vaginal prolapse

Anterior colporrhaphy, also known as anterior repair, is the most frequently performed operation for cystocele. Although this may work well for central support defects, a recurrence rate of up to 20% is described.[40] This is often because prolapse of the anterior vaginal wall may be due to lateral detachment from the ATFP. In this case, paravaginal repair, either performed vaginally or abdominally, may give better results but is a more complex procedure.

Prosthetic meshes have been introduced in order to augment the native tissue for the repair of this type of prolapse, in line with inguinal and abdominal hernia repairs. A variety of materials are used, including synthetic grafts, autologous fascial implants, and allografts.[41] Although anatomical results and recurrence rates may be improved, clinical data from randomized studies are currently lacking. High rates of vaginal erosions or infections with non-absorbable meshes are a matter of concern.[41] Furthermore, evidence of a significantly increased risk of dyspareunia in the sexually active has been found in some but not all studies.[42,43]

Women with a cystocele and urinary stress incontinence may be treated with a continence procedure such as a tension-free vaginal tape (TVT) at the same time as their prolapse repair. This may also be necessary for patients considered to be at high risk of developing incontinence postoperatively, when urethral kinking has been reversed and urethral sphincter incompetence unmasked (Figure 11.4).

Surgery for the posterior vaginal prolapse

The surgical options available to correct a posterior vaginal wall prolapse include the transanal, transvaginal, abdominal, and laparoscopic approaches. From the available literature, the transvaginal approach appears to be superior to

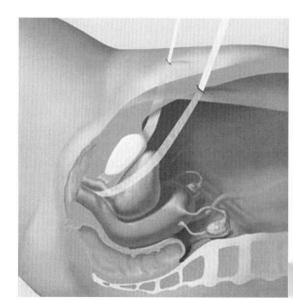

Figure 11.4 Tension-free vaginal tape.

the transanal approach, having better symptom improvement with less failure rates.[44]

Significant variations exist on the methods of the vaginal approach. The traditional surgical technique performed by gynecologists is posterior colporrhaphy, which consists of rectovaginal fascia reinforcement with side-to-side approximation and levator ani muscle plication. This technique, however, has been criticized for being associated with high rates of postoperative dyspareunia and bowel dysfunction. Levator ani plication between the rectum and vagina has also been implicated as a possible etiology for sexual dysfunction after standard posterior colporrhaphy, mostly attributable to atrophy and scarring of the levator ani muscles. Posterior colporrhaphy without levator ani plication is therefore preferred by some surgeons.

Richardson[45] attributed rectoceles to breaks in the rectovaginal fascia and advocated the repair of specific focal defects. Several surgeons describe favorable anatomical outcomes together with improved sexual activity using the defect-specific fascial plication,[44] but other reports show higher anatomical recurrence rates.[46]

In recent years, the introduction of mesh overlays was proposed to reinforce native tissue in posterior repairs. Short-term results show similar outcomes to the traditional surgical techniques, but long-term results from randomized trials are awaited, particularly in view of some concerns regarding complications such as vaginal erosions and dyspareunia.[44]

Several authors describe repair of anterior and/or posterior wall defects under local anesthetic with good results. This is obviously very important in elderly patients or patients with multiple medical disorders, as these patients might benefit from less side effects and a shorter hospital stay.[47]

Enterocele

An enterocele is a herniation of the small intestine into the vagina. It is therefore a true hernia, with a sac, a neck, and contents. The repair of an enterocoele can be performed vaginally, abdominally, or laparoscopically.

The vaginal approach, first described in 1922, involves a high ligation of the enterocele sac using a series of purse-string sutures. This technique gives good immediate postoperative results, but long-term results are poor. In 1957, the McCall cul-de-plasty was described using a series of continuous sutures which are being suspended to the uterosacral ligaments and then plicated in the midline, obliterating the redundant cul-de-sac.

Abdominal procedures such as the Moskowitz or Halban procedure are preferred by many gynecologists. These involve the obliteration of the cul-de-sac using either purse-string or roach sagittal sutures (a permanent suture in a continuous sagittal fashion) through the serosa of the sigmoid, the peritoneum of the cul-de-sac, and the back of the vaginal wall. Although the abdominal approach is associated with increased postoperative morbidity, various papers describe superior

results compared with the vaginal route. The abdominal procedures have also been adapted to a laparoscopic approach, but long-term results are lacking. Details of these procedures can be found in standard text books.[48]

Uterovaginal and vault prolapse

Definitive treatment for a uterine prolapse or prolapse of the vaginal vault after hysterectomy can only be achieved with surgery. These conditions are commonly associated with prolapse of the other vaginal compartments (cystocele, rectocele). Accordingly, gynecologists have developed a variety of techniques in order to approach this complex condition. Traditionally, women with vaginal vault prolapse were treated with an anterior and/or posterior or enterocele repair. For postmenopausal women with a uterus, a vaginal hysterectomy was also performed at the same time. However, poor outcomes with high failure rates and prolapse recurrence remain a significant problem and are generally poorly managed.

The vaginal sacrospinous colpopexy and the abdominal sacrocolpopexy have been developed to treat these complex conditions (Figure 11.5).

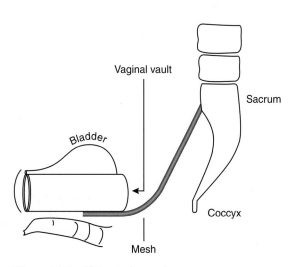

Figure 11.5 Abdominal sarcoplexy.

Vaginal sacrospinous fixation involves unilateral or bilateral fixation of the vaginal vault to the sacrospinous ligament and has the theoretical advantages of a shorter operating time, less postoperative pain, and less hospital stay. This would make this procedure more suitable for older, medically infirm patients. However, this approach can be complicated by injury to the pudendal nerve and vessels, with significant blood loss.

The abdominal sacrocolpopexy involves the attachment of the vaginal vault to the longitudinal ligament over the sacrum by a mesh. This can be performed during a laparotomy or, more recently, during a laparoscopic procedure with some good long-term follow-up results.[49]

For the elderly and medically frail patients who no longer wish to maintain their sexual function, vaginal obliterative procedures such as colpocleisis (from Greek *colpos* = vagina and *cleisis* = closure) are ideally suited as they are less invasive and provide good results. This procedure involves the fusion of the anterior and posterior vaginal walls, with or without concomitant hysterectomy.

In younger women wishing for uterine preservation, the following surgical options are available: Manchester repair, sacral hysteropexy (an abdominal approach), sacrospinous hysteropexy (a vaginal approach), or laparoscopic procedures (uterosacral suspension). Here again, the reader should refer to standard texts for operative details.[48]

CONCLUSION

With an aging population, increasing numbers of women present to their healthcare providers with pelvic floor disorders. A holistic approach, taking into account the severity of symptoms, medical history, and condition of the patient, together with a careful pelvic examination, are the first steps to be undertaken before making any therapeutic decisions. Each patient has different needs and expectations in life, and therefore treatment should be tailored to the individual patient. Advances in gynecological surgery presently offer a variety of effective and safe surgical options to alleviate most problems associated with prolapse.

REFERENCES

1. American College of Obstetricians and Gynaecologists. Pelvic organ prolapse. ACOG Technical Bulletin 214. Washington, DC: ACOG; 1995.
2. Bump RC, Mattiasson A, Bo K, et al. The standardization of terminology of female pelvic floor dysfunction. Am J Obstet Gynecol 1996; 175: 10–17.
3. Hall AF, Theofrastous JP, Cundiff GW, et al. Interobserver and intraobserver reliability of the proposed International Continence Society, Society of Gynecologic Surgeons, and American Urogynecologic Society pelvic organ prolapse classification system. Am J Obstet Gynecol 1996; 175: 1467–71.
4. Swift S, Woodman P, O'Bouyle A, et al. Pelvic Organ Support Study (POSST): the distribution, clinical definition, and epidemiologic condition of pelvic organ support defects. Am J Obstet Gynecol 2005; 192(3): 795–806.
5. Hendrix SL, Clark A, Nygaard I, et al. Pelvic organ prolapse in the Women's Health Initiative gravity and gravidity. Am J Obstet Gynecol 2002; 186: 1160–6.
6. Beck RP. Pelvic relaxational prolapse. In: Kase NG, Weingold AB, eds. Principles and Practice of Clinical Gynecology. New York: John Wiley & Sons; 1983: 677–85.
7. Olsen AL, Smith VJ, Bergstrom JO, Colling JC, Clark AL. Epidemiology of surgically managed

pelvic organ prolapse and urinary incontinence. Obstet Gynecol 1997; 89: 501–6.

8. DeLancey JO. Anatomic aspects of vaginal eversion after hysterectomy. Am J Obstet Gynecol 1992; 166(6 Pt 1): 1717–24; discussion 1724–8.

9. DeLancey JO. Pubovesical ligament: a separate structure from the urethral supports (pubourethral ligaments?). Neurourol Urodyn 1989; 8: 53–61.

10. Paramone RH. The uterus as a floating organ. In: Paramone RH, ed. The Statics of the Female Pelvic Viscera. London: Lewis; 1918: 12.

11. Nichols DH, Randall CL, eds. Vaginal Surgery, 4th edn. Baltimore: Williams and Wilkins; 1996.

12. Richardson AC, Lyon JB, Williams NL. A new look at pelvic relaxation. Am J Obstet Gynecol 1976; 126: 568–73.

13. Progetto Menopausa Italia Study Group. General and medical factors associated with hormone replacement therapy among women attending menopause clinics in Italy. Menopause 2001 Jul-Aug; 8(4): 290–5.

14. Slieker-ten Hove MCP, Vierhout M, Bloembergen H, Schoenmaker G. Distribution of pelvic organ prolapse (POP) in the general population; prevalence, severity, etiology and relation with the function of the pelvic floor muscles. ICS Congress, August 25–27, 2004, Paris.

15. Handa VL, Garrett E, Hendrix S, Gold E, Robins J. Progression and remission of pelvic organ prolapse: a longitudinal study of menopausal women. Am J Obstet Gynecol 2004; 190(1): 27–32.

16. Rinne KM, Kirkinen PP. What predisposes young women to genital prolapse? Eur J Obstet Gynecol Reprod Biol 1999; 84: 23–5.

17. Jack GS, Nikolova G, Vilain E, Raz S, Rodriguez LV. Familial transmission of genitovaginal prolapse. Int Urogynecol J Pelvic Floor Dysfunct 2005; 17: 498–501.

18. Norton PA, Baker JE, Sharp HC, et al. Genitourinary prolapse and joint hypermobility in women. Obstet Gynecol 1995; 85: 225–8.

19. Carley ME, Schaffer JI. Urinary incontinence and pelvic organ prolapse in women with Marfan or Ehlers–Danlos syndrome. Am J Obstet Gynecol 2000; 182: 1021–3.

20. Dietz HP. Do Asian women have less pelvic organ mobility than Caucasians? Int Urogynecol J Pelvic Floor Dysfunct 2003; 14: 250–3.

21. Kim S, Harvey MA, Johnston S. A review of the epidemiology and pathophysiology of pelvic floor dysfunction: do racial differences matter? J Obstet Gynaecol Can 2005; 27: 251–9.

22. Dwyer PL, Lee ETC, Hay DM. Obesity and urinary incontinence in women. Br J Obstet Gynaecol 1988; 95: 91–6.

23. Wingate L, Wingate MB, Hassanein R. The relation between overweight and urinary incontinence in postmenopausal women: a case control study. J North Am Menopause Soc 1994; 1: 199–203.

24. Nygaard I, Bradley C, Brandt D, for the Women's Health Initiative. Pelvic organ prolapse in older women: prevalence and risk factors. Obstet Gynecol 2004; 104: 489–97.

25. Wieslander CK, Word RA, Schaffer JI, et al. Smoking is a risk factor for pelvic organ prolapse. 26th Annual Scientific Meeting of the American Urogynecologic Society, September 15–17, 2005, Atlanta, Georgia.

26. Olsen AL, Smith VJ, Bergstrom JO, Colling JC, Clark AL. Epidemiology of surgically managed pelvic organ prolapse and urinary incontinence. Obstet Gynecol 1997; 89: 501–6.

27. Samuelsson EC, Victor FT, Tibblin G, Svardsudd KF. Signs of genital prolapse in a Swedish population of women 20 to 59 years of age and possible related factors. Am J Obstet Gynecol 1999; 180: 299–305.

28. Barber M, Walters M, Bump R. Association of the magnitude of pelvic organ prolapse and presence and severity of symptoms. J Pelvic Med Surg 2003; 9: 208.

29. Ellerkmann MR, Cundiff GW, Melick CF, et al. Correlation of symptoms with location and severity of pelvic organ prolapse. Am J Obstet Gynecol 2001; 185: 1332–8.

30. Burrows LJ, Meyn LA, Walters MD, et al. Pelvic symptoms in women with pelvic organ prolapse. Obstet Gynecol 2004; 104: 982–8.

31. Swift SE, Tate SB, Nicholas J. Correlation of symptoms with degree of pelvic organ support in a general population of women: what is pelvic organ prolapse? Am J Obstet Gynecol 2003; 189: 372–9.

32. Digesu SA, Khullar V, Cardozo L, Robinson D, Salvatore S. P-QOL: a validated questionnaire to assess the symptoms and quality of life of women with urogenital prolapse. Int Urogynecol J 2005; 16: 176–81.

33. Radley SC, Jones GL, Tanguy EA, et al. Computer interviewing in urogynaecology: concept, development and psychometric testing of an electronic pelvic floor assessment questionnaire in primary and secondary care. BJOG 2006; 113(2): 231–8.

34. Hextall A, Boos K, Cardozo L, et al. Videocystourethrography with a ring pessary in situ. A clinically useful preoperative investigation for continent women with urogenital prolapse. Int Urogynecol J Pelvic Floor Dysfunct 1998; 9: 205–9.

35. Davila GW, Bernier F. Multimodality pelvic physiotherapy treatment of urinary incontinence in adult women. Int Urogynecol J 1995; 6: 187–94.

36. Davila GW. Vaginal prolapse: management with nonsurgical techniques. Postgrad Med 1996; 99: 171–85.

37. Handa VL, Jones M. Do pessaries prevent the progression of pelvic organ prolapse? Int Urogynecol J 2002; 13: 349–52.

38. Fernando RJ, Thakar R, Sultan AH. Are vaginal pessaries as effective as surgery in symptomatic pelvic organ prolapse? Int Urogynecol J 2006; 17(Suppl. 2): S57–S100.

39. Sung VW. Effect of patient age on increasing morbidity and mortality following urogynaecologic surgery in the United States. J Pelvic Med Surg 2005; 11: 1.

40. Weber AM, Walters MD. Anterior vaginal prolapse: review of anatomy and techniques of surgical repair. Obstet Gynecol 1997; 89: 311–18.

41. Maher C, Baessler K. Surgical management of anterior vaginal wall prolapse: an evidence based literature review. Int Urogynecol J 2006; 17: 195–201.

42. Milani R, Salvatore S, Soligo M, et al. Functional and anatomical outcome of anterior and posterior vaginal prolapse repair with prolene mesh. BJOG 2005; 112(1): 107–11.

43. Dwyer PL, O'Reilly B. Dyspareunia following vaginal surgery for prolapse using polypropylene mesh. Re: paper by Milani et al. BJOG 2005; 112(8): 1164.

44. Maher C, Baessler K. Surgical management of posterior vaginal wall prolapse: an evidence-based literature review. Int Urogynecol J Pelvic Floor Dysfunct 2006; 17(1): 84–8.

45. Richardson AC. The rectovaginal septum revisited: its relationship to rectocele and its importance in rectocele repair. Clin Obstet Gynecol 1993; 36: 976–83.

46. Abramov Y, Gandhi S, Goldberg RP, et al. Site-specific rectocele repair compared with standard posterior colporrhaphy. Obstet Gynecol 2005; 105(2): 314–18.

47. Kuhn A, Gelman W, O'Sullivan S, Monga A. The feasibility, efficacy and functional outcome of local anaesthetic repair of anterior and posterior vaginal wall prolapse. Eur J Obstet Gynecol Reprod Biol 2006; 1: 88–92.

48. Zimmern PE, Stanton SL, eds. Female Pelvic Reconstructive Surgery. Heidelburg: Springer Verlag; 2003.

49. Higgs PJ, Chua HL, Smith AR. Long term review of laparoscopic sacrocolpopexy. BJOG 2005; 112(8): 1134–8.

Gynecological cancer 12

Jo Morrison and Sean Kehoe

INTRODUCTION

Changing demographics and improvements in life expectancy are such that by 2005 the average 70-year-old woman in the UK could expect to live another 15.2 years. Given these circumstances, our concept of what constitutes an elderly patient is rapidly changing.[1] As the risk of gynecological cancers rises with age (Figure 12.1), the demographic change in the female population is being accompanied by a rise in the overall incidence of several of these tumors, and these are becoming increasingly important factors in the health of women aged 70 and beyond.

As an increasingly elderly cohort of patients requiring treatment develops, it is of concern that the available evidence demonstrates that these individuals have less optimal survival rates following a diagnosis of gynecological cancer (Figure 12.2). There are a number of reasons for this including co-morbidity, the presence of more aggressive disease, and later presentation.[2] At the same time reported studies commonly indicate that treatment is often less aggressive, and thus less effective, in older women.[3,4] This could well be a physician-based phenomenon, with an assumption that survival prospects are poor and tolerance of

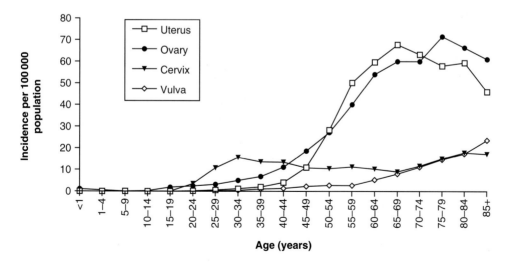

Figure 12.1 Incidence of gynecological malignancies by age group in England (2003). Figures from Office for National Statistics: www.statistics.gov.ukhttp://www.statistics.gov.uk/downloads/theme_health/MB1_34/MB1_34.pdf. (Reproduced with permission. Crown copyright.)

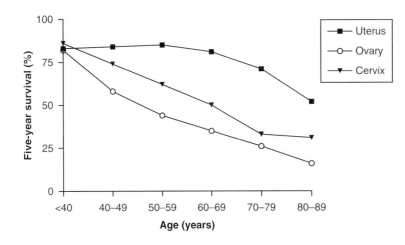

Figure 12.2 Five-year survival rates for ovarian, endometrial, and cervical cancer by age group, England (1999–2001): http://www.statistics.gov.uk/StatBase/Expodata/Spreadsheets/D8982.xls. (Reproduced with permission. Crown copyright.)

therapy reduced compared with younger patients. Although these may indeed be valid observations, a study of attitudes among older women diagnosed with a gynecological cancer found there were no differences in the desire for cure in women aged over 75 years compared with younger women.[5] In fact, older women were more prepared to undergo radical, disfiguring surgery and were less concerned about the effects of treatment on their femininity or sexuality than younger women. Thus, withholding radical, potentially curative, treatments for elderly women for paternalistic reasons may be based on the erroneous preconceptions of their younger caregivers.

Surgery is often the most effective treatment for solid cancers. In older women, where comorbidity, especially poor renal function, may limit chemotherapy, and complications from radiotherapy are more common, surgery may remain the best option. With advances in anesthetic techniques and aggressive preoperative correction of comorbidities, most women are able to undergo appropriate surgical treatment, with acceptable perioperative morbidity and mortality. One study evaluated the outcomes of 121 elderly women (>70 years old) undergoing surgery for gynecological cancer who had poor functional status (as defined by an American Society of Anesthesiologists (ASA) score of III and IV).[6] An equal number of controls, with an ASA score of I or II, were matched for age, site, and stage of cancer, surgical procedure, and year of operation. Although severe postoperative morbidities were more common in the poor performance status group (17% vs 5%; $p < 0.001$), this did not significantly prolong hospital stay, and complications were resolved without long-term sequelae. There were three postoperative deaths in the poor performance status group compared with none in the control group, although this was not statistically significant. Hence, 'frailty' as an indication for non-intervention should be an uncommon event; rather, maximizing health status with appropriate preoperative medical treatment should be a priority.

Having recognized that, elderly women have a slightly different spectrum of gynecological oncological diseases than their perimenopausal counterparts. This chapter explains the presentation and treatments of the more common gynecological cancers and how these may differ for those over 70 years of age.

ENDOMETRIAL CANCER

Incidence and etiology

Endometrial cancer is a disease of postmenopausal women, with 91% of cases worldwide occurring in women over 50 years old.[7] It is also a disease with varying global incidences, even after adjustment for age; the highest incidence is 22 per 100 000 women in North America, compared with 3.5 per 100 000 in Africa. These differences are largely due to differences in risk factors, which are associated with a so-called Western lifestyle. One of the main risk factors for endometrial cancer is unopposed estrogen. This may be exogenous, such as estrogen-only hormone replacement therapy (HRT), or endogenous, as with anovulatory cycles in polycystic ovarian syndrome. However, in postmenopausal women an important source of endogenous estrogen is adipose tissue. Also, tamoxifen, used as adjuvant therapy in the treatment of estrogen receptor-positive breast cancer, increases the risk of neoplasia through its estrogenic action on the endometrium.[8] Results from National Surgical Adjuvant Breast and Bowel Project P-1 Study demonstrated an increased incidence of endometrial cancer in the tamoxifen group (hazard ratio [HR] = 2.53; 95% confidence interval [CI] 1.35–4.97).[9] This was predominantly in women aged ≥50 years old, and endometrial cancer rates were higher following prolonged observation.[10] However, as these cancers were diagnosed at an early stage, tamoxifen-induced disease did not significantly increase mortality rates.

Many studies demonstrate an increase in obesity in developed countries. Adipose tissue expresses aromatase enzymes that convert androstenedione to estrone, which is then reduced to estradiol.[11] This peripheral aromatase activity is increased in postmenopausal women and accounts for significant levels of estrogen production, especially in obese women.[12]

Progestogens have a protective effect on the endometrium; increased progesterone levels, either physiologically, by placental production during pregnancy, or by exogenous delivery in the form of the contraceptive pill, reduce the incidence of endometrial cancer. Several population studies demonstrate how the combination of reduced parity, increased contraceptive use, increased obesity, and tamoxifen treatment contribute to increases in the incidence of endometrial cancer, especially in older women, whereas the incidence in the 40–45-year age group has declined.[13] Hence, it is likely that endometrial cancer rates will continue to rise, with an obese aging population of low parity.

Presentation and management

In the older woman, endometrial cancer normally presents with postmenopausal bleeding (PMB), but in this age group vaginal discharge and pyometra (pus within the endometrial cavity) is also highly suspicious of a cancer. Around 15% of women with PMB have a malignant or premalignant condition.[14] The severity of bleeding is not necessarily related to the likelihood of finding cancer, and all women with these symptoms require transvaginal ultrasonography to measure endometrial thickness, which will dictate the need for endometrial sampling, with either an outpatient sampling device (Pipelle) or hysteroscopy. Endometrial thickness of ≤4 mm on transvaginal ultrasound examination is very reassuring; false-negative rates for this technique are low.[15] However, irrespective of ultrasound findings, if bleeding is persistent, further endometrial evaluation is required.

Most women (75–80%) with PMB present with early stage disease (International Federation of Gynecology and Obstetrics (FIGO) stage I).[16] Standard treatment is a total hysterectomy and bilateral salpingo-oophorectomy. In more advanced disease (FIGO stage II and above), adjuvant radiotherapy (and occasionally chemotherapy) is administered to treat extrauterine spread. In earlier-stage disease, adjuvant radiotherapy does not improve overall survival, although it does reduce pelvic recurrences.[17] However, salvage rates for pelvic recurrences treated with radiotherapy are high, especially in patients who have not received it previously.

Whereas 5-year survival in women aged <60 years old is 80–85%, this falls for older women to just over 60% in women aged 70–79 years old; and only 46% in the over 80s.[18] Why is this so? In a retrospective study of 172 women with endometrial cancer, the pathological prognostic factors were compared between women under and over 70 years of age.[19] Equal numbers in both groups had FIGO[16] stage I disease (two-thirds of women), although older women had significantly deeper myometrial invasion compared with younger women (stage IC: 37% vs 21%; $p<0.01$)). In addition, older women had more high-grade tumors (grade 2 or 3: 75% vs 55%; $p<0.005$). In this relatively small study, older women had a greater tendency to present with clear cell carcinoma, which has a poorer prognosis, although numbers were small and did not reach significance (8% vs 4%). However, in a study of treatment of 180 women with advanced-stage endometrial cancer (FIGO stages III and IV), 103 had high-risk histology types (clear cell and serous papillary adenocarcinoma); younger women were more likely to have typical endometrioid adenocarcinoma of lower grade and had fewer clear cell and serous papillary adenocarcinoma compared with older women.[20]

Another larger study of women with endometrial cancer (FIGO stage IB-II) examined the role of age >70 years on outcome.[21] A total of 405 women (21% of whom were ≥70 years old) were treated with hysterectomy and adjuvant radiotherapy. Older women had a higher likelihood of deep myometrial invasion (i.e. more than 50% of the myometrium involved; 29% vs 13%; $p = 0.008$), but were otherwise well matched in terms of pathological features. Despite similar treatments, and correcting for deeper myometrial invasion, older women had poorer locoregional control and overall survival. These data are supported by the large multicenter trial of adjuvant radiotherapy for endometrial cancer – PORTEC.[16] Here, age of ≥60 years was an

independent predictor of death (HR = 3.1; 95% CI 1.2–8; $p = 0.02$). The PORTEC trial also found no significant difference in late complications from radiotherapy in women >70 years old compared with younger women. These data indicate that older women, despite adequate treatment, tend to do worse than younger women with endometrial cancer, for as-yet unknown reasons. However, they also support the proposition of treating older women adequately and using adjuvant treatment appropriately, as treatments are generally well tolerated in older women. Indeed, much of the current disparity in outcomes for older women outside clinical trials may be attributable to withholding of more aggressive treatments, perhaps inappropriately.[3,4]

OVARIAN CANCER

Incidence and etiology

In the UK, ovarian cancer is the predominant cause of death from gynecological malignancies. The majority (90%) arise from the epithelial layer of the ovary, which will be considered here. Other rare ovarian malignancies which arise from the ovarian stroma, such as granulosa cell tumors, are less of a health burden as they are more likely to present at an early stage due to symptoms caused by abnormal hormone production, e.g. postmenopausal bleeding in estrogen-secreting tumors, and are generally much less aggressive than epithelial tumors.

Currently, the lifetime risk of developing ovarian cancer (in England and Wales) is 1 in 48, although the incidence has been steadily rising over the past 25 years. This increase has been predominantly in women >65 years old, probably because this cohort of women have not benefited from the protective effect of the combined contraceptive pill (see below). In women >70 years, the incidence is around 70 new cases per

100 000 women per year.[17,22] The age-specific mortality rate mirrors the incidence rates, with a peak mortality rate in women aged 75–84 years (Figure 12.3). Overall, the 5-year survival rate for ovarian cancer is low (36%), as most tumors are not diagnosed until a late stage.

BRCA1 and BRCA2 are tumor suppressor genes and their gene products are involved in DNA repair, replication, and control of transcription. Inheritance of a mutation in these genes puts a woman at high risk of developing breast and/or ovarian cancer. Inherited BRCA1 mutations are found in 4–6% of patients with ovarian cancers, with BRCA2 mutations in 2–4%.[23,24] However, most of these women present at a younger age, and thus inherited BRCA mutations are less relevant in older women. Indeed, even in younger women, the majority of cases of ovarian cancer are not associated with known genetic mutations. Of equal importance, not every woman with a BRCA mutation will develop ovarian cancer. Thus, a combination of genetic and environmental factors predispose to ovarian cancer. Epidemiological data suggest that parity (odds ratio

[OR] = 0.61; 95% CI 0.46–0.81) and the oral contraceptive pill are protective (OR = 0.56; 95% CI 0.42–0.74).[25] Other protective factors include unilateral oophorectomy, early age of menopause, late age of first birth, and any pregnancy. Tubal ligation may also be protective.[26] Risk factors for ovarian cancer include use of talc in genital areas[27] and endometriosis.[28] Hypotheses for the cause of ovarian cancer include 'incessant ovulation', with damage to the ovarian epithelium during ovulation triggering carcinogenesis, and 'retrograde menstruation', which could act as an ovarian irritant. Whatever the initial trigger, recent experiments have shown that mutations of the tumor suppressor genes p53 and retinoblastoma (Rb) were sufficient to generate ovarian cancer in mice.[29]

Presentation and management

Regardless of their age, women subsequently diagnosed with ovarian cancer often present with a range of one or more symptoms: bloating; abdominal distention; weight loss or gain; abnormal bleeding; urinary symptoms; change in bowel habit;

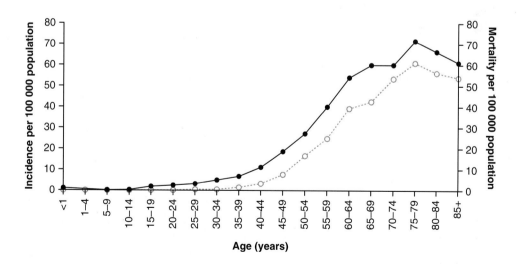

Figure 12.3 Incidence (●) and mortality rates (○) for ovarian cancer in England (incidence data 2003; mortality data 1999); adapted from Reference 17 and http://www.statistics.gov.uk/downloads/theme_health/MB1_34/MB1_34.pdf. Reproduced with permission. Crown copyright.)

or a pelvic mass is felt. Unfortunately, symptoms are vague and often misdiagnosed for more common conditions, such as diverticular disease and irritable bowel syndrome; indeed, up to 50% of women may initially present to a speciality other than gynecology. Because of this and other factors, over 75% of women present when the disease has spread throughout the abdominal cavity (FIGO stages III and IV),[19] with a poor 5-year survival rate at 30–40%.[22] One study suggested that a combination of these vague symptoms should arouse suspicion of ovarian cancer and that, in retrospect, they may be present for some time prior to diagnosis.[30] However, another UK study suggested that the duration of symptoms is relatively short, and that the majority of women (78%) presented to their general practitioner (GP) within 4 weeks of onset of symptoms.[31] In addition, in most cases (73%), they were referred for further investigation by their GP within 4 weeks.

Although preoperative imaging and elevated tumor markers (CA125) support a high index of suspicion of ovarian cancer, histological confirmation is required. This is normally performed as part of a staging laparotomy. The standard operation involves bilateral salpingo-oophorectomy, total hysterectomy, omentectomy, pelvic washings/ascites sampling, and pelvic lymph node sampling. The aim of surgery is to maximally debulk the tumor (currently defined as no residual macroscopic tumor) prior to adjuvant chemotherapy. Surgery may involve other organ systems as well, including bowel resection or splenectomy. However, no conclusive evidence exists to support the rationale of debulking surgery. Current practice is much influenced by a 1975 retrospective study of 102 women; those who had no deposit left >1.6 cm had improved survival.[32] An additional, but equally old, study also demonstrated improved survival in women who had optimal debulking.[33] However, these non-randomized studies only demonstrate that achievement of optimal surgery is a favorable prognostic factor,

and not necessarily directly therapeutic. Several prospective studies have shown that administering chemotherapy prior to, or instead of surgery, achieves equivalent survival rates for women with advanced disease (FIGO stages III and IV).[34–36] Two randomized controlled trials are presently recruiting to examine whether initial surgery is indeed the correct first-line treatment.[37,38]

In older women, the use of neoadjuvant chemotherapy is relatively attractive. Platinum chemotherapy can be relatively well tolerated, and results of prospective non-randomized trials suggested that chemotherapy prior to surgery may make surgery more achievable and enable maximal debulking surgery with less radical operations. However, debulking surgery is currently the standard of care for ovarian cancer. Appropriate treatment, outside of clinical trials, should be decided on the needs of the individual, and options should not be curtailed based on age alone.

Unfortunately, evidence is available which demonstrates that in practice this is not always the case.[3,4] Older women are more likely to present with more advanced disease.[39] However, even after correction for stage, residual disease, and performance status, women aged >70 years old have poorer survival rates than younger women. A large North American study, covering 10% of the population of the US, found that older women were less likely to receive combination surgery and chemotherapy than younger women.[4] Of equal importance, 40% of women aged ≥85 years old received no definitive treatment for their ovarian cancer. The 5-year survival rate for this age group, even after age adjustment for life expectancy, was just 8%, compared with 45% for the under 45 year olds. This is despite results from one of the few studies of gynecological surgery in older women that demonstrated that even those with poor ASA grade did well following surgery.[6]

Platinum-based chemotherapy is the standard first-line chemotherapy for ovarian cancer

Cisplatin was introduced in the late 1970s, followed shortly by carboplatin. Trials have demonstrated that cisplatin and carboplatin have equivalent efficacy, but that carboplatin has fewer side effects and is better tolerated. There is much controversy about the addition of paclitaxel to platinum agents in first-line treatment. Four different trials reported different results: two trials demonstrated improved survival with combination chemotherapy, whereas two trials found no difference. A meta-analysis of the four trials was difficult, owing to hetereogeneity in the treatment groups, but found a non-significant improvement in the platinum/paclitaxel group.[40] However, statistical testing of hypotheses for the different trial outcomes suggested that the differences were due to inadequate treatment in control arms in trials that had shown a benefit from additional paclitaxel.

Use of chemotherapeutic agents in older women is complicated by changes in pharmacokinetics and pharmacodynamics (see Chapter 9).[41] Carboplatin is excreted by the kidneys, and paclitaxel is also partially excreted through the kidneys. Thus, as glomerular filtration rate decreases with age, older women are more prone to the adverse chemotherapeutic sequelae unless these factors are fully taken into account when planning chemotherapy regimens. An additional complication is that women >70 years old are under-represented in chemotherapy clinical trials, and there are limited data as to their safety in this cohort, particularly regarding carboplatin/paclitaxel combination therapy. In view of the controversy surrounding evidence for the benefit of combination platinum/paclitaxel chemotherapy described above, in older women, who are more prone to complications from chemotherapy, first-line treatment should concentrate on giving adequate platinum-based chemotherapy, using carboplatin in preference to cisplatin. This axiom is supported by data from the largest platinum/paclitaxel combination study, ICON3.[42] Accepting the potential error in trial subgroup

analysis, this trial had 30% of patients aged >65 years old, and no benefit for combination chemotherapy was demonstrated for any age-defined subgroup.

CERVICAL CANCER

Cervical cancer is the second most common cancer in women worldwide, with 83% of cases occurring in developing countries.[7] Since the introduction of the national cervical screening programme in the 1980s, the incidence of cervical cancer deaths has fallen in the UK from approximately 4000 to 1000 cases per annum. Cervical cancer develops following persistent infection by high-risk oncogenic subtypes of the human papillomavirus (HPV, most commonly types 16 and 18), and risk factors are associated with sexual exposure to HPV (early age of first intercourse, multiple partners, non-barrier contraception) and a deficient immune response to infection (immunosuppression following organ transplantation and infection with the human immunodeficiency virus [HIV]). HPV is extremely prevalent; more than a third of women in their 20s have evidence of infection. However, most women will clear the infection and not go on to develop preinvasive changes or cervical cancer. HPV infection is therefore necessary, but alone insufficient for the development of cervical cancer. Other risk factors include cigarette smoking (squamous carcinoma), for which there is a strong dose–response effect, oral contraceptive use, and high parity, although separating these as independent factors from the risk of HPV infection is difficult. Cervical cancer has dual peaks of incidence of almost 20 per 100 000 women: the first peak occurs in the 30–39-year age group; the rates then fall somewhat, and rise again, with a second peak in the over 70s (Figure 12.4).

The mortality rate from cervical cancer worsens with increasing age, rising from 1.6 per

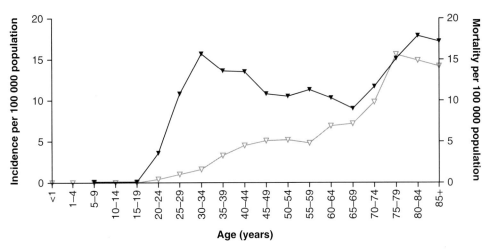

Figure 12.4 Incidence (▼) and mortality rates (▽) for cervical cancer in England (incidence data 2003; mortality data 1999); adapted from Reference 17 and http://www.statistics.gov.uk/downloads/theme_health/MB1_34/MB1_34.pdf. (Reproduced with permission. Crown copyright.)

100 000 women in the 30–34-year age group to 15.6 per 100 000 in the 75–79-year age group. Older women are less likely to present with microinvasive FIGO stage I disease and more frequently have later-stage disease, which confers a poorer prognosis. Data from a population-based study in the Netherlands found that only 5% of the over 70s had stage Ia disease, compared with 64% of women <50 years old.[43] Age was not an independent prognostic factor from multivariate analysis, but was associated with presentation at a more advanced stage; 5-year relative survival was only 49% for the over 70s compared with 81% for the under 50s. Treatment modalities in the different age groups were also different. More of the older age group had radiotherapy and were not treated with surgery. Although this may appear to be age-biased, a randomized controlled trial of 367 women compared radical surgery (Wertheim's hysterectomy and pelvic lymph node clearance) and pelvic radiotherapy for stage Ib and IIa cancer. Survival rates for the two groups were equivalent (84% in the surgical group and 88% in the radiotherapy group).[44] The side-effect profiles differed between the groups, however: 108 women in the surgery group required additional pelvic radiotherapy for positive lymph nodes and suffered the side effects of both treatment modalities. They also had poorer survival and higher complication rates than the pelvic radiotherapy group alone. Thus, dual treatment should be avoided and surgery reserved only for those who are likely (or found to have) negative lymph nodes; ideally, all women with stage IIb disease or more should be treated with primary radiotherapy. Hence, given that a higher proportion of older women have more advanced disease, it is therefore appropriate that they should receive more radiotherapy and less surgery, this treatment choice being based on clinical trials evidence.

VULVAL CANCER

The majority of vulval cancers are squamous cell carcinomas (>90%) and predominantly occur in older women. In a population study of 411 cases, the median age at diagnosis was 74 years.[4]

Under these circumstances, normative treatment is designed for women >70 years old. Vulval cancer commonly presents with a lump, often on a background of vulval dystrophy, so there may be a prolonged history of vulval itch or discomfort. Concerning features in a woman with vulval dystrophy include pain, bleeding, or a discharge. Unfortunately, symptoms may go unreported for some time, especially in older women, who may be inhibited about discussing vulval problems.

Older women are more likely to have squamous cell carcinoma of the vulva, which is often seen in the presence of lichen sclerosus, a chronic inflammatory condition of the perineal skin. In contrast, younger women have more basiloid and warty carcinomas, and vulval cancer is more often a consequence of HPV infection, occurring on a background of vulval intraepithelial neoplasia (VIN).[46]

En bloc dissection of the vulva and groins, the 'butterfly incision', was introduced in the early–mid 20th century and led to major improvements in survival[47,48] due to recognition for the need to treat involved groin lymph nodes. However, the operation was extensive and disfiguring, often needing to heal by secondary intention or requiring skin flaps/grafts, and led to prolonged hospitalization. The modified 'triple incision' vulvectomy was then introduced, with the aim of reducing morbidity without compromising clearance. Groin node dissection is performed through separate incisions (reviewed in Reference[49]). Lymphadenectomy is recommended if the depth of invasion of the primary tumor is >1 mm, due to the risk of groin node metastasis. However, if the lesion is unilateral, ipsilateral lymphadenectomy may be sufficient in conjunction with local excision of the vulval cancer. The trend in recent years has been to refine surgery, with the aim of reducing associated morbidity. Surgery can be performed using well-controlled regional anesthesia, which is useful in those with poor respiratory function. Good postoperative nursing care is essential, as women are at risk from problems with wound healing and may require prolonged hospital inpatient stays. This is one of the major reasons why this type of uncommon surgery should be performed at a regional cancer center that has appropriate expertise.

Although surgery for vulval cancer is fairly radical and often performed on frail and elderly women, it is important to recognize that lymphadenectomy, where indicated, is necessary. 'Sparing' someone from pelvic lymph node dissection may condemn them to groin recurrence. Unfortunately, recurrence in groin lymph nodes is difficult to treat and carries a very high mortality rate.[50]

Radiotherapy is used in vulval cancer both before and after surgery. Prior to surgery, radiation can shrink large tumors and so allow more conservative therapy, e.g. avoiding need for exenterative-type surgery. Following surgery, radiotherapy is used to treat women with positive groin nodes to prevent regional recurrence. Radiation therapy should not be used as an alternative to groin dissection. The Gynecologic Oncology Group (GOG) study, comparing surgical resection (plus radiotherapy if nodes were positive) with radiotherapy for groin nodes, was terminated early when 5 of 26 women in the radiation arm had groin recurrences, compared with none in the surgical arm.[51,52]

CONCLUSIONS

The incidence of many gynecological cancers increases with age and more women survive well into their 80s and 90s. Specific lifestyle changes, e.g. smaller families and increasing obesity, are also having an important impact on the incidence of many gynecological malignancies. It is therefore likely that larger numbers of older women will require treatment for gynecological malignancy. Unfortunately, adequate treatment often requires radical surgery, chemotherapy, and radio-therapy. Nonetheless, most elderly women have a strong desire for curative treatment and are likely to have significant improvement in their quantity and quality of life if treated appropriately. Older women have a poorer age-standardized prognosis from gynecological malignancies than a younger cohort. Evidence suggests this is often due to differences in care, rather than significant differences in tumor biology, although older women are more likely to present at later stages. It is therefore important to ensure that older women have comorbidities optimally managed to allow them to fully benefit from treatments with a curative intent. Currently, a multidisciplinary approach is used in the care of women with gynecological malignancies. With increasing numbers of elderly women requiring treatment, thought should be given to the routine inclusion of gerontologists and palliative care physicians in this team approach. Finally, as gynecological cancers are common in older women, there should be more effort to include these women in clinical trials, in order to optimize future care for this important age group.

REFERENCES

1. Penny D, ed. Annual Abstract of Statistics. Basingstoke, UK: Palgrave Macmillan; 2005.
2. Lawton FG, Hacker NF. Surgery for invasive gynecologic cancer in the elderly female population. Obstet Gynecol 1990; 76(2): 287–9.
3. Turner NJ, Haward RA, Mulley GP, Selby PJ. Cancer in old age – is it inadequately investigated and treated? BMJ 1999; 319(7205): 309–12.
4. Ries LA. Ovarian cancer. Survival and treatment differences by age. Cancer 1993; 71(2 Suppl): 524–9.
5. Nordin AJ, Chinn DJ, Moloney I, et al. Do elderly cancer patients care about cure? Attitudes to radical gynecologic oncology surgery in the elderly. Gynecol Oncol 2001; 81(3): 447–55.
6. Giannice R, Foti E, Poerio A, et al. Perioperative morbidity and mortality in elderly gynecological oncological patients (≥70 years) by the American Society of Anesthesiologists physical status classes. Ann Surg Oncol 2004; 11(2): 219–25.
7. Parkin DM, Bray F, Ferlay J, Pisani P. Global cancer statistics, 2002. CA Cancer J Clin 2005; 55(2): 74–108.
8. Gallo MA, Kaufman D. Antagonistic and agonistic effects of tamoxifen: significance in human cancer. Semin Oncol 1997; 24(1 Suppl 1): S1-71–S1-80.
9. Fisher B, Costantino JP, Wickerham DL, et al. Tamoxifen for prevention of breast cancer: report of the National Surgical Adjuvant Breast and Bowel Project P-1 Study. J Natl Cancer Inst 1998; 90(18): 1371–88.
10. Fisher B, Costantino JP, Wickerham DL, et al. Tamoxifen for the prevention of breast cancer: current status of the National Surgical Adjuvant Breast and Bowel Project P-1 study. J Natl Cancer Inst 2005; 97(22): 1652–62.
11. Bulun SE, Zeitoun K, Sasano H, Simpson ER. Aromatase in aging women. Semin Reprod Endocrinol 1999; 17(4): 349–58.
12. Misso ML, Jang C, Adams J, et al. Adipose aromatase gene expression is greater in older women and is unaffected by postmenopausal estrogen therapy. Menopause 2005; 12(2): 210–15.
13. Somoye G, Olaitan A, Mocroft A, Jacobs I. Age related trends in the incidence of endometrial cancer in South East England 1962–1997. J Obstet Gynaecol 2005; 25(1): 35–8.
14. Gredmark T, Kvint S, Havel G, Mattsson LA. Histopathological findings in women with postmenopausal bleeding. Br J Obstet Gynaecol 1995; 102(2): 133–6.
15. Karlsson B, Granberg S, Wikland M, et al. Transvaginal ultrasonography of the endometrium in women with postmenopausal bleeding –

Nordic multicenter study. Am J Obstet Gynecol 1995; 172(5): 1488–94.

16. Shepherd JH. Revised FIGO staging for gynaecological cancer. Br J Obstet Gynaecol 1989; 96(8): 889–92.

17. Creutzberg CL, van Putten WL, Koper PC, et al. Surgery and postoperative radiotherapy versus surgery alone for patients with stage-1 endometrial carcinoma: multicentre randomised trial. PORTEC Study Group. Post Operative Radiation Therapy in Endometrial Carcinoma. Lancet 2000; 355(9213): 1404–11.

18. Quinn M, Babb P, Brock A, Kirkby L, Jones J. Cancer Trends in England and Wales. London: The Stationery Office; 2001.

19. Bellino R, Arisio R, D'Addato F, et al. Pathologic features of endometrial carcinoma in elderly women. Anticancer Res 2001; 21(5): 3721–4.

20. Sutton G, Axelrod JH, Bundy BN, et al. Whole abdominal radiotherapy in the adjuvant treatment of patients with stage III and IV endometrial cancer: a gynecologic oncology group study. Gynecol Oncol 2005; 97(3): 755–63.

21. Alektiar KM, Venkatraman E, Abu-Rustum N, Barakat RR. Is endometrial carcinoma intrinsically more aggressive in elderly patients? Cancer 2003; 98(11): 2368–77.

22. Walsh P, Cooper N. Ovary. In: Office of National Statistics editor. Cancer Atlas of the United Kingdom and Ireland 1991–2000. Basingstoke: Palgrave Macmillan; 2005: 193–200.

23. Berchuck A, Heron KA, Carney ME, et al. Frequency of germline and somatic BRCA1 mutations in ovarian cancer. Clin Cancer Res 1998; 4(10): 2433–7.

24. Rubin SC, Blackwood MA, Bandera C, et al. BRCA1, BRCA2, and hereditary nonpolyposis colorectal cancer gene mutations in an unselected ovarian cancer population: relationship to family history and implications for genetic testing. Am J Obstet Gynecol 1998; 178(4): 670–7.

25. Riman T, Dickman PW, Nilsson S, et al. Risk factors for invasive epithelial ovarian cancer: results from a Swedish case-control study. Am J Epidemiol 2002; 156(4): 363–73.

26. Narod SA, Sun P, Ghadirian P, et al. Tubal ligation and risk of ovarian cancer in carriers of BRCA1 or BRCA2 mutations: a case-control study. Lancet 2001; 357(9267): 1467–70.

27. Cramer DW, Liberman RF, Titus-Ernstoff L, et al. Genital talc exposure and risk of ovarian cancer. Int J Cancer 1999; 81(3): 351–6.

28. Brinton LA, Lamb EJ, Moghissi KS, et al. Ovarian cancer risk associated with varying causes of infertility. Fertil Steril 2004; 82(2): 405–14.

29. Flesken-Nikitin A, Choi KC, Eng JP, Shmidt EN, Nikitin AY. Induction of carcinogenesis by concurrent inactivation of p53 and Rb1 in the mouse ovarian surface epithelium. Cancer Res 2003; 63(13): 3459–63.

30. Vine MF, Calingaert B, Berchuck A, Schildkraut JM. Characterization of prediagnostic symptoms among primary epithelial ovarian cancer cases and controls. Gynecol Oncol 2003; 90(1): 75–82.

31. Kirwan JM, Tincello DG, Herod JJ, Frost O, Kingston RE. Effect of delays in primary care referral on survival of women with epithelial ovarian cancer: retrospective audit. BMJ 2002; 324(7330): 148–51.

32. Griffiths CT. Surgical resection of tumor bulk in the primary treatment of ovarian carcinoma. Natl Cancer Inst Monogr 1975; 42: 101–4.

33. Griffiths CT, Fuller AF. Intensive surgical and chemotherapeutic management of advanced ovarian cancer. Surg Clin North Am 1978; 58(1): 131–42.

34. Ansquer Y, Leblanc E, Clough K, et al. Neoadjuvant chemotherapy for unresectable ovarian carcinoma: a French multicenter study. Cancer 2001; 91(12): 2329–34.

35. Kuhn W, Rutke S, Spathe K, et al. Neoadjuvant chemotherapy followed by tumor debulking prolongs survival for patients with poor prognosis in International Federation of Gynecology and Obstetrics Stage IIIC ovarian carcinoma. Cancer 2001; 92(10): 2585–91.

36. Kayikcioglu F, Kose MF, Boran N, Caliskan E, Tulunay G. Neoadjuvant chemotherapy or primary surgery in advanced epithelial ovarian carcinoma. Int J Gynecol Cancer 2001; 11(6): 466–70.

37. Phase III randomized study of neoadjuvant chemotherapy followed by interval debulking surgery versus upfront cytoreductive surgery followed by chemotherapy with or without interval debulking surgery in patients with IIIc or IV ovarian epithelial, peritoneal or fallopian tube cancer. Protocol EORTC-55971. http://www.ncrn.org.uk/portfolio/data.asp?ID=921

38. CHORUS (Chemotherapy or Upfront Surgery). A randomised feasibility trial to determine the impact of timing of surgery and chemotherapy in newly diagnosed patients with advanced epithelial ovarian, primary peritoneal or fallopian tube carcinoma. ISRCTN number: 74802813. http://www.ctu.mrc.ac.uk/studies/documents/protocol.pdf

39. Yancik R. Ovarian cancer. Age contrasts in incidence, histology, disease stage at diagnosis, and mortality. Cancer 1993; 71(2 Suppl): 517–23.

40. Sandercock J, Parmar MK, Torri V, Qian W. First-line treatment for advanced ovarian cancer: paclitaxel, platinum and the evidence. Br J Cancer 2002; 87(8): 815–24.

41. Balducci L, Beghe C. Pharmacology of chemotherapy in the older cancer patient. Cancer Control 1999; 6(5): 466–70.

42. Paclitaxel plus carboplatin versus standard chemotherapy with either single-agent carboplatin or cyclophosphamide, doxorubicin, and cisplatin in women with ovarian cancer: the ICON3 randomised trial. Lancet 2002; 360(9332): 505–15.

43. de Rijke JM, van der Putten HW, Lutgens LC, et al. Age-specific differences in treatment and survival of patients with cervical cancer in the southeast of The Netherlands, 1986–1996. Eur J Cancer 2002; 38(15): 2041–7.

44. Landoni F, Maneo A, Colombo A, et al. Randomised study of radical surgery versus radiotherapy for stage Ib-IIa cervical cancer. Lancet 1997; 350(9077): 535–40.

45. Rhodes CA, Cummins C, Shafi MI. The management of squamous cell vulval cancer: a population based retrospective study of 411 cases. Br J Obstet Gynaecol 1998; 105(2): 200–5.

46. Toki T, Kurman RJ, Park JS, et al. Probable nonpapillomavirus etiology of squamous cell carcinoma of the vulva in older women: a clinicopathologic study using in situ hybridization and polymerase chain reaction. Int J Gynecol Pathol 1991; 10(2): 107–25.

47. Taussig F. Cancer of the vulva: an analysis of 155 cases. Am J Obstet Gynecol 1940; 40: 764–70.

48. Way S. Carcinoma of the vulva. Am J Obstet Gynecol 1960; 79: 692–9.

49. DiSaia PJ. The case against the surgical concept of en bloc dissection for certain malignancies of the reproductive tract. Cancer 1987; 60(8 Suppl): 2025–34.

50. Monaghan JM, Hammond IG. Pelvic node dissection in the treatment of vulval carcinoma - is it necessary? Br J Obstet Gynaecol 1984; 91(3): 270–4.

51. Phillips GL, Bundy BN, Okagaki T, Kucera PR, Stehman FB. Malignant melanoma of the vulva treated by radical hemivulvectomy. A prospective study of the Gynecologic Oncology Group. Cancer 1994; 73(10): 2626–32.

52. Stehman FB, Bundy BN, Dvoretsky PM, Creasman WT. Early stage I carcinoma of the vulva treated with ipsilateral superficial inguinal lymphadenectomy and modified radical hemivulvectomy: a prospective study of the Gynecologic Oncology Group. Obstet Gynecol 1992; 79(4): 490–7.

Section V
Promoting healthy living

Multidisciplinary day services for the older woman

13

James David Price

INTRODUCTION

Day hospitals are outpatient health facilities that provide care from one to several days weekly, for several hours but not overnight, to community-dwelling people. Services provided vary greatly, but day hospitals usually have either a predominantly medical, psychiatric, or social approach, and may focus primarily on acute, subacute, or chronic illness.

Usually there is no formal age restriction, but given the nature of needs, services usually cater predominantly for older people. Similarly, although most services make no distinction on grounds of gender, older women form the majority of consumers of day hospital services.

The evidence base for day services is patchy, and does not permit robust gender-specific recommendations or conclusions to be made. However, reflecting health needs, most trials in this area recruit a majority of older women, and arguments against the application of trial evidence to the older woman cannot be supported.

CONTEXT

The clinically and cost-effective provision of health services for the older person is an issue of increasing importance. There is yearly increase in the numbers of people admitted to hospital emergently and in their average age. The future of inpatient emergency care looks increasingly to be the care of the older person.

The age-related increase in comorbidity and disability is complicated by particularly high prevalence of conditions such as frailty, a complex syndrome of decreased ability to withstand illness without loss of function, or a reduced functional homeostasis.[1]

Women have greater longevity but greater morbidity than men, have higher hospitalization rates, and are more frequently affected by chronic conditions and disability, including immobility. Accentuating these issues, disabled women have lower incomes and are more likely to live alone.[2]

This increase in the numbers of older women, their complexity and vulnerability, makes the optimal design and implementation of healthcare services for them of the highest importance. The search for the optimal model of care for the older person has been a serial task for geriatricians since the specialty arose in the 1940s.

There is a growing appreciation of the need to develop integrated systems of care for older people that support the shifting emphasis from institutional to domiciliary long-term care and incorporate:

- smooth, efficient flows from community to hospital care
- smooth, efficient flows from hospital to community care

- appropriate, integrated use of specialist care
- coordinated multidisciplinary (interprofessional) services.

Multidisciplinary day services have been and remain at the interface between community and hospital, and are well placed to assist in meeting these challenges.

THE GERIATRIC PROCESS (COMPREHENSIVE GERIATRIC ASSESSMENT)

Marjory Warren is considered a forerunner of the specialty of geriatric medicine. In 1935, her hospital in London took on the responsibility for hundreds of dependent, poorly evaluated, and poorly treated frail older people residing in the local workhouse. Through a systematic evaluation of these patients – of their medical, social, functional, and psychological needs – she identified those who might benefit from medical rehabilitation. Numerous readily recognizable and treatable problems were attended to and, in many cases, discharge to the patient's home was possible.[3]

With time, the elements and principles of best-quality care for older people were developed and agreed upon. This comprehensive, systematic, and multistage method can be described simply as the geriatric process or geriatric rehabilitation, or the less helpful but more contemporary 'comprehensive geriatric assessment'.

However, the process is more than only a diagnostic process that identifies needs. It includes also the specification, management, and delivery of treatments to address needs. Such interventions are almost always multifaceted, but their dominant aim is the restoration of function and independence.

The principles of the geriatric process are distilled in Table 13.1; the emphasis is always on functional goals that are agreed by both patient and clinical multidisciplinary team.

Comprehensive geriatric assessment is complex, and involves many subprocesses and skills. This 'black box' intervention includes both overt and concealed elements, many of which are not easily codified into a protocol or guideline. The ways in which it can be delivered reflect that complexity. However some elements – professional skills, care processes, and facilities – are seen in most programs, and their delivery differs more in style than in substance across trials.[5] A breakdown of the components of this 'black box' of inpatient care is shown in Table 13.2.

The multidisciplinary team is an essential component: a group of experienced professionals from medical, nursing, and allied health professions who share responsibility for assessment and for the formulation and implementation of treatment plans. Key in most trials has been the roles of doctor, nurse, therapists (physiotherapy and occupational therapy), and social worker (care manager).

Many trials specify particular experience and training in the care of older people with complex needs. However, the key element is a set of skills rather than a particular professional background, and programs have at times delivered effective services through the use of generic workers (e.g. therapists who combine both a physical and occupational therapy role), or else have leveraged the expertise of professionals through the use of assistants who have more limited training. In practice, team constitution owes much to differences in resource and broad models of healthcare delivery.

Comprehensive geriatric assessment can be performed in many different settings, including the day hospital. There is a consensus that it should be performed following significant functional change and certainly following a step-up in the level of care required, e.g. when admission to long-term care is being considered (Table 13.3).

Table 13.1   The geriatric process

A multidimensional, interdisciplinary process that determines an older person's medical, psychological, and functional capability in order to develop and deliver a coordinated, integrated plan for treatment and long-term maintenance.

A. Assessment
Health (diagnosis, prognosis)
Function (physical, cognitive)
Resources (e.g. social, economic)

B. Objectives of care
What does the patient want?
What is feasible?
Team and patient agreement

C. Specify the management plan
Objectives. Close the 'ecological gap' between what the patient can do and what the environment demands
Therapeutic changes – aim to improve the patient
Prosthetic changes – aim to reduce environmental demands
Environmental changes – bring the environment closer to the patient

D. Regular review
Is progress as expected?
Does the plan need modifying?
Looking ahead – when should the patient be discharged, or transferred to a more appropriate facility?

Adapted from References 4 and 5.

Models of comprehensive geriatric assessment

Several models have been described. Inpatient services may be bed-based services or services delivered by a mobile consulting team consisting of key members of the multidisciplinary team.[5]

Bed-based services are delivered typically from specific wards that have a permanent and dedicated multidisciplinary team. Such services are clearly effective: at 6 months, for every 100 patients treated, 4 extra patients (95% confidence interval [CI] 1–7 patients) would be alive and at home.[5]

Consultation teams visit and assess patients, and formulate treatment plans. However, trial evidence to support this approach has been inconsistent. Combining studies of adequate quality, no significant effect is seen.[5]

Differences in effectiveness may arise as treatment recommendations are implemented incompletely or ineffectually, a fact which argues strongly for a *combined* assessment and treatment role for geriatric teams and the importance of *specialist* nurses and therapists in treatment delivery.

Services for outpatients are more heterogeneous. The complex nature of the intervention and the breadth of skill set required renders comprehensive assessment in the home difficult if not impossible. However, a more focused set of treatment goals can be delivered at home after comprehensive assessment centrally. This central clinical, diagnostic, and treatment focus of resource

Table 13.2   Elements of the geriatric process

Core team members	Processes of care
Geriatrician or primary care doctor with specialist skills	Comprehensive assessment
Specialist nursing	Frequent multidisciplinary team meetings
Physiotherapy	Patient-centered goal setting
Occupational therapy	Treatment plan
Social work	Use of generic assessment tools
Easy access to other allied health professionals: e.g. dietetics, pharmacy, speech and language therapy, audiology, dentistry, psychiatry, pastoral care	Appropriate ward environment
Easy access to other medical specialist teams: e.g. neurology, respiratory	Therapy space and equipment
	Case conferences with patient and family

Table 13.3   Possible benefits of comprehensive geriatric assessment

Enhanced precision of diagnosis
Optimization of treatment
Improved (restored) and maintained function
Improved mental status (cognition, mood)
Improved quality of life
Improved survival
Reduced medication (especially drugs associated with confusion, falls, immobility)
Whole system cost reductions (societal: social and health)

may be in day hospitals or day centers, in therapy or medical outpatient facilities, or in other healthcare settings.

Comprehensive geriatric assessment is expensive, and should be targeted on those most likely to benefit, thus excluding those who will return to good health without the intervention and those who will remain dependent despite receiving it. The most common targeting criteria are old age, physical disease, geriatric syndromes, impairment of functional ability, and social problems.[5]

EARLY HISTORY OF THE DAY HOSPITAL

It is more than 50 years since the first geriatric day hospital opened, closely followed by the first purpose-built day hospital, developed by Lionel Cosin in Oxford, UK.[6]

The numbers of day hospitals then grew very rapidly, reflecting the brisk development of geriatric services for the frail older person designed to prevent institutionalization and to reduce the number of hospital inpatients. By 1969, there were 90 geriatric day hospitals and by 1995 there were 600, of which 200 were psychogeriatric.[4,7]

Day hospitals are a component of a multifaceted system – at its most developed format 'comprehensive geriatric service' that included, at a minimum, inpatient beds, outpatient services, and home consultations (domiciliary visiting).[8] The quest for early and effective detection and management of disability in older people led also to community-orientated initiatives, some filling gaps in primary care and since rendered unnecessary by improvements in general practice.

For two decades, older people's services were generally separate from those of younger adults. The first geriatricians developed rehabilitation facilities, working the 'traditional' model of geriatrics, largely responsible for patients chosen for them by other referring teams. However, patients referred for 'long-stay care' were noted to have suffered functional decline, potentially avoidable if they had received more effective management earlier in their illness. Geriatricians therefore sought influence over acute as well as rehabilitative and long-term care of older people, leading in the 1970s to the emergence of two geriatric medical models in the UK:

1. The 'age-defined' model. Separate parallel hospital medical services for patients above and below an arbitrary age.
2. The 'integrated' model. Geriatric and acute teams share diagnostic and therapeutic facilities, but separate specialist rehabilitation facilities are retained.[4]

This extension of the geriatric medical model into more acute services was reflected in an evolution of the work of day hospitals towards more acute aspects of care.

As population aging has continued, day hospitals and programs aimed specifically at older frail adults have been developed worldwide. In many cases, models of care developed in Europe have been adopted. There is ongoing controversy as to the function, effectiveness, and efficiency of day hospitals, but their evolution continues.

MULTIPLE ROLES OF THE MODERN DAY HOSPITAL

The primary purpose of day hospitals is to prolong healthy and independent living in the community.[9] This comes through helping older people *regain* and *maintain* independence and quality of life. The focus is particularly on people who are frail and who have complex problems that require the intervention of several health professionals.

Effective day hospital care should therefore reduce case fatality, reduce dependency and institutionalization, and prevent hospital admissions. Impairment, disability, and handicap should be impacted and mental health (cognition, mood) improved. The burden on caregivers, especially informal carers (e.g. family members) should be reduced.

Day hospitals have had multiple roles that have evolved with time and are the result of local history, local needs, and the nature of coexisting inpatient and outpatient services. A major strength of day hospitals is their potential for flexibility of function in meeting a wide range of patient needs in a developing service context.

Traditionally, the day hospital in the UK served a primarily rehabilitative role for people who were medically stable and already assessed either as inpatients or outpatients. More recently, the focus has shifted towards more acute care, providing an assessment facility aimed at preventing hospital admissions. Some have suggested (but it has rarely been implemented) a twin day hospital model for any particular service: one acute and another longer term, resourced and structured accordingly.

There has been a reducing cohort of patients who attend day hospital indefinitely for indications such as respite or maintenance of function. Those functions are increasingly being delivered by services in or close to the home, such as care homes and health centers with a primarily social function. Other functions have developed in line with service needs and increasing subspecialty interests of geriatricians.

The British Geriatrics Society[10] recommends that provision should include:

- Comprehensive geriatric assessment of frail older people.
- Crisis intervention and subacute assessment, with the possibility of preventing hospital admission and/or subsequently promoting early discharge.
- Integrated assessments of health and care needs, e.g. associated with decisions regarding institutional care placement or chronic disease management programs in the community.[11]
- Treatment and rehabilitation, in particular for complex multifaceted problems as part of community-based rehabilitation and intermediate care.[11]
- Specialist nursing and medical procedures.
- Speciality outpatient clinic venues, particularly where multidisciplinary assessment is required.
- 'Rapid access' ('admission avoidance') clinics.
- Health education for the third age.

Few day hospitals fulfil all these roles, but many perform several of them. Flexibility is essential, as is an ability to manage a wide breadth of dependency of patient.

There is mostly a focus on medical and physical functional problems, and comprehensive geriatric assessment of frail older people remains a key role, although some day hospitals have been developed by psychiatric teams for the management of older people with dementia, depression, and other psychogeriatric problems[12,13] (see Chapter 5).

Crisis intervention and subacute assessment

Emergency hospital admission rates for older people are rising, and there are multiple factors that can reduce (or stem the rise in) admission rates and lengths of hospital stay. Geriatric day hospitals are being used increasingly as acute treatment and assessment centers (admission avoidance) for older people at risk of hospital admission.[14,15]

Patients who present, typically to primary health services, with either organ-specific or non-specific symptoms, can be referred to and seen by a multidisciplinary team the same or next day. A potent stimulus to the development of such services in England was the National Service Framework (NSF) for Older People[16] that encouraged local health and social care organizations to develop effective crisis response methods. Such services have also a particular role to play as part of intermediate care provision, through providing a comprehensive assessment of people whose function has declined, requiring a step-up of care.[17]

Older people often become ill in different ways to younger people.[18] Commonly, the older person suffers multiple pathologies, atypical presentations of common diseases, and a combination of psychiatric and physical diseases. Recovery may be delayed and inconsistent. Acute organ-specific illness such as respiratory infection is made more sinister and more difficult to manage by the occurrence of complications distant from the primary pathology such as the geriatric syndromes of acute confusion (delirium), immobility, and incontinence. Despite these features, much illness and disability in old age is treatable and reversible, although it may respond best to multifaceted and multidisciplinary interventions whose complexity reflects that of the presentations themselves.[19]

Despite these accepted features of illness in older people, there is debate about the need for involvement of specialist multidisciplinary geriatric services in the care of the older person who has sustained acute functional decline. However, an audit of an admission avoidance scheme[15] demonstrated that many people were acutely unwell with, for example, infection, dehydration, and delirium. One-third were referred on immediately for acute hospital admission, many others required immediate diagnostic tests, and many were scheduled for tests (e.g. gastroscopy, ultrasound, brain imaging) performed only in an acute general hospital.

The requirements for such a service are therefore appropriate specialist medical and nurse staffing and prompt access to a range of diagnostic tests and treatments.[10] On-site (or point-of-care) plain radiography, blood testing, urinalysis, and electrocardiogram could be considered a minimum diagnostic suite for any day hospital accepting non-specifically unwell people.

To provide an urgent or emergent service, occupancy rates must be less than 100%, mandating a high turnover of patients, with active management and prompt discharge. Identifying patients at the borderline between outpatient and inpatient treatment is difficult. Given this, and the frailty and consequent clinical instability of many patients, the option to escalate assessment and treatment to an inpatient level must always be immediately available. It is expected that this option will be exercised in a significant minority of patients.[15]

Early supported discharge (accelerated discharge, post-discharge support)

There is no doubt of the need for geriatric multidisciplinary team input to patients in an acute general hospital setting. For example, one census of all inpatients in a large UK teaching hospital complex over six sites showed that, at one time point, 69% of 1324 patients had multidisciplinary needs.[20] Such needs often delay discharge, and services that can meet those needs outside hospital can speed discharge to the patient's own home.

Historically, in the UK and elsewhere, convalescence (passive recuperation) and rehabilitation of older people following acute medical illness or surgery has taken place mostly in hospitals. Recent policy emphasizes the potential role of services with a more community or domiciliary setting. A range of services with the collective name 'intermediate care' (between home and acute hospital) have been proposed and established: some new and some renamed and reconfigured.[16] However, there is concern that such services may be inferior to existing hospital services,[21] and driven by cost-cutting and political principle rather than evidence-based service improvement.

Chronic disease management

Recent changes in emphasis in healthcare reflect wider appreciation of the burden of chronic disease both on the patient and the healthcare system. Much of that disease burden falls on older people, many of whom live with more than one chronic condition.[22]

Chronic disease management targets cost-effectiveness as well as improved patient-centered outcomes. Programs are usually complex systems of coordinated healthcare interventions in which important elements are self-care (monitoring and initiation of treatment by patient or carer), provision of information, broad use of condition-specific guidelines, regular review and monitoring, anticipation of and planning for functional decline and acute illness, and better coordination of care between agencies.

The development of chronic disease management programs is complex. Important success factors are clinical involvement, and joint development of local solutions with meaningful cooperation between primary and secondary care, leading to whole system change and service redesign.[11] There should be integrated performance monitoring and evaluation.

Day hospitals may have a particular role to play, especially those located closer to the community, in community hospitals rather than acute general hospitals. Roles may include case finding, monitoring, and, particularly, early multidisciplinary assessment and intervention during the immediate pre-crisis period (admission avoidance).

One model that has developed in the US is PACE (Program of All-inclusive Care for the Elderly),[23] a comprehensive finance, healthcare, and social care program. Comprehensive multidisciplinary care for life is free of charge for older people who meet state funding criteria. PACE is delivered from a comprehensive day hospital, often purpose-built. Most care is on an outpatient or day care basis, but often there are attached residential beds, and other options are domiciliary care or admission to an acute hospital. Claimed positive outcome measures include reduced institutional care, reduced use of higher-level medical services, and cost savings.

Subspecialist services

Geriatricians have been very much involved in the development of multidisciplinary approaches to management of acute and chronic conditions in the setting of the day hospital. Specialist services may include services focusing on patients with falls, stroke (or transient ischaemic attack), leg ulcers, Parkinson's disease, cognitive impairment ('memory clinics'), diabetes mellitus, urinary incontinence, or heart failure.

STRUCTURE AND PROCESS

The major advantage of day hospitals is the effective delivery, to a complex and vulnerable group of older people, of a 'one-stop-shop' service. Patients are seen who could otherwise require multiple visits to different hospital departments or else, multiple home visits from several health professionals, with associated costs, delays, and information-sharing issues.

Although medical staff continue often to play a team leader role, there is in general a move away from the traditional medical model of care to one where all team members have an important decision-making role. There may be a defined care manager or key worker who, with the team, develops and reviews the care plan. The care manager may most appropriately be the professional who is most involved in achieving treatment goals.

Typically, for patients undergoing comprehensive geriatric assessment, the first visit will include assessments and the definition – agreed with the patient and/or carer – of an individual treatment plan. Later sessions will involve individual or group therapy programs. Goal-setting and regular review and, if necessary, revision are an essential part of the process, and team decisions are facilitated by continual sharing of information at multidisciplinary review meetings. Goals should be specific, realistic, time-based and achievable while appropriately stretching both patient and therapist. Once full potential has been realized – whether initial goals have been achieved or not – then discharge from the unit should follow.

Patients usually attend for the greater part of a day (4–6 hours), and return home for the evening and night. A midday meal is usually provided. Frail patients can find the day grueling – with assessments, tests, and therapies as well as two possibly prolonged journeys. Inactive time for rest, social interaction, and meals may be beneficial.

although the more able patients find the inevitable fallow periods frustrating. Attendance frequency varies from once to five times weekly. Total attendances also vary according to need, from a total of one or two visits to a much more intensive and prolonged therapy program that may involve multiple weekly attendances for several months.

Most day hospitals are on sites with a range of other health facilities, but others may be within community health centers or facilities without a primary health function such as shopping centers. Where possible, facilities should be custom-built to suit the ambulant but frail person. In the UK, most are located within acute (district) general hospitals, although some are in community hospitals. Desirable design features include:

- large indoor spaces for communal activities, including group physical therapy
- facilities to assess activities of daily living (ADLs), e.g. adapted kitchen
- adapted toilets, washing, and bathing facilities
- easy access from outside, including for ambulance access
- easy access to other diagnostic and therapeutic facilities, e.g. radiology.

The quality of transport to the site is important, and can determine acceptability and success. Key aspects include journey reliability and timing, in order to permit adequate team assessment and therapy. Travel sickness and fatigue may deter attendance, especially in rural areas.

There are several potential weaknesses, some integral to the process and others the product of poor professional skill. For example:

- attendance schedules and treatment programs may be unfocused or non-specific

- agreed goals may not be measurable, may provide insufficient stretch, or may be unrealistically optimistic
- the process itself or the physical/social environment may be unacceptable to the patient
- periods of inactivity can be considerable
- attendance rates are often poor – e.g. due to poor treatment concordance or transport difficulties.

The correct skill mix is essential to clinical- and cost-effectiveness and should reflect the purposes of the unit, although evidence of the most effective mix is lacking. Staff may be part of a clinical department delivering a comprehensive geriatric service, with job plans that reflect that complexity: i.e. temporally and geographically disparate responsibilities. Core team members reflect the dominant role of the day hospital in comprehensive geriatric assessment. In addition, prompt and easy access to other professionals is highly desirable: e.g. psychologists, dieticians, podiatrists. Medical care may be provided by either primary or secondary care doctor(s) with specialist interests and skills in managing older people.

Specific eligibility criteria for day hospital attendance are uncommon. Most patients are frail and old. Stroke, Parkinson's disease, fractures, arthritis, and osteoporosis are common disease processes. Other patients have sustained a broad functional decline, with deconditioning of cardiopulmonary, muscular, and other systems due to acute or subacute illness such as sepsis syndrome. Most have premorbid impaired function, but live in their own homes, often alone. Some have psychiatric illness, the most common being depression or dementia. Dementing patients may, however, benefit from rehabilitation, due both to physical reconditioning and some preservation of the ability to learn.[24]

Sources of referrals are broad, and include primary care, hospital (usually geriatric), or intermediate care teams. Following referral, agreement to enroll may itself be a multidisciplinary process. It is vital that the patient's usual clinical team are kept informed of enrollment, outcomes, and treatment changes.

Ensuring fitness for purpose

The clinical audit scheme for geriatric day hospitals of the Royal College of Physicians of England[25,26] provides useful guidance as to the processes of care and audit that will optimize quality of service:

- Each patient must have a care plan with clear goals and an agreed schedule of interventions agreed by team, patient, and carer. The care manager should review the plan regularly.
- Non-attendance should be followed up and patients should be discharged promptly when objectives have been achieved.
- Staff levels and mix must be appropriate to the workload of the unit and patient needs.
- Performance and costs must be monitored, through audit of structure, process, patient characteristics, and satisfaction.
- Periodic service reviews with key stakeholders should consider current service provision as well as possible innovations: e.g. weekend attendance, dual daily sessions (morning or afternoon), attendance by inpatients (complementing or intensifying inpatient interventions), outreach domiciliary rehabilitation, and use as a training resource or demonstration center.

Day hospitals vs day centers for older people

Day services can be divided, somewhat arbitrarily, into those delivered by day *centers* and those delivered by day *hospitals*. The heterogeneity of services precludes a clear distinction, but in general, day centers deliver services with greater focus on socialization and caregiver relief and less on acute medical illness and active rehabilitation.[27]

There may commonly be a progression or handover of care from an inpatient rehabilitation facility to a day hospital and thence to day center. General distinctions are summarized in Table 13.4.

EVIDENCE

It is of the utmost importance that innovations in service delivery are evaluated as rigorously as other healthcare interventions. Cost-effectiveness, and the magnitude and nature of beneficial and adverse clinical effects, should be determined before services are reconfigured according to preordained and prejudicial national policy. Despite its importance in many areas of health service research, such evaluation is missing.

There is no doubt that experimental studies of day services for older people are difficult. Aggregating disparate trial evidence – not least the interpretation of studies of complex interventions in widely differing international healthcare settings – is also challenging. However, the magnitude of the aggregated clinical and societal impact of effective intervention is enormous and thus demands greater attention.

Broadly, there is a considerable descriptive literature on day hospital care. However, relatively few high-quality controlled trials have been published, and the evidence for clinical- and cost-effectiveness is weaker. Reflecting the difficulties of research, and the inadequacies of studies, benefits have not been consistently demonstrated across studies and settings. Evaluation of what characterizes the more successful programs is essential.

Table 13.4 Typical characteristics of day hospitals and day centers

Characteristic	Day hospital	Day center
Primary function	Complex geriatric (acute and rehabilitation) assessment	Socialization of patient Caregiver relief ('respite')
Activities	Rehabilitation bias	Social bias
Staff:patient ratio	Higher	Lower
Specialist medical input	Usual	Uncommon
Specialized nursing input	Usual	Uncommon
Specialist therapy input	Usual	Uncommon
Relationship with hospital (e.g. as source of referrals)	Usually close	Less common
Affiliation with healthcare institution	Usual	Less common
Functional status	Improvement targeted and expected	Greater maintenance and monitoring role

Comprehensive geriatric assessment

Despite widespread belief in and enthusiasm for comprehensive geriatric assessment, and the rapid growth of services delivering it, prior to systematic review and meta-analysis,[28] there was inconsistent trials' evidence of its effects when delivered in any setting. A total of 28 trials of adequate quality addressed the research question, randomizing almost 10 000 older people. Both bed-based and domiciliary services were effective. Bed-based services were most successful, with a combined odds ratio (OR) of benefit (alive at home at long-term follow-up) of 1.68 (95% CI 1.17–2.41). Additional service characteristics associated with enhanced effectiveness were having control over the implementation of assessment recommendations and offering extended follow-up (day hospital or domiciliary). Bed-based services with those characteristics

were usually provided by a geriatric multidisciplinary team.

One comprehensive systematic review[29] sought randomized prospective controlled studies of comprehensive geriatric assessment in a medical (cf. psychiatric) day hospital. Day center studies were not included. Desirable outcomes were reductions in death, dependency, and institutionalization. Specified subgroup comparisons were of day hospital care vs comprehensive elderly care (inpatient or outpatient), vs domiciliary rehabilitation, and vs usual care (i.e. no comprehensive assessment or rehabilitation). Twelve satisfactory studies were found, recruiting 2867 patients.

In comparison to those receiving usual care, the combined adverse outcome of institutionalization or death was significantly less common (OR = 0.53, 95% CI 0.36–0.79; $p < 0.001$), as was a deterioration in ADLs (OR = 0.6;

0.38–0.97; $p < 0.05$). In both cases, however, outcomes were similar to other forms of care.

There was a trend towards fewer survivors requiring long-term institutional care (OR = 0.77; 0.52–1.13), which reached significance in the subgroup receiving usual care (OR = 0.50; 0.26–0.96; $p < 0.05$). On this basis, 15 (95% CI 10–34) patients would need to attend day hospital to prevent one admission to long-term care. There were non-significant reductions in hospital bed use.

The conclusion was that day hospital outcomes are comparable to alternative comprehensive elderly care services (inpatient, outpatient, and domiciliary) for which there is considerable evidence.[28] If other elements of a comprehensive geriatric service are in place, the benefits are less unclear.

Early supported discharge

There is reasonable evidence that intermediate care services, of which day hospitals can form a part, can be clinically effective in some circumstances, especially for step-down care that follows more acute – usually inpatient – healthcare. However, many of the recently initiated services have been poorly evaluated and the evidence where it exists can be contradictory, although unifying explanations of disparate results are possible.

For example, a whole system analysis of the effect of domiciliary intermediate care for supported discharge from geriatric service beds (Leeds, UK)[30] showed increased hospital bed days and costs, whereas a home-based multidisciplinary rehabilitation and care program delivered to patients from surgical and medical wards (Nottingham, UK),[31] showed reduced hospital use and trends towards lower institutionalization and death at 3 months, preserved to some extent at 12 months. The difference in effect may be the result of the dilution of effect of the intervention by the universal provision of comprehensive geriatric assessment prior to discharge on the geriatric service.

There is much better evidence for the effectiveness of early supported discharge in the case of stroke. More broadly, stroke patients receiving rehabilitation are the largest patient group treated in geriatric day hospitals. Stroke is a major public health problem: e.g. at least 5% of healthcare resources are dedicated to stroke, mostly due to care of disabled persons in hospital: most patients are old and, of survivors, half have significant residual disability.

Coordinated inpatient stroke unit care improves functional ability after stroke, and early supported discharge appears safe and effective,[32] although most evidence exists for trials of services recruiting patients with less severe disability. Both hospital-based outreach and community-based inreach services appeared equally effective. For most services, however, day hospital care was not a key service component.

A randomized controlled trial of day hospital vs domiciliary rehabilitation after stroke[33] showed broadly similar clinical outcomes, although there were non-significant trends towards improved outcomes for domiciliary care in the less-disabled patient. Rehabilitation costs and total health service costs were similar, but greater home care inputs to the domiciliary group led to higher social and overall costs. Broadly, the domiciliary service was as effective as day hospital care. However, the study was underpowered to determine whether less-common adverse health events might be avoided by regular assessments in a medical day hospital.

Perhaps patients who stand to benefit more from day hospital care include those who have needs that are particularly complex, challenging, or time-consuming, those with severe disability, and those where there is strong carer or patient preference, perhaps due to benefits of respite.

A mixed model of day hospital and domiciliary therapy may be the most cost-effective policy for community rehabilitation of older people following stroke, contingent upon local services and specific patient characteristics (Table 13.5).

Table 13.5 Theoretical advantages of home- and day hospital-based rehabilitation

Home	Day hospital
Greater involvement of informal caregiver(s)	Clustering of professional expertise facilitates education, networking, and informal referral
Assessment and rehabilitation in the patient's usual environment	Potential for improved coordination
Avoidance of patient travel	Seamless specialist medical referral and monitoring
Separate home visit assessments unnecessary	Opportunities for group activities and social interaction
Reduced infrastructure costs	Reduced professional travel

Specialist interventions

There is reasonable evidence that, in some circumstances, interventions can be delivered as, or more, effectively from a day hospital setting than other settings. However, the evidence base is patchy and reflects the usual difficulties.

For example, in falls prevention in community dwelling older people, a cluster randomized controlled trial of usual care vs community nurse assessment vs multidisciplinary assessment in a day hospital showed a 50% reduction of repeat falls in the day hospital group.[34]

However, in patients with Parkinson's disease, a 6-week individualized multidisciplinary rehabilitation program in a day hospital was no more effective at 6 months than an education program alone. Explanations offered included that existing management may have been satisfactory, therapy input may not have been sufficient, continued input may be necessary, and outcome measures may be inappropriate.[35]

Other services

Reflecting the dominant service (post-acute comprehensive geriatric assessment) provided by day hospitals, there is little evidence of clinical- or cost-effectiveness of day hospital care at the extremes of the acuity spectrum. Crisis intervention (admission avoidance) is an attractive model of care, but high-quality experimental evidence of its effects is very weak, as is the evidence for long-term care (e.g. respite care, or maintenance of function). Studies must seek appropriate outcomes – e.g. in trials of long-term interventions, absence of deterioration, or reductions in rate of decline may be appropriate and desirable criteria.

Costs

The debate around cost-effectiveness is less about the benefits in a day hospital setting than about its benefits compared with other forms of care delivery. Comprehensive geriatric assessment is expensive, not least due to the clustering of a team of experienced specialist health professionals and a relatively high staff to patient ratio. There are few recent data of high quality. The consensus[29] is that day hospital treatment is as expensive or more expensive than comparator non-bed-based treatments. It is cheaper, however, than inpatient treatment, although patients may have to bear social and other costs that may tip the overall cost balance in favor of the day hospital. Most studies do not include the costs of long-term social care; thus, the front-loaded higher (health) spend may be recouped in the longer term by lower social care spend.

One quasi-experimental study[36] has assessed functional autonomy at admission to and discharge from a geriatric day hospital and estimated the cost benefit from a societal perspective. For every $1 spent within the geriatric day hospital, there was $2.14 (95% CI 1.72–2.56) benefit for the health and social system.

Further and more stringent costing analyses are required to assess the extent to which higher costs may be offset by reduced demands on hospital and institutional care resources. Pending this, the day hospital should be used flexibly and efficiently, and day hospital attendance should be carefully audited and justified.

It may be that a contingency approach is needed, according to specific patient needs, the nature of existing services, and their geographical configuration. For example, in urban areas, clustering of medically complex and unstable patients in day hospital care may be more clinical- and cost-effective, whereas more stable patients in sparsely populated areas may be best served by domiciliary services (Table 13.6).

Table 13.6 Issues and difficulties in health services research in frail older populations

---

Service considerations
- Evaluation of a service often begins early, when performance is atypical (e.g. teambuilding and operational difficulties; initial flush of enthusiasm)
- Multicenter studies for complex interventions are difficult to set up (local interest and organizational factors are key factors and are not universal)
- Interventions are delivered and described in different international healthcare settings
- Interventions are delivered and described over prolonged time periods (>30 years), during which healthcare systems have evolved, and the applicability of results to the modern context will have diminished

Study populations
- Often highly heterogeneous, both within studies (e.g. 'stroke' – breadth of age, function, comorbidity) and between studies
- Often described imprecisely. Standardization of patient descriptors and assessment instruments is necessary
- Exclusions may reduce the applicability of study findings: e.g. dementia, communication difficulties

Interventions
- Treatment and control interventions in trials of complex healthcare ('black box') must be precisely described. What distinctions define the intervention? What personnel were involved, how often, and for what period of time?
- In seeking to aggregate studies for analysis, treatment and control interventions may be found to be heterogeneous

Outcomes
- Assessors of outcome (usually patients or staff) can rarely be blinded to the intervention. Hard indicators (e.g. death, long-term institutionalization, resource use, costs) are therefore desirable
- Outcome measures may be imprecise, poorly evaluated, or insensitive (e.g. ceiling effects of instruments more appropriate to an inpatient setting)
- Combining results of studies is often difficult, as differing outcome measures are used, and variance measures not quoted
- More sophisticated instruments – e.g. measures of general health, handicap, goal attainment scoring – are now available and should be used where appropriate
- Perspectives on desirable outcome measures commonly differ (patients, carers, staff, care providers, funders)
- Cost assessment should be comprehensive and include health and social services (including home social care and institutional care), transport (of patients and therapists), healthcare professionals, and overheads

---

THE FUTURE

Inpatient populations are becoming more aged and medically complex. As conditions such as cardiovascular and cerebrovascular disease are managed more effectively, so the epidemic of physical and cognitive frailty may come to be dominant. The population as a whole is aging, dependency ratios are growing, and the portfolio of effective but expensive medical interventions continues to grow.

It is understandable therefore that policy agendas are dominated by an emphasis on cost-containment through approaches such as chronic disease management, admission avoidance, intermediate care, and other non-hospital-based services.

New models of care for older people must be developed that leverage the skills of the MDT specializing in care and assessment of older people to deliver effective care that has cost benefits for the whole health/social care system.

Geriatricians and other health professionals with specialist knowledge cannot directly provide care for all older people. However, they have a responsibility to ensure adequate standards of care and adequate access to appropriate specialist input and multidisciplinary services, through, for example, the expansion and development of liaison services, and the development of educational programs for the non-specialist.

Further research, utilizing larger or more focused randomized controlled trials, and well-evidenced predictors of outcome such as frailty indicators, may permit targeting of particular day hospital interventions at patients with particular characteristics. Given the diversity of older people, of possible interventions and settings, such trials should either be large and multi-center, offering the possibility of subanalyses, or else address more focused questions than has hitherto been the case.

REFERENCES

1. Rockwood K, Stolee P, McDowell I. Factors associated with institutionalization of older people in Canada: testing a multifactorial definition of frailty. J Am Geriatr Soc 1996; 44: 578–82.

2. DesMeules M, Turner L, Cho R. Morbidity experiences and disability among Canadian women. BMC Womens Health 2004; 4(Suppl 1): S10.

3. Matthews DA. Dr Marjory Warren and the origin of British geriatrics. J Am Geriatr Soc 1984; 32: 253–8.

4. Grimley Evans J. Geriatric medicine: a brief history. BMJ 1997; 315: 1075–7.

5. Ellis G, Langhorne P. Comprehensive geriatric assessment for older hospital patients. Br Med Bull 2005; 71: 45–59.

6. Cosin L. The place of the day hospital in the geriatric unit. Practitioner 1954; 172: 552–9.

7. Brocklehurst J. Geriatric day hospitals. Age Ageing 1995; 24: 89–90.

8. Grimley Evans J. Integration of geriatric with general medical services in Newcastle. Lancet 1983; 1: 1430–3.

9. Donaldson C, Wright KG, Maynard AK, Hamill JD, Sutcliffe E. Day hospitals for the elderly: utilisation and performance. Community Med 1987; 9: 55–61.

10. Geriatric (medical) day hospitals for older people. British Geriatrics Society Compendium document 4.4: http://www.bgs.org.uk/Publications/Compendium/compend_ 4-4.htm.

11. Clinicians, Services and Commissioning Chronic Disease Management in the NHS. The need for co-ordinated management programmes. Report of a joint working party of the Royal College of Physicians of London, the Royal College of General Practitioners and the NHS Alliance. London: Royal College of Physicians of London; 2004.

12. Marshall M, Crowther R, Almaraz-Serrano AM, Tyrer P. Day hospital versus out-patient

care for psychiatric disorders. Cochrane Database Syst Rev 2001; (2): CD003240.

13. Marshall M, Crowther R, Almaraz-Serrano A, et al. Day hospital versus admission for acute psychiatric disorders. Cochrane Database Syst Rev 2003; (1): CD004026.

14. Black DA. Emergency day hospital assessments. Clin Rehabil 1997; 11: 344–6.

15. Black DA. An audit of outcomes in day hospital-based crisis intervention. Age Ageing 2003; 32: 360–1.

16. National Service Framework for Older People. London: Department of Health; 2001.

17. Our Health, Our Care, Our Say: A New Direction for Community Services. London: Department of Health; 2006.

18. Management of the older medical patient. Working Party Report. Royal College of Physicians; 2000: http://www.rcplondon.ac.uk/pubs/books/momp/index.htm.

19. Inouye SK, Bogardus ST, Charpentier PA, et al. A multicomponent intervention to prevent delirium in hospitalized older patients. N Engl J Med 1999; 340: 669–76.

20. Hubbard RE, O'Mahony MS, Cross E, et al. The ageing of the population: implications for multidisciplinary care in hospital. Age Ageing 2004; 33: 479–82.

21. Grimley Evans J, Tallis R. A new beginning for care for elderly people? BMJ 2001; 322: 807–8.

22. Focus on Older People. London: Office for National Statistics; 2005.

23. Eng C, Pedulla J, Eleazer GP, McCann R, Fox N. Program of All-inclusive Care for the Elderly (PACE): an innovative model of integrated geriatric care and financing. J Am Geriatr Soc 1997; 45: 223–32.

24. Huusko TM, Karppi P, Avikainen V, Kautiainen H, Sulkava R. Randomised, clinically controlled trial of intensive geriatric rehabilitation in patients with hip fracture: subgroup analysis of patients with dementia. BMJ 2000; 321: 1107–11.

25. Day hospitals: Their Role and Guidelines for Good Practice. London: Royal College of Physicians; 1994.

26. Clinical Audit Scheme for Geriatric Day Hospitals. London: Royal College of Physicians; 1994.

27. Currie A, McAllister-Williams RH, Jacques A. A comparison study of day hospital and day centre attenders. Health Bull (Edinb) 1995; 53: 365–72.

28. Stuck AE, Siu AL, Wieland GD, Adams J, Rubenstein LZ. Comprehensive geriatric assessment: a meta-analysis of controlled trials. Lancet 1993; 342: 1032–6.

29. Forster A, Young J, Langhorne P, Day Hospital Group. Medical day hospital care for the elderly versus alternative forms of care. Cochrane Database Syst Rev 1999; (3): CD001730.

30. Young JB, Robinson M, Chell S, et al. A whole system study of intermediate care services for older people. Age Ageing 2005; 34: 577–83.

31. Cunliffe AL, Gladman JR, Husbands SL, et al. Sooner and healthier: a randomised controlled trial and interview study of an early discharge rehabilitation service for older people. Age Ageing 2004; 33: 246–52.

32. Early Supported Discharge Trialists. Services for reducing duration of hospital care for acute stroke patients. Cochrane Database Syst Rev 2005; (2): CD000443.

33. Roderick P, Low J, Day R, et al. Stroke rehabilitation after hospital discharge: a randomized trial comparing domiciliary and day-hospital care. Age Ageing 2001; 30: 303–10.

34. Spice C, Morotti W, Dent T, et al. The Winchester Falls Project: a randomised controlled trial of secondary falls prevention. Oral presentation. British Geriatrics Society Spring Meeting, 2005.

35. Wade DT, Gage H, Owen C, et al. Multidisciplinary rehabilitation for people with Parkinson's disease: a randomised controlled study. J Neurol Neurosurg Psychiatry 2003; 74: 158–62.

36. Tousignant M, Hebert R, Desrosiers J, Hollander MJ. Economic evaluation of a geriatric day hospital: cost-benefit analysis based on functional autonomy changes. Age Ageing 2003; 32: 53–9.

Diet

14

Margaret Rees and Rossana Salerno-Kennedy

INTRODUCTION

The nutritional requirements of older women are of increasing interest as more are living into their 80s and beyond. Nevertheless, there is a paucity of research conducted in the elderly and, in particular, in women.[1]

Older people are more vulnerable to inadequate nutrition than younger adults and have a higher risk of nutrient deficiencies.[2] Undernutrition in the elderly leads to the 'anorexia of aging' and gradual weight loss. Poor nutritional status is associated with increased demands on health services, lengthier hospital stays, and immune dysfunction, and is recognized as an important predictor of morbidity and mortality.[1]

Undernutrition in the elderly has been found in a variety of settings: community, care home, and hospital residents. In particular, the prevalence of malnutrition is 5–10% of independently living older individuals, 30–60% of institutionalized patients, 35–65% of hospitalized patients,[3–5] and ≤85% of nursing home patients.[6] These circumstances have led to the development of guidelines and policy initiatives on treating and preventing malnutrition.[7–9]

This chapter will examine individual dietary components, factors which can contribute to poor nutrition in the elderly, and strategies for improvement.

DIETARY COMPONENTS

Macronutrients

Macronutrients encompass carbohydrate, protein, and fat, and dietary reference intakes are detailed in Table 14.1.

Carbohydrate

The World Health Organization has recommended that 55–75% of energy input should come from carbohydrate, with less than 10% from free sugars.[10] Amongst British older adults, although carbohydrate intakes are close to recommendations, the proportion coming from non-milk extrinsic sugars (NMES), from foods such as sugar, preserves, sweet spreads, sugary drinks and confectionery, were higher, particularly amongst those older adults living in institutions.[11] As diets high in NMES may reduce intake of foods that are more nutrient-dense, these should be eaten in moderation. More emphasis is needed on other carbohydrate-rich foods (such as wholegrain breakfast cereals, grains and breads, and bakery products), which also would provide fiber and a number of B vitamins. Furthermore, diets high in grains are associated with a lower risk of developing metabolic syndrome.[12]

Table 14.1 Dietary reference intakes (DRIs) for older adults: macronutrients

RDA or AI[1]	Energy[2] (kcal)	Protein[3] (g)	Carbohydrates[4] (g)	Total fat[5,6] (%kcal)	ω-6 PUFA (g)	ω-3 PUFA (g)	Total fiber (g)	Drinking water, beverages, water in food (L)
Age 51–70								
Male	2204	**56**	**130**		14★	1.6★	30★	3.7★
Female	1978	**46**	**130**		11★	1.1★	21★	2.7★
Age 70+								
Male	2054	**56**	**130**		14★	1.6★	30★	2.6★
Female	1873	**46**	**130**		11★	1.1★	21★	2.1★
ADMR[7]		10–35%	45–65%	20–35%	5–10%	0.6–1.2%		

1. Recommended dietary allowances (RDAs) in **bold type**, Adequate intakes (AIs) in ordinary type followed by an asterisk (★).

2. The RDA for protein equilibrium in adults is a minimum of 0.8 g/kg body weight for reference body weight.

3. The RDA for carbohydrate is the minimum adequate to maintain brain function in adults.

4. Because percent of energy consumed as fat can vary greatly and still meet energy needs, an Acceptable macronutrient distribution ranges (AMDR) is provided in the absence of AI, Estimated average requirements (EAR), or RDA for adults.

5. Values for mono- and saturated fats and cholesterol not established as 'they have no role in preventing chronic disease, thus not required in the diet'.

6. Acceptable macronutrient distribution ranges (AMDRs) for intakes of carbohydrates, proteins, and fats expressed as percent of total calories.

7. AMDR is the range of intake for a particular energy source that is associated with reduced risk of chronic disease while providing intakes of essential nutrients. If an individual consumes in excess of the AMDR, there is a potential of increasing the risk of chronic diseases and/or insufficient intakes of essential nutrients.

The values for this table were derived from the Institute of Medicine, Dietary Reference Intakes: Applications in Dietary Assessment, 2000 and Dietary Reference Intakes for Energy, Carbohydrates, Fiber, Fat, Protein and Amino Acids (Macronutrients) 2002.[24]

Protein

Protein is an important nutrient for the elderly. Current recommendations are 10–15% of total energy intake. As lean body mass decreases with age, intuitively it would seem that protein requirements would decline, but instead they increase to maintain nitrogen equilibrium. Demand further increases in wound healing (including fractures), infection, and restoring muscle mass lost from immobility.[1]

Fat

The World Health Organization has recommended that total fat intake should account for 15–30% of total energy intake, with saturated fats accounting for <10% and polyunsaturated fats for 6–10%.[10] Although the main message in the past has been to limit the total amount of fat, particular types such as ω-3 fatty acids, which are found mainly in oily fish, may be more important than previously recognized. The Women's Health Initiative randomized controlled trial (RCT) examined the effect of reduction of total fat intake on the risk of breast and colorectal cancer and cardiovascular disease.[13–15] In this study 16 541 women were assigned to a diet with reduced total fat intake (20% total energy) and increased intakes of vegetables, fruits, and grains. The comparison group of 29 294 women did not have any dietary changes, and mean follow-up was 8.1 years. The dietary intervention had no effect.

Much of the interest in the association between ω-3 fatty acids and cardiovascular disease follows studies with Greenland Inuits, who traditionally have low mortality from coronary heart disease despite a diet rich in fat.[16] Omega-3 fatty acids have been studied in relation to cardiovascular disease and dementia. A systematic review has found no cardiovascular benefit, but this observation may reflect the characteristics of the populations in the included trials.[17] On the other hand, seafood intake, as found in both a European and a North American study, may protect against Alzheimer's disease and dementia, and this protection may be mediated by ω-3 fatty acids.[18,19]

Micronutrients

Micronutrients encompass vitamins and minerals. Low nutrient status has been noted amongst older adults; e.g. in the British National Diet and Nutrition Survey (NDNS).[11] The significant micronutrients that may be associated with deficiencies in elderly women include vitamin B_{12}, vitamin A, vitamin C, vitamin D, calcium, zinc, and other trace minerals. Low levels of calcium and vitamin D are associated with poor skeletal health and osteoporotic fractures.[20] Low intakes of a range of micronutrients, such as iron, folate, and vitamin B_{12}, can cause a number of anemias and a range of other problems (such as neuropathies and dementia).[21] Unfortunately, whereas these facts are well known by the medical profession, little specific information exists regarding micronutrient requirements for elderly women. The nutrition recommendations provided by the dietary reference intakes (DRIs) and recommended dietary allowances (RDAs) are not generally helpful when it comes to providing advice to old and very old women, although in the most recent publications there are separate recommendations for individuals over age 70 (Table 14.2).[22–24] With the exception of vitamin D, it would appear that the other major vitamin groups are dosed at the same level, regardless of age.

Table 14.2   Dietary reference intakes (DRIs): recommended vitamin intakes in women

Age (years)	Vitamin A[1] (μg/day)	Vitamin C (μg/day)	Vitamin D[2,3] (μg/day)	Vitamin E[4] (μg/day)	Folate[5] (μg/day)	Cobalamin (μg/day)
31–50	700	75	5	15	400	2.4
51–70	700	75	10	15	400	2.4
>70	700	75	15	15	400	2.4

1. As Retinol activity equivalents (RAEs). 1 RAE = 1 μg retinol, 12 μg β-carotene, 24 μg α-carotene, or 24 μg β-cryptoxanthin. The RAE for dietary provitamin A carotenoids is twofold greater than retinol equivalents (REs), whereas the RAE for preformed vitamin A is the same as RE.

2. As cholecalciferol. 1 μg cholecalciferol = 40 IU vitamin D.

3. In the absence of adequate exposure to sunlight.

4. As α-tocopherol.

5. As Dietary folate equivalents (DFEs). 1 DFE = 1 μg food folate = 0.6 μg of folic acid from fortified food or as a supplement consumed with food = 0.5 μg of a supplement taken on an empty stomach.

Adapted from Food and Nutrition Board, Institute of Medicine, National Academies: http://www.iom.edu/Object.File/Master/21/372/0.pdf.

Vitamin A

Vitamin A has many roles in the maintenance of health. It is important for normal vision, cell differentiation, immune function, and genetic expression.[25] Lower levels of α-carotene have been linked to atherosclerosis in older adults and low levels of α-carotene and β-carotene correlate with higher risk of coronary artery disease in adult women.[26] The Women's Health and Aging Study has shown that low levels of α- and β-carotene and total carotenoids increase levels of the inflammatory cytokine interleukin-6 (IL-6).[26] Vitamin A recommendations for older adults have been lowered from previous editions of the RDAs. Present suggested levels are 700 μg retinol activity equivalents (RAEs) for women.[23]

One consequence of high vitamin A intake is its association with a higher risk for fractures. Vitamin A is a vitamin D and calcium antagonist, and a high intake of vitamin A over long periods of time may adversely affect bone health.[27] Obtaining supplemental vitamin A in its precursor form, β-carotene, appears to be considerably safer, more effective, and has not been associated with adverse or unanticipated side effects. Consuming a diet rich in fruits and vegetables is a reasonable way to meet vitamin A needs in older adults as well as providing a good source of dietary fiber.[25]

Calcium and vitamin D

Supplementation with calcium and vitamin D particularly may be relevant when evidence of insufficiency exists, especially in elderly people. Provision of adequate dietary or supplemental calcium and vitamin D is an essential part of the management of the treatment and prevention of osteoporosis (Table 14.3). In northern latitudes, cutaneous synthesis of vitamin D occurs only in the summer months, and the national diet in the

Table 14.3 Calcium content of some foods

Food	Calcium content (mg)
Full-fat milk (250 ml)	295
Semi-skimmed milk (250 ml)	300
Skimmed milk (250 ml)	305
Low-fat yogurt (100 g)	150
Cheddar cheese (50 g)	360
Boiled spinach (100 g)	159
Brazil nuts (100 g)	170
Tinned salmon (100 g)	93
Tofu (100 g)	480

UK lacks sufficient amounts of this vitamin for adequate intake in the absence of solar exposure.[20] Other countries, such as the US, fortify foods by adding vitamin D to dairy products.

Most studies show that about 1.5 g of elemental calcium is necessary to preserve bone health in postmenopausal women and elderly women who are not taking hormone replacement therapy (HRT). This figure has been reinforced by the National Institutes of Health in the US. In women who use HRT, 1 g/day is sufficient to maintain calcium balance.[28] However, use of HRT in women over 70 is low.

The effects of calcium and vitamin D supplements alone or in combination on fracture, however, are contradictory and may depend on the study population. For example, people in sheltered accommodation or residential care may be more frail, have lower dietary intakes of calcium and vitamin D, and are at higher risk of fracture than those living in the community.

Calcium A meta-analysis of 15 trials representing 1806 participants showed that calcium alone was more effective than placebo in reducing rates of bone loss after ≥2 years of treatment.[29] The pooled difference in percentage change from baseline was 2.05% (95% CI 0.24–3.86%)

for total body bone density, 1.66% (95% CI 0.92–2.39%) for the lumbar spine at 2 years, 1.60% (95% CI 0.78–2.41%) for the hip, and 1.91% (95% CI 0.33–3.50%) for the distal radius. The relative risk (RR) of fractures of the vertebrae was 0.79% (95% CI 0.54–1.09%) and of non-vertebral fractures was 0.86 (95% CI 0.43–1.72%). Calcium supplementation alone thus has a small positive effect on bone density. The data show a trend towards a reduction in vertebral fractures, but whether calcium reduces the incidence of non-vertebral fractures is unclear.

Vitamin D   Vitamin D supplementation has been reported to reduce the risk of fracture and falls, but, again, the evidence is conflicting. A meta-analysis of 12 RCTs involving 19 114 participants found that a dose of vitamin D alone of 700–800 IU/day reduced the RR of hip fracture by 26% (RR = 0.74; 0.61–0.88) and of any non-vertebral fracture by 23% (RR = 0.77; 0.68–0.87) vs calcium or placebo.[30] No significant benefit was observed for RCTs that used 400 IU/day vitamin D (RR for hip fracture = 1.15; 0.88–1.50; RR for any non-vertebral fracture 1.03; 0.86–1.24). The authors thus concluded that oral supplementation of vitamin D at a dose of 700–800 IU/day seems to reduce the risk of hip and any non-vertebral fractures in ambulatory or institutionalized elderly people. An oral dose of vitamin D of 400 IU/day is not sufficient for fracture prevention.

Calcium and vitamin D   Combined calcium and vitamin D supplements have also been reported to reduce the risk of fracture, but, again, the evidence is conflicting. An early French study had shown a 30% lower risk of hip fracture in elderly women given 1.2 g of elemental calcium and 800 IU of vitamin D.[31] Bone mineral density at the hip increased, and secondary hyperparathyroidism present in many women at the outset was reversed in the active treatment group but

continued in the placebo group. A significant reduction was also seen in all long bone fractures in women treated for 18 months. More recent studies in community-dwelling women or as a secondary prevention, however, show no benefit.[32–34] Furthermore, the Women's Health Initiative Study showed an increase in kidney stones in low-risk women taking calcium and vitamin D supplements.[34]

Vitamin B12 (cobalamin) and folate

Vitamin B_{12} (cobalamin) deficiency occurs in about 20% of elderly patients.[35] Causes of the deficiency include, most frequently, food–cobalamin malabsorption syndrome (>60% of all cases), pernicious anemia (15–20%), insufficient dietary intake, and malabsorption. Dietary sources of vitamin B_{12} are primarily meats and dairy products. A typical Western diet provides approximately 3–30 μg of vitamin B_{12} daily, much more than the recommended daily allowance of 2–5 μg. Normally, humans maintain a large vitamin B_{12} reserve, which can last 2–5 years even in the presence of severe malabsorption. Nevertheless, nutritional deficiency can occur in the elderly, especially in those relying on so-called 'tea and toast' or 'cooked cereal' diets. The primary clinical manifestations of cobalamin deficiency are highly polymorphic and vary in severity, ranging from milder conditions, such as the common sensory neuropathy and isolated anomalies such as macrocytic anemia, to severe disorders, including combined sclerosis of the spinal cord and hemolytic anemia.

Folates are found in fruit and fresh vegetables. Insufficient food intake of folate is a common cause of low folate levels. The elderly are at increased risk of low folate intake, but there are no exact figures on the prevalence or incidence of folate deficiency.[36] Deficiency may also lead to macrocytic anemia and neurological problems. It is important to distinguish between cobalamin and folate deficiency, since supplementation with folate may delay the diagnosis and worsen the sequelae of cobalamin deficiency. Cobalamin and folate are involved in homocysteine metabolism. High homocysteine levels have been suggested as risk factors for cognitive decline, dementia, cardiovascular disease, and osteoporotic fracture.[37,38] Gender differences may exist in that lower bone mineral density has been associated with higher homocysteine levels in women but not in men.[37]

Vitamins E and C

The antioxidant vitamins E and C protect the body from damage from free radicals. Free radicals are produced during normal metabolism, but they may be associated with disease and the aging process. Several epidemiological studies have shown that people with high intakes of fruit and vegetables may have a lower risk of chronic disease than those with low intakes.[39] The benefits of high intakes of fruits and vegetables are hypothesized to result from their antioxidant content. However, data in elderly women are contradictory. Supplementation with vitamin E does not prevent cancer or major cardiovascular events in healthy women and may increase the risk for heart failure in those with vascular disease or diabetes.[40,41] Also, all-cause mortality is associated with high-dose vitamin E supplements.[42]

With regard to vitamin C, low blood concentrations of the vitamin in men and women aged 75–84 years old are predictive of mortality.[43] Vitamin C status is generally related to dietary intake. Newer data set the recommendations for vitamin C at 90 mg/day for males and 75 mg/day for females over age 50.[1] Lowered intake is often associated with chronic disease, including atherosclerosis, cancer, senile cataracts, lung diseases, cognitive decline, and organ degenerative diseases.[1] However, high intake of vitamin C

from supplements is associated with an increased risk of mortality from cardiovascular disease in postmenopausal women with diabetes.[44]

In addition, antioxidant vitamin supplements that contain both vitamins E and C do not provide cardiovascular benefit in postmenopausal women.[45]

Trace elements

The DRIs for trace elements are shown in Table 14.4.

Table 14.4 Dietary reference intakes (DRIs) for trace elements

Nutrient	Age group#	RDA/AI★ (g/day)	UL^a
Boron (mg/day)	a	ND	20
	b	ND	20
	c	ND	20
Calcium (mg/day)	a	1,000★	2,500
	b	1,200★	2,500
	c	1,200★	2,500
Chromium (μg/day)	a	25★	ND
	b	20	ND
	c	20	ND
Copper (μg/day)	a	**900**	10,000
	b	**900**	10,000
	c	**900**	10,000
Fluoride (mg/day)	a	3★	10
	b	3★	10
	c	3★	10
Iodine (μg/day)	a	**150**	1,100
	b	**150**	1,100
	c	**150**	1,100
Iron (mg/day)	a	**18**	45
	b	**8**	45
	c	**8**	45

(Continued)

Table 14.4   (Continued)

Nutrient	Age group#	RDA/AI* (g/day)	UL[a]
Magnesium	a	**320**	350
(mg/day)	b	**320**	350
	c	**320**	350
Manganese	a	1.8*	11
(mg/day)	b	1.8*	11
	c	1.8*	11
Molybdenum	a	**45**	2,000
(μg/day)	b	**45**	2,000
	c	**45**	2,000
Nickel (mg/day)	a	ND	1.0
	b	ND	1.0
	c	ND	1.0
Phosphorus	a	**700**	4,000
(mg/day)	b	**700**	4,000
	c	**700**	4,000
Selenium (μg/day)	a	**55**	400
	b	**55**	400
	c	**55**	400
Vanadium	a	ND	1.8
(mg/day)	b	ND	1.8
	c	ND	1.8
Zinc (mg/day)	a	**8**	40
	b	**8**	40
	c	**8**	40

#Age group: a, 31–50 years old; b, 50–70 years old; c, >70 years old.

The table is adapted from the DRI reports (2001): see www.nap.edu. It represents recommended dietary allowances (RDAs) in **bold type**, adequate intakes (AIs) in ordinary type followed by an asterisk (*), and tolerable upper intake (ULs)[a]. RDAs and AIs may both be used as goals for individual intake. RDAs are set to meet the needs of almost all (97–98%) individuals in a group.

ULa = the maximum level of daily nutrient intake that is likely to pose no risk of adverse effects. Unless otherwise specified, the UL represents total intake from food, water, and supplements. Due to lack of suitable data, ULs could not be established for vitamin K, thiamine, riboflavin, vitamin B_{12}, pantothenic acid, biotin, or carotenoids. In the absence of ULs, extra caution may be warranted in consuming levels above recommended intakes.

ND = not determinable due to lack of data of adverse effects in this age group and concern with regard to lack of ability to handle excess amounts. Source of intake should be from food only to prevent high levels of intake.

Selenium   Selenium is an essential nutrient that enhances immune function and increases antioxidant activity. Its level in food reflects the soil in which it was grown and therefore varies worldwide. Its deficiency has been reported among institutionalized elderly, particularly those who have multiple pathologies.[46] The Women's Health and Aging Study has shown that low levels of selenium were associated with increased risk of all-cause mortality over a period of 5 years.[26] Selenium deficiency is associated with a host of inflammatory tissue responses and with disease progression, including coxsackievirus- and human immunodeficiency virus (HIV)-induced myocarditis, thyroid dysfunction, arthritis, cancer, depression, and cardiovascular disease.[26] Low selenium intake is also associated with anxiety, depression, and tiredness, and selenium therapy alleviates these symptoms.[47,48] There is an upper limit of 400 μg of selenium/day, which, if exceeded, may lead to toxicity.[1] Symptoms of toxicity include nausea, vomiting, hair and nail brittleness and loss, irritability, peripheral neuropathy, and fatigue.

Magnesium   Hypomagnesemia has been considered as a possible factor in depressed immune function, muscle atrophy, osteoporosis, hyperglycemia, hyperlipidemia, and other neuromuscular, cardiovascular, or renal dysfunctions.[46,49] The role of magnesium (Mg) in dementia and other degenerative disorders has been a recent focus of attention. Low Mg intake over generations may be involved in the pathogenesis of substantia nigra degeneration, and therefore in Parkinson's disease.[50] Low Mg levels are found in the brain of patients with Alzheimer's disease and it has been hypothesized that use of Mg with memantine, which acts via this ion channel, could be of benefit.[51]

Recommendations for magnesium intake are 320 mg/day, and there is no indication that the elderly have different needs from younger adults.[1]

Selected food sources are green leafy vegetables, unpolished grains, nuts, meat, starches, and milk.

Zinc

Zinc is another essential trace nutrient: it is essential for neurogenesis and plays an important role in neurotransmission.[52] Consequences of poor zinc status may include reduced immune function, dermatitis, loss of taste acuity, impaired wound healing, and impaired cognitive function.[1] Malabsorption, physiological stress, trauma, and muscle wasting, which are common situations in older women, will all contribute to inadequate zinc status. Phytates, from grains, cereals, rice, and legumes, may also interfere with zinc absorption; zinc found in vegetables may be less bioavailable than that from animal sources.[1] Dietary zinc supplementation can correct deficiencies and also improve cognitive function.[49] Selected food sources are fortified cereals, red meats, and certain seafood.

FACTORS AFFECTING NUTRITION IN ELDERLY WOMEN

The causes of nutritional deficiency in older people are likely to be multifactorial: age-related changes, chronic and acute medical conditions and also environmental, social, financial, and functional barriers may interfere with adequate dietary intake[54] (see Table 14.5).

Changes in body composition and nutrient intake

Aging is associated with changes in body composition: the most notable are decreases in intracellular fluid and lean body mass and an increase in the amount of and change in the distribution

Table 14.5 Factors affecting nutrition in elderly women

Aging:
- Changes in body composition – sarcopenia
- Changes to the gastrointestinal tract
- Oral changes and food intake
- Atrophic gastritis
- Changes in sensory function
- Changes in fluid and electrolyte regulation

Chronic illness

Medication and hospitalization

Drug–diet interactions

Social and economic determinants

of fat stores.[53] These changes predispose older people to dehydration, reduced basal metabolism, falls and injury, and central weight gain. Nutrition plays a role in the progression and attenuation of these changes.[54–56] The major age-related physiological change in older people is a decline in skeletal muscle mass, known as sarcopenia.[54,55] The nutritional consequences of a reduced lean body mass are reduced metabolic rate, together with a proportional decline in total energy requirements.[56] Energy requirements decline with age in both sexes. For example NHANES III data show that energy intakes between ages 25 and 70 years fell by 600–800 kcal/day for women.[57] By age 80, 1 in 10 women consumed less than 750 kcal/day. A reduction in energy expenditure is also associated with sedentary behavior and a loss of mobility related to systemic (e.g. cardiovascular, pulmonary) or bone and joint disease.[54] Reduced energy intakes can lead to inadequate consumption of protein, vitamins, and minerals. NHANES III data also show potentially important decreases with age in median protein and zinc intakes as well as intakes of calcium, vitamin E, and other nutrients.[57] Also, the nutrient density of the diet (i.e. consumption of a given nutrient expressed per 1000 kcal) falls with age. Low nutrient density and inadequate intakes of protein, vitamins, and minerals are thus important areas of concern.

Gastrointestinal changes

Aging has been associated with altered sensations of thirst, hunger, and satiety. Alterations in satiety may be mediated by neuroendocrine changes such as an increase in levels of cholecystokinin. Inflammatory disorders, such as rheumatoid arthritis, that result in the release of cytokines may also lead to age-associated anorexia.

Poor nutritional status is also related to decreased efficiency of the gastrointestinal tract.[58] Nutrients may not be well digested and absorbed due to atrophic gastritis, a decrease in hormone and enzyme production, senescent changes in the cells of the bowel surface, and interactions among drugs and nutrients.[59,60]

Chewing and swallowing may also be impaired for a variety of reasons.[60] Poor oral health, edentulousness, dentures that may not fit properly, or lesions in the oral cavity will interfere with consumption of a well-balanced diet.[61] Mortality is increased, as evidenced by a study of 829 women aged 70–79 years old in Baltimore.[62] Women who used dentures and reported difficulty chewing or swallowing had lower 5-year survival (HR = 1.43, 95% CI 1.05–1.97). Up to 40% of older people complain of having a dry mouth. Although this might be due to medical conditions, medication, inadequate fluid intake, and/or dehydration, 80% of the medications most commonly used by older people reduce salivary secretion.[56,63,64] The observed deficits in taste and smell may also lead to a reduced sensory enjoyment of foods, and therefore to the adoption of a restricted diet.

Compounding these changes is the effect of both chronic and acute illness.[65] As the elderly have to take more drugs, interactions between drugs and diet are more likely to cause them additional problems. Drugs can affect nutrition by altering appetite, absorption, metabolism, action on target tissues, or excretion of macronutrients and micronutrients, thereby causing a deficiency.[66] Malnutrition may also affect drug metabolism and hence the required dosage and possible toxicity[66] (see Chapter 9).

Social and economic factors

Dietary intakes in elderly women may also decrease due to challenges associated with their environment, social and financial status, and their level of functional ability. Social determinants include facilities for food storage and preparation, opportunities for and access to shopping, and the ability to prepare food and eat with the company of others.[8] Many of them have been widowed, have had their children move to other geographical areas, are living on a fixed income, and/or experience disability. Cooking for one may not be a motivating activity after years of shopping and preparing food and meals for a family and spouse. Surveys of independently living older people indicate that those living alone, or eating alone, eat less and are at higher risk of poor nutritional status.[67] Limited income has its own financial challenges, leading to prioritization of expenditure, which may not include food as a main concern. Thus, overall dietary quality decreases. The elderly are more likely to consume foods which fall into the category of 'favorite and comfort', and are frequently those that are high in fat and carbohydrate. The challenge is to obtain an adequate nutrient intake and, in particular, sufficient amounts of micronutrients, within the complex nature of the human aging process.[61]

STRATEGIES TO IMPROVE NUTRITION

Strategies to improve nutrition range from changing dietary components to reducing social isolation as well as health promotion (Table 14.6).

Table 14.6 Strategies to improve nutrition

Functional foods:
- Probiotics
- Prebiotics
- Synbiotics
- Nutraceuticals
- Fiber

The Mediterranean diet
Reducing social isolation
Improving nutrient density
Multivitamin and mineral supplements
Health promotion

Functional foods

Functional foods generally are defined as foods that confer a 'benefit' to the host beyond simple nutrition.[68] Five main types of functional foods show promise in women's health:

- probiotics
- prebiotics
- synbiotics
- nutraceuticals
- fiber.

Probiotics

A probiotic is defined as a 'live microbial food supplement which beneficially affects the host animal by improving its intestinal balance'. Currently, the best-studied probiotics are the lactic acid bacteria, particularly *Lactobacillus* spp. and *Bifidobacterium* spp. These can be combined with food products such as cereals, bio yoghurts, and drinks. Increasing evidence shows the potential of probiotics in benefiting gastrointestinal conditions (such as diarrhea and irritable bowel syndrome) and non-gastrointestinal tract conditions (such as candidiasis and urinary tract and respiratory tract infections).

Prebiotics

Prebiotics are 'non-digestible food ingredients which selectively stimulate a limited number of bacteria in the colon, to improve host health'. The emphasis of prebiotic research, therefore, is to enhance the indigenous probiotic flora. This includes strategies to develop specific prebiotics for individual probiotic organisms, as well as aiding persistence of prebiotic effects throughout the gastrointestinal tract. They may be involved in calcium absorption.

Synbiotics

Synbiotics contain complementary probiotic and prebiotic ingredients that interact to provide a synergistic effect towards the maintenance of a desirable microbial population in the intestinal microbiota. This is a developing area of functional foods, and few clinical studies of their impact on human health have been performed to date.

Nutraceuticals

Nutraceuticals are natural components of foods (such as isoflavones and phytoestrogens) that may be released during digestion and therefore become bioavailable. Such compounds may have a direct health effect on the host or an indirect health effect via the microflora, or both.

Fiber

Dietary fiber consists of plant substances that resist hydrolysis by digestive enzymes in the small bowel and is an extremely complex group of substances.[69] Fiber can be classified according to its solubility and fermentability by bacteria: a soluble fiber is readily fermentable by colonic bacteria and an insoluble fiber only slowly fermentable. Fibers may act in several ways, including through gel-forming effects in the stomach and small intestine, fermentation by colonic bacteria, a 'mop and sponge' effect, and concomitant changes in other aspects of the diet. These actions lead to potentially beneficial effects in the gastrointestinal tract and, systemically, by lowering levels of cholesterol in serum and improving glycemic control.

The Mediterranean diet

Studies consistently support the view that the Mediterranean diet is compatible with healthier aging and increased longevity. It may also lower the risk of Alzheimer's disease.[70] The Mediterranean diet is characterized by a high intake of vegetables, legumes, fruits, and cereals (in the past largely unrefined); a moderate to high intake of fish; a low intake of saturated lipids but a high intake of unsaturated lipids, particularly olive oil; a low to moderate intake of dairy products, mostly cheese and yoghurt; a low intake of meat; and a modest intake of alcohol, mostly as wine (Figure 14.1). Mediterranean and modified Mediterranean diets are associated with reductions in mortality.[71,72] The benefit of the diet does not seem to be limited to Mediterranean countries and can be exported to others.[72]

Reducing social isolation

The eating environment and fellowship at meal times affect appetite, with studies being mainly undertaken in hospitals and residential and nursing homes.[73] Older acute care patients in hospital who eat in a supervised dining room improve their food intake but not their weight in comparison to those eating from a tray at the bedside.[74] Buffet-style dining in long-term care improves older residents' satisfaction with meals but yielded no significant difference in weight or biochemical markers of nutritional status.[75] A cluster quasi-randomized trial of family-style dinners vs tray service in nursing home residents with an average age of 77 years old found that quality of life, physical functioning, energy intake, and body weight were improved in the former group.[75]

Improving nutrient density

Increasing nutrient density with nutritional supplements can lead to weight gain and improved wound healing, especially in those at risk of undernutrition.[76–78] Provision of a nutrient-dense protein–energy liquid supplement and encouragement to improve intake from other foods was studied in 83 elderly people (mean age = 80 ± 7 years) receiving community home-care services and at high risk for undernutrition.[76] The intervention resulted in significant improvement of nutritional status with respect to energy and nutrient intake and weight gain. Weight loss stopped and in some cases reversed; however, increased physical activity may also be required to improve health and functional status. Similar findings have been found in nursing home residents.[78]

Meta-analysis of 55 trials concluded that oral nutritional supplements can improve nutritional status and seem to reduce mortality and complications for undernourished elderly hospital patients. However, the evidence did not support routine supplementation for older people at home or for well-nourished older patients in any setting.[79]

Multivitamin and mineral supplements

Whether there is a need to supplement the dietary intake of vitamins and trace elements with some form of commercial artificial supplement is one of the hottest topics in nutritional research

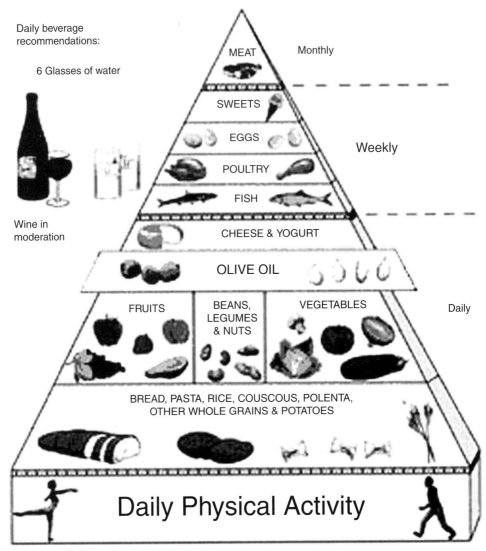

Daily beverage recommendations:

6 Glasses of water

Wine in moderation

MEAT — Monthly

SWEETS

EGGS

POULTRY — Weekly

FISH

CHEESE & YOGURT

OLIVE OIL

FRUITS | BEANS, LEGUMES & NUTS | VEGETABLES — Daily

BREAD, PASTA, RICE, COUSCOUS, POLENTA, OTHER WHOLE GRAINS & POTATOES

Daily Physical Activity

Figure 14.1 The Mediterranean diet pyramid.

in the developed world. The data available are controversial.[80–82] The main conclusions are:

1. Individual micronutrient supplements are beneficial where there is evidence of a deficiency state.
2. A multiple supplement may be beneficial in certain specific risk groups and those with known inadequate intakes, e.g. institutionalized elderly.
3. There is little evidence to support the use of supplements to reduce the risk of heart disease or cancer in the general population.
4. High intakes should only be used in the few situations where there is proof of benefit, since such intakes may be harmful.

However, the evidence presented in this chapter regarding deficiency is so compelling, that, in the absence of readily available and cost-effective tests for specific deficiencies, practitioners could consider routine multivitamin supplementation in the elderly. As many older individuals only have access to the dietary advice that can be obtained from the media, it seems prudent therefore for supplements to be discussed with a health professional to avoid any adverse effects. For example it is essential to distinguish between cobalamin and folate deficiencies and avoid vitamin A excess (see above).

Health promotion

Health promotion is part of healthcare. Reluctance to develop health promotion programs for older adults exists because of a perception that they would not follow such plans or change their lifestyles. Longitudinal studies have shown that health promotion activities extend the number of years of health in older people, although the relationship weakens in older age.[83] Changes in diet and exercise patterns are most effective when they are instituted early in life, particularly in the prevention of nutrition-related conditions, but positive effects can occur at any age. Good nutrition is ageless and the message to older people must be that the quality of their nutrition is basic to the quality of their life. Therefore, more information should be given on how to improve the nutritional intake of elderly people, particularly to those suffering from limited income, disability, and institutionalization.

CONCLUSION

Good nutrition is essential to the health, self-sufficiency, and quality of life of the elderly. Nutritional status of many older individuals lacks balance; they fail to get the amounts and types of food necessary to meet essential energy and nutrient needs. Thus, undernutrition, leading to the 'anorexia of aging', is a major concern. Maintaining good nutrition is an essential part of medical care and should be promoted by health professionals, and research needs to be expanded to identify the most effective and acceptable interventions.

REFERENCES

1. Chernoff R. Micronutrient requirements in older women. Am J Clin Nutr 2005; 81(5): 1240–5S.
2. Jensen GL, McGee M, Binkley J. Nutrition in the elderly. Gastroenterol Clin North Am 2001; 30: 313–34.
3. Chen CC, Schilling LS, Lyder CH. A concept analysis of malnutrition in the elderly. J Adv Nurs 2001; 36: 131–42.
4. Gilford A, Khun RK. Development of nutritional risk screening in the community. Br J Community Health Nurs 1996; 1: 335–6.
5. Vellas B, Lauque S, Andrieu S, et al. Nutrition assessment in the elderly. Curr Opin Clin Nutr Metab Care 2001; 4: 5–8.
6. Mion LC, McDowell JA, Heaney LK. Nutritional assessment of the elderly in the ambulatory care setting. Nurse Pract Forum 1994; 5: 46–51.
7. National Institute for Clinical Excellence. Nutrition support in adults: oral nutrition support, enteral tube feeding and parenteral nutrition; 2006. www.nice.org.uk/pdf/ CG032NICE guideline.pdf: accessed May 1, 2006.
8. NHS Quality Improvement Scotland. Food, fluid and nutritional care. Clinical Standards. Glasgow: NHS Quality Improvement Scotland; 2003. http://www.nhshealthquality.org/: accessed May 1, 2006.

9. Council of Europe. Food and nutritional care in hospitals: how to prevent under-nutrition. Report and recommendations of the Committee of Experts on Nutrition, Food Safety and Consumer Protection. Strasbourg: Council of Europe Publishing; 2002.

10. Diet, nutrition and the prevention of chronic diseases Report of the joint WHO/FAO expert consultation. 2003 WHO Technical Report Series, No. 916 (TRS 916). http:// www.who.int/dietphysicalactivity/publications/trs916/en/

11. Finch S, Doyle W, et al. National Diet and Nutrition Survey: People Aged 65 Years and Over. Volume 1: Report of the Diet and Nutrition Survey. London: HMSO; 1998.

12. Sahyoun NR, Jacques PF, Zhang XL, Juan W, McKeown NM. Whole-grain intake is inversely associated with the metabolic syndrome and mortality in older adults. Am J Clin Nutr 2006; 83(1): 124–31.

13. Prentice RL, Caan B, Chlebowski RT, et al. Low-fat dietary pattern and risk of invasive breast cancer: the Women's Health Initiative Randomized Controlled Dietary Modification Trial. JAMA 2006; 295: 629–42.

14. Beresford SAA, Johnson KC, Ritenbaugh C, et al. Low-fat dietary pattern and risk of colorectal cancer: the Women's Health Initiative Randomized Controlled Dietary Modification Trial. JAMA 2006; 295: 643–54.

15. Howard BV, Van Horn L, Hsia J, et al. Low-fat dietary pattern and risk of cardiovascular disease: the Women's Health Initiative Randomized Controlled Dietary Modification Trial. JAMA 2006; 295: 655–66.

16. Din JN, Newby DE, Flapan AD. Omega 3 fatty acids and cardiovascular disease – fishing for a natural treatment. BMJ 2004; 328(7430): 30–5.

17. Hooper L, Thompson RL, Harrison RA, et al. Risks and benefits of omega 3 fats for mortality, cardiovascular disease and cancer: systematic review. BMJ 2006; 332: 752–60.

18. Barberger-Gateau P, Letenneur L, Deschamps V, et al. Fish, meat, and risk of dementia: cohort study. BMJ 2002; 325: 932–3.

19. Morris MC, Evans DA, Tangney CC, Bienias JL, Wilson RS. Fish consumption and cognitive decline with age in a large community study. Arch Neurol 2005; 62: 1849–53.

20. Reginster JY. The high prevalence of inadequate serum vitamin D levels and implications for bone health. Curr Med Res Opin 2005; 21: 579–86.

21. Robinson B. Cost of anemia in the elderly. J Am Geriatr Soc 2003; 51(3 Suppl): S14–17.

22. Institute of Medicine. Dietary Reference Intakes for Thiamin, Riboflavin, Niacin, Vitamin B6, Folate, Vitamin B12, Pantothenic Acid, Biotin, and Choline. Washington, DC: National Academy Press; 2001: 1–564.

23. Institute of Medicine. Dietary Reference Intakes for Vitamin A, Vitamin K, Arsenic, Boron, Chromium, Copper, Iodine, Manganese, Molybdenum, Nickel, Silicon, Vanadium, and Zinc. Washington, DC: National Academy Press; 2001.

24. Institute of Medicine. Dietary Reference Intakes for Energy, Carbohydrates, Fiber, Fat, Fatty Acids, Cholesterol, Protein, and Amino Acids. Washington, DC: National Academy Press; 2002: 1–450.

25. Olson JA. Vitamin A. In: Rucker RB, Suttie JW, McCormick DB, Machlin LJ, eds. Handbook of Vitamins. New York: Marcel Dekker; 2001: 1–50.

26. Walston J, Xue Q, Semba RD, et al. Serum antioxidants, inflammation, and total mortality in older women. Am J Epidemiol 2005; 163 (1): 18–26.

27. Lips P. Hypervitaminosis A and fractures. N Engl J Med 2003; 348: 347–9.

28. Optimal Calcium Intake. National Institutes of Health. Consensus Development Conference Statement June 6–8, 1994. http://consensus.nih.gov/1994/1994OptimalCalcium097html.htm

29. Shea B, Wells G, Cranney A, et al. Calcium supplementation on bone loss in postmenopausal women. Cochrane Database Syst Rev 2004; (1): CD004526.

30. Bischoff-Ferrari HA, Willett WC, Wong JB, et al. Fracture prevention with vitamin D

supplementation: a meta-analysis of randomized controlled trials. JAMA 2005; 293:2257–64.

31. Chapuy MC, Arlot ME, Duboeuf F, et al. Vitamin D₃ and calcium to prevent hip fractures in the elderly women. N Engl J Med 1992; 327: 1637–42.

32. Porthouse J, Cockayne S, King C, et al. Randomised controlled trial of calcium and supplementation with cholecalciferol (vitamin D₃) for prevention of fractures in primary care. BMJ 2005; 330: 1003–6.

33. Grant AM, Avenell A, Campbell MK, et al; RECORD Trial Group. Oral vitamin D₃ and calcium for secondary prevention of low-trauma fractures in elderly people (Randomised Evaluation of Calcium or vitamin D, RECORD): a randomised placebo-controlled trial. Lancet 2005; 365: 1621–8.

34. Jackson RD, LaCroix AZ, Gass M, et al; Women's Health Initiative Investigators. Calcium plus vitamin D supplementation and the risk of fractures. N Engl J Med 2006; 354: 669–83.

35. Andres E, Loukili NH, Noel E, et al. Vitamin B₁₂ (cobalamin) deficiency in elderly patients. CMAJ 2004; 171(3): 251–9.

36. Lokk J. News and views on folate and elderly persons. J Gerontol A Biol Sci Med Sci 2003; 58(4): 354–61.

37. Gjesdal CG, Vollset SE, Ueland PM, et al. Plasma total homocysteine level and bone mineral density: the Hordaland Homocysteine Study. Arch Intern Med 2006; 166(1): 88–94.

38. Selhub J. The many facets of hyperhomocysteinemia: studies from the Framingham cohorts. J Nutr 2006; 136(6): 1726S–30S.

39. Frazier AL, Li L, Cho E, Willett WC, Colditz GA. Adolescent diet and risk of breast cancer. Cancer Causes Control 2004; 15: 73–82.

40. Lee IM, Cook NR, Gaziano JM, et al. Vitamin E in the primary prevention of cardiovascular disease and cancer: the Women's Health Study: a randomized controlled trial. JAMA 2005; 294: 56–65.

41. Lonn E, Bosch J, Yusuf S, et al. Effects of long-term vitamin E supplementation on cardiovascular events and cancer: a randomized controlled trial. JAMA 2005; 293: 1338–47.

42. Miller ER III, Pastor-Barriuso R, Dalal D, et al. Meta-analysis: high-dosage vitamin E supplementation may increase all-cause mortality. Ann Intern Med 2004; 142: 1–11.

43. Fletcher AE, Breeze E, Shetty PS. Antioxidant vitamins and mortality in older persons: findings from the nutrition add-on study to the Medical Research Council Trial of Assessment and Management of Older People in the Community. Am J Clin Nutr 2003; 78(5): 999–1010.

44. Lee DH, Folsom AR, Harnack L, et al. Does supplemental vitamin C increase cardiovascular disease risk in women with diabetes? Am J Clin Nutr 2004; 80: 1194–200.

45. Waters DD, Alderman EL, Hsia J, et al. Effects of hormone replacement therapy and antioxidant vitamin supplements on coronary atherosclerosis in postmenopausal women: a randomized controlled trial. JAMA 2002; 288: 2432–40.

46. Vaquero MP. Magnesium and trace elements in the elderly: intake, status and recommendations. J Nutr Health Aging 2002; 6(2): 147–53.

47. Benton D, Cook R. The impact of selenium supplementation on mood. Biol Psychiatry 1991; 29: 1092–8.

48. Salerno-Kennedy R, Cashman KD. Relationship between dementia and nutrition-related factors and disorders: an overview. Int J Vitam Nutr Res 2005; 75(2): 83–95.

49. Lindeman RD. Mineral requirements. In: Chernoff R, ed. Geriatric Nutrition: The Health Professional's Handbook, 3rd edn. 2006, Boston: Jones & Bartlett (in press).

50. Ozturk S, Cillier AE. Magnesium deficiency over generations in rats with special references to the pathogenesis of the Parkinsonism-dementia complex and amyotrophic lateral sclerosis of Guam. Neuropathology 2006; 26(2): 115–28.

51. Ozturk S, Cillier AE. Magnesium supplementation in the treatment of dementia patients. Med Hypotheses 2006; 67(5): 1223–5.

52. Bhatnagar S, Taneja S. Zinc and cognitive development. Br J Nutr 2001; 85: S139–45.

53. Brownie S. Why are elderly individuals at risk of nutritional deficiency? Int J Nurs Pract 2006; 12: 110–18.

54. Evans WJ. Exercise, nutrition and aging. Clin Geriatr Med 1995; 11: 725–34.

55. Haller J. The vitamin status and its adequacy in the elderly: an international overview. Int J Vitam Nutr Res 1999; 69: 160–8.

56. Jensen GL, McGee M, Binkley J. Nutrition in the elderly. Gastroenterol Clin North Am 2001; 30: 313–34.

57. Wakimoto P, Block G. Dietary intake, dietary patterns and changes with age: epidemiological perspective. J Gerontol A Biol Sci Med Sci 2001; 56 Spec No. 2: 65–80.

58. Blechman MB, Gelb AM. Aging and gastrointestinal physiology. Gastroenterology 1999; 15: 429–38.

59. Pilotto A. Aging and the gastrointestinal tract. Ital J Gastroenterol Hepatol 1999; 31: 137–53.

60. Kim YI, Saltzman JR. The aging gut. In: Chernoff R, ed. Geriatric Nutrition: The Health Professional's Handbook, 3rd edn. 2006, Boston: Jones & Bartlett (in press).

61. Martin WE, Saunders MJ. Oral health in the elderly. In: Chernoff R, ed. Geriatric Nutrition: The Health Professional's Handbook, 3rd edn. 2006, Boston: Jones & Bartlett (in press).

62. Semba RD, Blaum CS, Bartali B, et al. Denture use, malnutrition, frailty, and mortality among older women living in the community. J Nutr Health Aging 2006; 10(2): 161–7.

63. Finkelstein JA, Schiffman SS. Workshop on taste and smell in the elderly: an overview. Physiol Behav 1999; 66: 173–6.

64. Rolls BJ, Phillips PA. Aging and disturbances of thirst and fluid balance. Nutr Rev 1990; 48: 137–44.

65. Suter PM. Vitamin metabolism and requirements in the elderly: selected aspects. In: Chernoff R, ed. Geriatric Nutrition: The Health Professional's Handbook, 3rd edn. 2006, Boston: Jones & Bartlett (in press).

66. Neuvonen PJ, Kivistö KT. The clinical significance of food–drug interactions: a review. Med J Aust 1989; 150: 36–40.

67. Wright L, Hickson M, Frost G. Eating together is important: using a dining room in an acute elderly medical ward increases energy intake. J Hum Nutr Diet 2006; 19: 23–6.

68. Smejkal C. Functional foods. In: Rees M, Mander T, eds. Managing the Menopause without Oestrogen. London: RSM Press; 2004.

69. James SL, Muir JG, Curtis SL, Gibson PR. Dietary fibre: a roughage guide. Intern Med J 2003; 33: 291–6.

70. Salerno-Kennedy R, Cashman KD. The role of nutrition in dementia: an overview. J Br Menopause Soc 2006; 12(2): 44–8.

71. Knoops KT, de Groot LC, Kromhout D, et al. Mediterranean diet, lifestyle factors, and 10-year mortality in elderly European men and women: the HALE project. JAMA 2004; 292: 1433–9.

72. Trichopoulou A, Orfanos P, Norat T, et al. Modified Mediterranean diet and survival: EPIC-elderly prospective cohort study. BMJ 2005; 330: 991.

73. Wikby K, Fägerskiöld A. The willingness to eat. Scand J Caring Sci 2004; 18: 120–7.

74. Remsburg RE, Lukin A, Baran P, et al. Impact of a buffet-style dining program on weight and biochemical indicators of nutritional status in nursing home residents. J Am Diet Assoc 2001; 101: 1460–3.

75. Nijs KA, de Graaf C, Kok FJ, van Staveren WA. Effect of family-style mealtimes on quality of life, physical performance, and body weight of nursing home residents: cluster randomised controlled trial. BMJ 2006: 332: 1180–3.

76. Payette H, Boutier V, Coulombe C, Gray-Donald K. Benefits of nutritional supplementation in free-living, frail, undernourished elderly people: a prospective randomized community trial. J Am Diet Assoc 2002; 102(8): 1088–95.

77. Lauque S, Arnaud-Battandier F, Mansourian R, et al. Protein-energy oral supplementation in malnourished nursing-home residents. A controlled trial. Age Ageing 2000; 29(1): 51–6.

78. Collins CE, Kershaw J, Brockington S. Effect of nutritional supplements on wound healing in home-nursed elderly: a randomized trial. Nutrition 2005; 21(2): 147–55.

79. Milne AC, Avenell A, Potter J. Meta-analysis: protein and energy supplementation in older people. Ann Intern Med 2006; 144(1): 37–48.

80. Bender DA. Daily doses of multivitamin tablets. BMJ 2002; 325: 173–4.

81. Fletcher RH, Fairfield KM. Vitamins for chronic disease prevention in adults: clinical applications. JAMA 2002; 287: 3127–9.

82. Shenkin A. Micronutrient intake in the UK – when to supplement? In: Carr T, Descheemaeker K, eds. Nutrition & Health Current Topics 3. Antwerp: Garant; 105–14.

83. Chernoff R. Nutrition and health promotion in older adults. J Gerontol A Biol Sci Med Sci 2001; 56 Spec No. 2: 47–53.

Home, residential, and palliative care

15

Liv Wergeland Sørbye

INTRODUCTION

Worldwide, the size of the older population is increasing more than that of the overall population and will increase further as the 'baby boomer' generation born between 1945 and 1954 ages, leading to concerns about securing good care for older people.[1] Traditional patterns of care of the elderly are changing and more are electing and wish to live independently of their families, either in their own homes or in residential care (see Chapter 1). The pattern of provision of care is also shifting, with more emphasis on home than residential care. Increased life expectancy is accompanied by a rise in disability-free life expectancy and years lived with disability and their relative proportions vary in different countries.[2,3] The ways in which care of the elderly, both with and without disability, can best be delivered is of great concern to governments, and in the UK has been most recently addressed by the Wanless Report published in 2006.[1]

This chapter focuses on common challenges for care of women over 70 in three settings: home, residential, and palliative. Their needs and how they can be met in their own homes, as well as ensuring acceptable quality of life in a residential setting, are examined. The implications of new technologies such as telecare and dedicated housing are discussed, as well as the needs and support required for both formal and informal carers.

HOME CARE

The major database used in the section on home care is the European Aged in Home Care project (AdHOC).[4] It consists of 4010 people receiving home care services in urban settings in 11 European countries, with a mean age of 82 years, of whom 74.2% are women. In Europe, women 70+ receiving formal home care are on average aged 84.[5] Younger women either manage themselves or obtain informal care from relatives, neighbors, or friends. Important differences exist between individual countries: in Scandinavia, the Netherlands, and the UK less than 10% of elderly women live with one of their children, but in Italy it is 35% (Table 15.1).

Assessing need

Older people in need of home care often have multiple problems related to functional decline caused by aging and disease. The main disability-causing diseases are dementia and depression, coronary heart disease, stroke, arthritis, sensory problems (vision and hearing), and incontinence. A standard way to assess need resulting from disability and impairment is in terms of people's ability to carry out basic activities of daily living (ADLs).[1] The following is a list of widely used (self-care) ADLs:

- get up and down stairs or steps
- go out of doors and walk down the road

Table 15.1 Socioepidemiological data (women 70+; $N = 2826$)

Country and sample size	Average age: mean ($\pm SD$)	Living alone	Living with a child	Primary informal helper: (child / child-in-law)	Hours of informal help weekdays	Hours of informal help weekends
Czech Republic, 321	82.7 ± 5.9	71%	10%	46%	10.1 ± 18.9	5.5 ± 9.4
Denmark, 364	85.3 ± 6.3	82%	1%	60%	2.8 ± 8.5	0.9 ± 3.4
Finland, 140	83.3 ± 6.3	89%	4%	36%	6.6 ± 22.9	2.6 ± 9.9
France, 257	84.0 ± 7.1	46%	23%	67%	18.3 ± 24.2	7.2 ± 9.3
Germany, 423	83.0 ± 6.6	70%	13%	53%	18.9 ± 35.4	7.7 ± 14.4
Iceland, 288	82.8 ± 5.8	75%	7%	65%	8.7 ± 22.9	4.2 ± 9.7
Italy, 236	83.3 ± 7.0	18%	35%	69%	19.9 ± 17.1	8.2 ± 6.9
Netherlands, 147	80.8 ± 6.3	66%	3%	55%	11.4 ± 22.6	4.5 ± 9.1
Norway, 271	84.6 ± 5.8	83%	2%	61%	5.5 ± 16.2	2.2 ± 6.6
Sweden, 174	85.2 ± 6.1	86%	1%	71%	3.7 ± 13.4	1.9 ± 6.1
UK, 205	83.7 ± 6.6	72%	7%	60%	31.2 ± 4.9	13.0 ± 19.4
Total, 2826	83.6 ± 6.5	69%	10%	59%	12.1 ± 25.9	5.2 ± 10.7

Adapted from Sørbye et al.[5]

- get around indoors (except steps)
- wash face and hands
- bath, shower, or wash all over
- transfer: get in and out of bed (or chair)
- use toilet
- get dressed and undressed
- feed self.

People are asked whether they can usually manage these tasks: on their own without help; on their own with difficulty; only with someone else's help; or not at all. The latter two possibilities can be combined to define an ADL failure. Four core ADLs are: transfer, use toilet, get dressed and undressed, and feed self. The AdHOC study showed that the majority of the older women living at home were still able to move around and get to the toilet independently.[4]

In addition to ADLs, the ability to perform instrumental activities of daily living (IADLs) can be assessed. These activities include shopping, cleaning, laundry, preparation of hot meals, and managing personal affairs (e.g. paying bills). Problems with functioning may have both physical and cognitive causes. Cognitive impairment not only limits ability to carry out ADLs but also leads to concerns about an individual's safety. There are a number of instruments for measuring cognitive functioning, which generally combine memory, awareness, and reasoning tests.[6] In categorizing the results, it is usual to distinguish between mild and severe cognitive impairment.

Once need has been assessed, care plans can be formulated. They need to be individualized and should give a structure and timetable which can be adhered to. An individual care plan consists of

1. Client requirements: activities and services
2. Type of support provided by different services (home care, meals, equipment, respite care, etc.).
3. Service providers and how they should be organized.

4. Time schedules.
5. Methods of evaluation to ensure the service is appropriate.
6. Overall responsibility for the service.

Common health problems

Older women staying in the community may suffer pain, depression, loneliness, cognitive impairment, urinary incontinence (see Chapter 7) and unintended weight loss due to poor nutrition (see Chapter 14) (Table 15.2). These need to be regularly evaluated by carers.[7]

Pain

Pain is a frequent problem for home care recipients. Onder et al, using the AdHOC database, found that those with pain were more likely to be women, and this was associated with depression.[8]

Oral health

Oral health is important not only for self-esteem but also a key factor for the maintenance of an adequate diet (see Chapter 14). Cognitive impairment and reduced physical health can lead to

Table 15.2 Selected conditions in home care clients (N = 2826)

Conditions	N (%)
Daily pain	1271 (45.0)
Use of incontinence pads	1242 (43.9)
Problem with short-term memory	947 (33.5)
Self-rated bad health	845 (29.9)
Loneliness	639 (22.6)
Use of antidepressants	412 (14.6)
Unintended weight loss	370 (13.1)
Signs of abuse	127 (4.5)

Adapted from Sørbye et al.[5]

inadequate oral care and side effects of medication may result in dry mouth.

Pressure ulcers

Pressure ulcers may result from reduced mobility, cardiovascular disease, malnutrition, and incontinence. The most common sites are the sacrum, heels, hips, ankles, elbows, and occiput. Most pressure damage can be prevented, and guidelines are available such as those developed by the European Pressure Ulcer Advisory Panel.[9]

Fatigue

Fatigue can reduce motivation, impair physical activity, and cause depression. Different assessment tools have tried to identify symptoms of fatigue and this may be supplemented with a diary.[10]

Cognitive impairment

In the AdHOC study, 33.5% of women had problems with short-term memory.[4] In the five Nordic countries, relatively few older women with serious cognitive impairment lived alone in their own homes. This is due mainly to the high provision of residential care. For those who wish to live in their own homes, the main problems are accidents such as fires or wandering and not knowing where they are: here, new technologies may be of help (see below). For example, heat or smoke detectors can detect fires and GSM (Global System for Mobile communications) bracelets monitored via assisted global positioning system (GPS) can be used to notify carers if the wearer wanders outside a predefined 'secure zone.'

Frailty

Frailty represents a state of reduced homeostasis and resistance to stress. Cohen et al surveyed

1388 frail patients with a mean age of 74 years.[11] They suggest that risk of frailty is present if two or more of the following markers are found:

- inability to perform one or more basic ADL functions in the 3 days prior to assessment
- a stroke in the past 3 months
- depression
- dementia
- a history of falls
- one or more unplanned admissions in the past 3 months
- difficulty in walking
- malnutrition
- prolonged bed rest
- incontinence.

Frail people need close follow-up and documentation that basic needs are being met by their carers.

Problems with home care

The key issues are ensuring security and preventing accidents and falls, as well as ascertaining that the individual is still alive. An important concern is that elderly people who rarely go out of their homes may be dead for some time, even several months, before anybody notices. A common whistleblower is the postman who finds unemptied mail boxes. In Copenhagen, a study of the death certificates in 1994 showed that 13% of the women and 15% of the men were found dead – alone in their apartments. The age distribution showed that the rate increased with advancing age, the mean for women was 77 years and that for men 61 years.[12]

Older people tend to live in old dwellings, which are harder and more expensive to heat than newer ones. Hypothermia may aggravate concurrent medical conditions, leading to death,

and excess winter mortality is well documented[13] (see Chapter 2).

Older women, and particularly those living alone, know that they are vulnerable to crime. Organizations to provide volunteers to accompany women when they go out or security alarms may be helpful. On average, 35% of the women aged over 70 years in the AdHOC study who lived alone had a security alarm, but this varied from country to country, ranging from 73% in Norway to 5% in Italy and none in the Czech Republic.[15]

Some older women may be abused by carers. At least one indicator of possible abuse (unexplained injuries, fractures, or burns) was present in 4.4 % of the women 70+ in the AdHOC population.[4] Abuse was more frequently registered in countries where older people mainly lived with relatives and had little intervention from formal services.

New influences on care

Climate tourism

In the US there are examples of villages for older people, especially in Florida and California. Older people from the northern states and Canada move south to enjoy a warmer climate. In Europe, older people from northern countries settle in the south, especially in Spain, during the winter season.[14] Modern housing stock is available. However, lack of community-based home care has resulted in elderly Nordic people returning home.

Housing and extra care housing

The rising number of older people, combined with increased longevity, will create a much greater need for properties suitable for the impaired and as such a need exists for assistive technologies such as stairlifts, and/or ground floor bedrooms and bathrooms. Extra care housing (also referred to as very sheltered housing) with round the clock care and support on offer, sometimes with nursing support and a meals service, is another option.[1] These housing complexes may be communities specifically for older people.

Leisure World Laguna Hills is one example of a community for retired people.[15] Leisure World is located about 50 miles south of Los Angeles and has about 18 000 residents with an average age of 77, and a minimum age requirement of 55. It is of modern design and has good security and staff to deal with emergencies. Consequently, older people who seek alternative accommodation due to isolation or loneliness may increase their social contact and well-being in a retirement village.[16] However, as frailty increases, loneliness and depression occur.[17] Also, living in an elderly community reduces exposure to younger generations and could potentially be restrictive.

Telecare and related technology

'Telecare' describes any service bringing health and social care directly to a user, generally in their own homes, supported by information and communication technology.[1,18] The principle of telecare is that data are collected through sensors, fed into a home hub, and sent electronically to a call or monitoring center. Basic telecare units include fall alarms, safety sensors for risks such as gas leaks and bath floods, and 'wander' monitors for people with dementia. More sophisticated 'intelligent' systems are designed to recognize changes in activity levels, such as visits to the toilet or fridge, which may indicate changes in a person's condition. Interventions can then be implemented early, with the emphasis on prevention. 'Telehealth' can be defined as the remote monitoring of vital signs, such as temperature and blood pressure, which can then be assessed by health professionals.

A potential disadvantage of these technologies is they could reduce interaction with carers and increase loneliness. The counterargument is that telecare can allow redeployment of carer time, with a shift of resources towards more meaningful activities.

Cost-effectiveness of these interventions is a major issue. Various pilot studies are beginning to offer evidence that providing telecare can prevent a move into residential care by an older person who feels unsafe and vulnerable in the community.[19]

In the UK the biggest telecare pilot study is the 'Opening Doors for Older People' project in West Lothian which started in 1999.[1] The council is providing technology packages for its 'Home Safety Service' to everyone in the district aged ≥60 (about 10 000 households). The aim is to increase the level of care as needs increase, rather than moving the person into increasingly intensive care settings. Smart technology is being used in newly built housing developments designed to offer 'Housing with Care' with an onsite staff team for those who cannot manage in their own homes. By February 2006, there were 1950 Home Safety Service households with a package consisting of:

- a 'lifeline' unit, which links sensors to the call center when triggered
- two passive infrared (PIR) detectors to monitor activity and potential intruders
- two flood detectors, activated by leaking pipes, overflowing baths, etc.
- one heat sensor, sensitive to both high and low temperatures
- one smoke detector.

About 10% of participating households had additional technology such as falls detectors, falls alarms, medication reminders, and bed occupancy monitors. The whole project is supported by an intensively trained care team. In an interim evaluation, nearly all the respondents reported the positive impact of the smart technology, which had been important in relieving worries about falling and about home security, and this has also been found by others.[20,21] However, there are ethical issues with people feeling that they are being controlled by others.[22]

RESIDENTIAL CARE

Moving from home to residential care

Increasing disability leads to the need for residential care. Table 15.3 shows the reasons given by social workers for admissions to care homes. The leading causes are physical and mental health problems.[23]

More women than men live in residential care, and the proportion varies worldwide. In the

Table 15.3 Reasons for admission of older people to care homes

Reason for admission	Percentage
Physical health problems	69
Mental health problems	43
Functional disablement	42
Stress on carers	38
Lack of motivation	22
Present home physically unsuitable	15
Family breakdown (including loss of carer)	8
Need for rehabilitation	6
Fear of being the victim of crime	4
Abuse	2
Loneliness or isolation	2
Homelessness	1
Number of individuals	2573

Note: multiple answers possible so percentages add up to more than 100%.

UK, 5.2% of women aged 75–84 live in residential care, compared with 3.2% of men in the same age group.[24] A comparison between 10 countries from three continents showed that between 2 and 5% of elderly people lived in nursing homes.[25] In Norway, 15.4% of individuals aged ≥80 live in a nursing home.[26] In the US, 44% of the women are admitted to nursing homes from a hospital and in the Netherlands the corresponding value is 50%.[25] In the US, 33% of the women had lived in their own home until some acute illness occurred or complications of a chronic disease required hospital admission; the corresponding value for the Netherlands is 35%.[27,28]

Characteristics of residential care residents

The principal database referred to in this section is the 1997 US National Nursing Home Survey, which has information on 10 929 women in residential care.[27] In the US, 89% of women in residential care were aged over 75.[29] The average length of stay for women is 5 months longer than for their male counterparts. Dependency in toilet use, eating, and use of a wheelchair is more common in residential care than in those living at home. Whereas residential care may be short term for rehabilitation after an accident or an acute illness, the majority will stay for the rest of their lives. On average, this is 2.5 years for women.

Mental illness

The prevalence of dementia and depression in residential care homes varies widely. For Alzheimer's disease or other types of dementias, it ranges from 50 to 80% in different nursing home populations. An international comparison of depression among nursing home residents showed that the prevalence in Canada and the Netherlands was about 30%, whereas the corresponding value was 18% in Sweden and 14% in the US.[30]

Delivering residential care

The quality of care and vulnerability of residents to potential physical and mental abuse are areas of major concern. Most countries have developed measures to address quality. For example in the UK, The Care Standards Act 2000 introduced a set of National Minimum Standards for Care Homes and also established a General Social Care Council to regulate the training and conduct of social care staff.[31] In the US, the 1987 Federal Nursing Home Reform Act from the Omnibus Budget Reconciliation Act (OBRA) created a national minimum set of standards of care and rights for people living in registered nursing facilities.[32] Thus, inspections can be conducted to ensure that official guidelines are followed. OBRA '87 led to implementation of Resident Assessment Instrument (RAI) quality indicators (QIs) to identify standards of care.[33] QIs are markers of potentially poor or good care practices and are the starting point for evaluating quality of care; they can provide information for those looking for a residential care home. Jensdóttir et al undertook an international comparison of QIs in the US, Iceland, and Canada.[34] They found great variation in the use of feeding tubes, prevalence of incontinence, pressure ulcers, falls, and use of antipsychotic drugs.

OBRA '87 focused on abuse and neglect in nursing homes. Neglect is 'failure of a person having the care or custody of an elderly person or dependent adult to exercise that degree of care which a reasonable person in a like position would exercise'.[35] Unreasonable physical restraint or inappropriate use of antipsychotics should be avoided. Persistent poor–quality care is associated with low staffing levels, and restraints tend to be used for patients with behavior problems, dementia, or low ADL functioning.[35] The reasons given for their use are protection of the patient or other individuals or a need to undertake essential care or treatment. It is of concern that protocols for quality assurance about the use of restraint are lacking, as was found in a study of Norwegian nursing homes.[36] Older women living in nursing homes are often severely functionally and cognitively impaired; they need trained staff. Not surprisingly, nursing home quality depends on the ratio of carers to residents as well as training home support.[37–39]

PALLIATIVE CARE

The World Health Organization defines palliative care as:

> an approach that improves the quality of life of patients and their families facing the problems associated with life-threatening illness, through the prevention and relief of suffering by means of early identification and impeccable assessment and treatment of pain and other problems, physical, psychosocial and spiritual.[40]

Palliative care provides relief from pain and other distressing symptoms, affirms life and regards dying as a normal process, and intends neither to hasten nor to prolong death. Palliative care integrates the psychological and spiritual aspects of patient care, and offers a support system to help patients live as actively as possible until death. It also offers a support system to help the family cope during the patient's illness and in their own bereavement. Using a team approach, palliative care addresses the needs of patients and their families, including bereavement counseling if necessary.

Palliative care and hospice programs have grown rapidly in recent years in response to an increasing proportion of the population living with chronic, debilitating, and life-threatening illness. Hospital is still the most common place to die in countries with developed public health systems. However, the average length of stay has decreased mainly due to the increase in home care nursing.[41,42]

Palliative care has traditionally been associated with cancer. However, older people with multiple health problems (cardiovascular disease, dementia) also need palliative care. This care can be delivered in a variety of settings, such as hospitals, nursing homes, and the community, but availability varies between countries.[43] Whatever the setting, it is essential that care is delivered by trained health professionals to the same high standard.

Clinical guidelines

Different interest groups have developed guidelines to meet the challenges of palliative care. Ferrell compared six models of end-of-life care and found three common domains: physical, psychological, and social.[44] The most comprehensive guidelines are published by the National Consensus Project for Quality Palliative Care (NCP) in the US in 2004.[45] Eight domains were identified as the framework for these guidelines:

- Structure and Processes
- Physical Aspects of Care
- Psychological and Psychiatric Aspects of Care
- Social Aspects of Care
- Spiritual, Religious, and Existential Aspects of Care
- Cultural Aspects of Care
- Care of the Imminently Dying Patient
- Ethical and Legal Aspects of Care.

It is hoped that widespread adoption of guidelines such as these will help establish palliative care as an integral component of the healthcare of persons with life-threatening and debilitating chronic illness.

Place of death

Most studies have found that around 75% of respondents would prefer to die at home.[43]

However, 75–80% of elderly Europeans die in an institution.[46,47] Peters and Sellick examined two groups of cancer patients.[48] They concluded that terminally ill cancer patients receiving home-based care have better health status and quality of life than those cared for in an inpatient setting, and patients cared for at home have greater control over their illness. Cancer patients who die in nursing homes tend to be older, not living with a spouse, and more functionally impaired.[49] To provide home-based palliative care, additional support by informal carers is also required, as shown in a study undertaken in the Netherlands by Klinkenberg et al.[50] They found that patients receiving informal as well as formal home care had an increased possibility of dying at home. Consequently, it seems important that formal caregivers are supported by informal caregivers, and vice versa. Informal care could be provided by relatives, friends, or volunteers, but may not always be available.

CARING FOR CARERS

Care can be provided by either formal or informal carers. Caring may be stressful for carers, as they are dealing with people with physical and cognitive impairments. Training and support for carers is essential for the provision of good-quality care for the elderly.

Formal care

Large numbers of people are involved in providing care for older people. It has been estimated that in 2003/4 in England, 680 000 people were working in services for older people.[51] The voluntary sector accounts for a minority of the workforce, being about 11%. Recruitment and retention of staff remains a big challenge, since other sectors pay higher salaries and the work is stressful. In the UK, much of the social care workforce is minimally qualified and poorly trained. Lack of financial incentives and time constraints may explain the relatively low level of qualification in social care.[1]

Informal care

The provision of long-term care for older people relies very heavily on the contribution from informal carers. It is estimated that in 2000 in England, there were around 3–4 million people providing care to those aged over 65.[52] More than one-fifth of carers who are living with the care recipient provide care for $\geq$100 hours a week. The tasks performed by informal carers reflect those performed by formal carers, but vary in the proportions devoted to different types of support. Tasks such as personal care and medication make up the majority of formal carers' work but are provided by smaller proportions of informal carers.[52] Informal carers devote most time to practical care tasks such as shopping and laundry. Large numbers of carers also see a key role in providing company and supervision. This task is particularly important when the care recipient is cognitively impaired.

Of carers in total, the highest numbers are children (and children-in-law) of the care recipient (filial carers) (Table 15.4). Married or cohabiting adults appear to be more likely to be carers than those who are single or previously married (19% compared with 10% and 12%, respectively).[52]

Being a carer is also significantly linked to age and gender. The probability of becoming a carer increases with age.[53] In 2000, 16% of people over the age of 65 were providing some form of care. The role of caring has traditionally been performed by women. Thus, women >70 should not be considered solely as care recipients, since they may also be providing care. Whereas in recent years the gender division with regard to care provision has changed, care tends still to be

Table 15.4 Relationships of carer to care recipient in Great Britain

Relationship of carer to care recipient	Great Britain (%)[a]	Great Britain (millions)[b]
Spouse	18	1.2
Child/child in law	52	3.5
Friend/neighbor	21	1.4
Other	30	2.0

[a] Percentages add up to more than 100, because some carers were looking after more than one person and are therefore counted more than once in these figures.
[b] Estimate, Wanless Review.[1]
Based on figures in Maher and Green.[52]

administered by more women than men (11% vs 7%).[52,54] Also, in both spousal and filial relationships, more women perform the caring role than men. However, in their later years (70+), a high proportion of male spouses are carers.

Health of carers is of great concern. The Princess Royal Trust for Carers indicated that 85% of carers said that caring had a negative impact on their health.[55] The main self-reported problems experienced by carers, which have been attributed to some extent to caring responsibilities, include:

- feeling both tired and stressed (20%)
- being short-tempered (17%)
- feeling depressed (14%)
- disturbed/loss of sleep (14%).[52]

This is in addition to other problems and conditions that have been associated with caring, particularly when for long hours and over extended periods.[55,56] These can include anxiety, depression, and psychiatric illness, lowered social functioning, increased susceptibility to physical illness, increased rates of chronic diseases during episodes of caring, and general negative impacts on physical well-being. These problems have been documented in other countries. In the AdHOC study

23% of carers looking after women aged over 70 were stressed, and this was significantly higher if they lived with the person they were caring for.[4] However, in spite of a high prevalence of care burden stress in countries such as Italy, care-givers felt that the relative would not be better off elsewhere.[13] The predisposition to having health problems as a result of caring varies with a range of factors, including severity and duration of need and the intensity and nature of caring. The characteristics of the carer also matter (age, sex, relationship with care recipient).[52,55,56] The effects can be compounded by a lack of support or respite for carers generally or poor access to healthcare.[57] The insecurity and fear that family caregivers have lived through for years does not disappear when the relative dies. Lim and Zebrack state, after a critical review of caregiver literature, that we know too little about the outcomes of stress–related variables over time.[58]

In addition, there are other effects such as social exclusion and erosion of personal relation-ships.[55] Various types of support are available for carers to reduce carer stress, such as respite care, day care services, and carer support groups, but availability varies between countries. Also, older carers may not be aware of them.[59] Formal carers should be able to give advice about support networks for informal carers such as Help the Aged and Age Concern in the UK.[60,61]

CONCLUSIONS

Caring for an aging population is an important public health issue. The elderly may not just be care recipients but also informal carers for a rela-tive, and these tend to be women. Traditional family structures have changed, with a greater wish for independent living. Governments need to plan the future of care. Decisions need to be made about the range and type of services, the size of the workforce providing care, the implications for housing, and the use of technology to assist people to live with more control.

ACKNOWLEDGMENTS

I am grateful for the help provided by my collaborators represented by Roberto Bernabi, Italy, for the AdHOC Project Research Group founded by the European Commission Vth Frame-work Programme, contract number QLRT-2000-00002.

REFERENCES

1. Wanless D. Securing good care for older people. Taking a long term view. Wanless social care review. http://www.kingsfund.org.uk/resources/publications/securing_good.html. Accessed August 7, 2006.
2. Aijanseppa S, Notkola IL, Tijhuis M, et al. Physical functioning in elderly Europeans: 10 year changes in the north and south: the HALE project. J Epidemiol Community Health 2005; 59(5): 413–19.
3. Mathers C. International trends in health expectancies: Do they provide evidence for expansion or compression of morbidity?. In: Compression of Morbidity (Department of Health and Aged Care Occasional Papers Series no 4). Canberra: Department of Health and Aged Care; 1999.
4. Carpenter I, Gambassi G, Topinkova E, et al. Community care in Europe. The Aged in Home Care project (AdHOC). Aging Clin Exp Res 2004; 16(4): 259–69.
5. Sørbye LW. Characteristics of Urban Women Aged 70+ in 11 European Countries. The Aged in HOme Care project (AdHOC). Oslo: Diakonhjemmet University College; December 2006.

6. Comas-Herrera A, Wittenberg R, Pickard L, Knapp M. Cognitive impairment in older people: its implications for future demand for services and costs. PSSRU discussion paper No. 1728. London: Alzheimer's Research Trust; 2003.

7. Morris JN, Fries BE, Steel K, et al. Comprehensive clinical assessment in community setting: applicability of the MDS-HC. J Am Geriatr Soc 1997; 45: 1017–24.

8. Onder G, Landi F, Gambassi G, et al. Association between pain and depression among older adults in Europe: results from the Aged in Home Care (AdHOC) project: a cross-sectional study. J Clin Psychiatry 2005; 66(8): 982–8.

9. European Pressure Ulcer Advisory Panel: www.equap.org. Accessed August 7, 2006.

10. Loge JH, Ekeberg Ø, Kaasa S. Fatigue in the general Norwegian population: normative data and associations. J Psychosom Res 1998; 1: 53–65.

11. Cohen HJ, Feussner JR, Weinberger M, et al. A controlled trial of inpatient and outpatient geriatric evaluation and management. N Engl J Med 2002; 346: 905–12.

12. Smith E, Larsen DF, Rosdahl N. [To die alone in a big city]. Ugeskr Læger 2001; 163: 3069–73. [in Danish]

13. Healy JD. Excess winter mortality in Europe: a cross country analysis identifying key risk factors. J Epidemiol Community Health 2003; 57(784): 789.

14. Mathers C. International trends in health expectancies: do they provide evidence for expansion or compression of morbidity? Compression of Morbidity Workshop Papers, Occasional Papers Series No. 4, Department of Health and Ageing, Canberra 2006; 33–55.

15. http://www.cnn.com/US/9903/03/leisure.world.01/. Accessed March 2006.

16. Buys LR. Life in a retirement village: implications for contact with community and village friends. Gerontology 2001; 47(1): 55–9.

17. Adams KB, Sanders S, Auth EA. Loneliness and depression in independent living retirement communities: risk and resilience factors. Aging Ment Health 2004; 8(6): 475–85.

18. Audit Commission. Older People: Implementing Telecare. London: Audit Commission; 2004.

19. Lansley P, McCreadie C, Tinker A. Can adapting the homes of older people and providing assistive technology pay its way? Age Ageing 2004; 33(6): 571–6.

20. Bowes A, McColgan G. Smart Technology at Home: users' and carers' perspectives, interim report. Stirling: West Lothian Council and the University of Stirling; 2005.

21. Tinker A, Lansley P. Introducing assistive technology into the existing homes of older people: feasibility, acceptability, costs and outcomes. J Telemed Telecare 2005; 11(Suppl 1): 1–3.

22. Marshall M. Technology is the shape of the future for dementia care. J Dementia Care 1995; 3: 12–14.

23. Bebbington A, Darton R, Netten A. Care Homes for Older People: Volume 2, Admissions, Needs and Outcomes. The 1995/96 National Longitudinal Survey of Publicly-Funded Admissions. London: Personal Social Services Research Unit; 2001.

24. England and Wales: National Statistics. Census 2001: People Resident in Communal Establishments. State Base S126. http://www.oft.gov.uk/NR/rdonlyres/6131BFAF-F8E8-4B19-B44A-97FCE93D98D3/ 0/oft780c.pdf. Accessed August 16, 2006.

25. Ribbe MW, Ljunggren G, Steel K, et al. Nursing homes in 10 nations: a comparison between countries and settings. Age Ageing 1997; 26(Suppl 2): 3–12.

26. Statistics of Norway. Statistical Yearbook. Oslo: The Norwegian Central Bureau of Statistics; 2005. www.ssb.no.

27. Gabrel CS. Characteristics of elderly nursing home current residents and discharges: data from the 1997 National Nursing Home Survey. Adv Data 2000; (312): 1–15. http://www.cdc.gov/nchs/data/ad/ad312.pdf.

28. Achterberg W. Project: caring for quality. The use of Minimum Data Set (MDS) for research into quality of care and patient functioning in nursing homes. University of Amsterdam; 2004.

29. Arias E. United States Life Tables 2002. National Vital Statistic Report, 2002; 53(6). http://www.cdc.gov/nchs/data/nvsr/nvsr53/nvsr53_06.pdf.

30. Holtkamp CM. Effects of the resident assessment on quality of life in nursing home. Amsterdam: Faculty of Health, University of Amsterdam; 2003.

31. General Social Care Council (GSCC). Code of Practice for Social Care Workers and Code of Practice for Employers of Social Care Workers. London: GSCC; 2002.

32. Federal Nursing Home Reform Act. http://www.ltcombudsman.org/uploads/OBRA87summary.pdf. Accessed August 8, 2006.

33. InterRAI Welcome to interRAI. http://www.interrai.org. Accessed August 8, 2006.

34. Jensdóttir AB, Rantz M, Hjaltadottir I, et al. International comparison of quality indicators in United States, Icelandic and Canadian nursing facilities. Int Nurs Rev 2003; 50(2): 79–84.

35. Castle NG. Nursing homes with persistent deficiency citations for physical restraint use. Med Care 2002; 40(10): 868–78.

36. Kirkevold O, Engedal K. A study into the use of restraint in nursing homes in Norway. Br J Nurs 2004; 13(15): 902–5.

37. Lee CL, Liu TL, Wu LJ, Chung UL, Lee LC. Cost and care quality between licensed nursing homes under different types of ownership. J Nurs Res 2002; 10(2): 151–60.

38. Rantz MJ, Hicks L, Grando V, et al. Nursing home quality, cost, staffing, and staff mix. Gerontologist 2004; 44(1): 24–38.

39. Fossey J, Ballard C, Juszczak E, et al. Effect of enhanced psychosocial care on antipsychotic use in nursing home residents with severe dementia: cluster randomised trial. BMJ 2006; 332(7544): 756–61.

40. World Health Organization. WHO Definition of Palliative Care. http://www.who.int/cancer/palliative/definition.html. Retrieved March 21, 2005.

41. Higginson IJ. End-of-life care: lessons from other nations. J Palliat Med 2005; 8(Suppl 1): S161–73.

42. Sørbye LW. A longitudinal study on dying in a Norwegian hospital. Int J Palliat Nurs 2000; 6(2): 71–9.

43. Davies E, Higginson IJ. Better palliative care for older people. WHO Europe 2004. www.euro.who.int/. Accessed August 8, 2006.

44. Ferrell BR. Overview of the domains of variables relevant to end-of-life care. J Palliat Med 2005; 8(Suppl 1): S22–9.

45. National Consensus Project. Clinical Practice Guidelines for Palliative Care; 2004. www.nationalconsensusproject.org. Accessed August 8, 2006.

46. Cohen J, Bilsen J, Hoort P, et al. Dying at home or in an institution using death certificates to explore the factors associated with place of death. Health Policy 2006; 78: 319–29.

47. Jordhoy MS, Fayers P, Saltnes T, et al. A palliative-care intervention and death at home: a cluster randomised trial. Lancet 2000; 356(9233): 888–93.

48. Peters L, Sellick K. Quality of life of cancer patients receiving inpatient and home-based palliative care. J Adv Nurs 2006; 53(5): 524–33.

49. Jordhoy MS, Saltvedt I, Fayers P, et al. Which cancer patients die in nursing homes? Quality of life, medical and sociodemographic characteristics. Palliat Med 2003; 17(5): 433–44.

50. Klinkenberg M, Visser G, van Groenou MI, et al. The last 3 months of life: care, transitions and the place of death of older people. Health Soc Care Community 2005; 13(5): 420–30.

51. Eborall C. The State of the Social Care Workforce 2004: The second Skills Research & Intelligence Annual Report and Statistical Appendix. Leeds: Skills for Care; 2005.

52. Maher J, Green H. Carers 2000. London: The Stationery Office; 2002.

53. Hirst M. Transitions to informal care in Great Britain during the 1990s. J Epidemiol Community Health 2002; 56: 579–87.

54. Office for National Statistics 2004. Marriages and Divorces 1950–2001. 2004. www.statistics.gov.uk/statbase. Accessed August 9, 2006.

55. Keeley B, Clarke M. Carers Speak Out Project: Report on Finding and Recommendations.

London: The Princess Royal Trust for Carers; 2002.

56. Hirst M. Carer distress: a prospective, population-based study. Soc Sci Med 2005; 61: 697–708.

57. Arksey H, Hirst M. Unpaid carers' access to and use of primary care services. Primary Health Care Res Devel 2005; 6(2): 101–16.

58. Lim JW, Zebrack B. Caring for family members with chronic physical illness: a critical review of caregiver literature. Health Qual Life Outcomes 2004; 2: 50.

59. Rees J, O'Boyle C, MacDonagh R. Quality of life: impact of chronic illness on the partner. J R Soc Med 2001; 94: 563–6.

60. Help the Aged: www.helptheaged.org.uk.

61. Age Concern: www.ageconcern.org.uk.

Keeping sex alive in later years   16

Kathleen E Walsh, Laura A Berman, and Stephanie Wai

INTRODUCTION

Elderly sexuality should not be viewed as an oxymoron. A healthy sexuality is a right that every woman possesses, in all stages of her life. Regardless of age, an individual's sexuality has an enormous impact on their quality of life. Sexual experience and relationships are strongly associated with emotional well-being, safety, and intimacy. All individuals, particularly the elderly, can experience the negative potential of illness, medications, and life stressors on their sexual interest and function. The United Kingdom has an aging population. The overall population grew by 7%, from 55.9 million in 1971 to 59.8 million in mid-2004. This growth, however, has not taken place evenly across all age groups. The percentage of the population aged ≥65 increased from 13% to 16%, but within the population aged ≥65, the proportion of people aged ≥85 has increased from 7% in mid-1971 to 12% in mid-2004.[1] Research in female sexuality at both the basic and social sciences levels, including older age cohorts, has burgeoned over the past several years. It is not possible to recognize and treat the effects of aging on sexuality without understanding the psychosocial and physiological changes that occur with aging and their effects on sexual desire and response. As sexual health is very much a 'couple phenomenon', male problems must not be ignored.

SEXUALITY AND THE OLDER WOMAN

Sexuality is an important component of a woman's overall health and well-being. Her sexual experiences underpin how she feels and how she defines herself. Many different factors impact on the sexual experience of the aging woman, as shown in Figure 16.1. Combinations of physical, psychological, emotional, societal, and relational experiences create a unique sexual blueprint for each woman. These factors change as a woman ages, and it is important to address all aspects in a comprehensive manner when attending to the aging woman's sexual health.

Contrary to general societal beliefs, older women have an interest in and need for maintaining sexual activity.[2] Regardless of age, a satisfying sex life is strongly associated with improved relationship satisfaction and higher quality of life.[3–8] Although the types and frequencies of sexual acts may change with age, satisfaction can indeed remain high.[9,10] A number of studies show that women can continue to enjoy meaningful sexual relations in their older years, especially if they enjoyed fulfilling sexual relations earlier in life.[10,11] This holds true for women in their 90s and even centenarians who continue to engage in sexual contact.[9]

Despite such encouraging findings, until recently, elderly sexuality was viewed as a trivial topic in the medical and psychological fields.

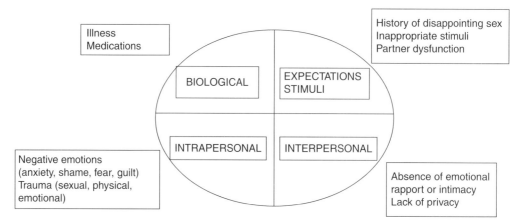

Figure 16.1 Factors affecting sexual well-being.

Cultural stereotypes glorifying an inflated value of youth and depicting the elderly as helpless and asexual contribute to the neglect of this issue by many health professionals.[12] It is important, however, that clinicians recognize the legitimacy of older women's sexual concerns and the value of providing this heterogeneous population with open and unbiased care.

This chapter provides an overview of the medical and psychological concerns that elderly females face in addressing their sexuality.

ATTITUDES TOWARD SEXUALITY AND THE OLDER WOMAN

Attitudes toward sexuality in the elderly play a significant role in affecting the sexual identities of older women. Unfortunately, many cultural attitudes are internalized by the elderly and are ultimately manifested in their behaviors. Thus, contemporary societal stereotypes making sexuality a taboo for older women constrain their behavior.

Today's most pervasive viewpoint of sexuality is that it is reserved for the young. In our youth-obsessed society, aging is commonly viewed as tragic and the elderly are falsely assumed to be asexual.[12,13] Societal attitudes toward female sexuality have become more open as a result of

more liberal attitudes in the media, and many people now characterize a woman's sexual expression as a healthy and pleasurable part of life. However, older women are generally excluded from this belief. A premium is placed on the perceived benefits of being young, such as physical strength and attractiveness, independence, potential for growth, ability to earn a living, and sexual freedom.[14] The implications of such widespread conceptions can be particularly damaging for the older woman, who may be retired, physically disabled, or who no longer fits cultural standards of physical beauty. Such women may come to regard themselves as insignificant members of society or a burden to others.[12] Moreover, many otherwise happy and well-adjusted aging women may internalize negative stereotypes that the elderly are non-sexual, making them reluctant to verbalize their sexual desires for fear of being ridiculed or viewed as depraved.[15]

Sadly, many older adults in assisted-living institutions and convalescent homes are given insufficient or no support and information whatsoever about sexual health. Staff members at residential care homes often find it difficult to address the sexual concerns of their patients, reporting feelings of confusion, embarrassment, helplessness, and negativity when confronted with sexual situations.[16] One study investigated groups of nurses and found that many of them did not even believe that older adults in their 70s had sexual relations at all.[17] Clearly, this finding may not be isolated, and it is important to provide nursing home staff with adequate information and training around facilitating the sexual health of the elderly in their care. At the same time, clinicians should work toward unravelling these preconceptions of sexuality with their patients. A permissive attitude toward sex and a positive, trusting, and empathetic relationship between patient and practitioner can be useful in building a greater sense of self-worth and sexual self-esteem in elderly women.[18,19]

Having recognized that, it is important to note that many practitioners exhibit strong negative emotional reactions when discussing sexuality with their older patients. Clinicians must be cognizant of their own attitudes and reactions in order to take appropriate steps to avoid transferring their own discomfort onto their patients.[12] By recognizing personal biases and misconceptions, the practitioner can maintain objectivity and neutrality when treating older women with sexual challenges.

ANATOMICAL AND PHYSIOLOGICAL CHANGES

The older woman experiences numerous changes to her genitourinary system as she approaches and proceeds through menopause and beyond (Table 16.1). The changes in hormone levels, in particular the decrease in estrogen, are believed to cause a significant number of these physical changes. As a prime example, the vaginal epithelium is highly estrogen-dependent, and when estrogen levels decrease, there is a loss of glycogen, which leads to flattening and decreased elasticity of the epithelium. Women with vaginal atrophy commonly complain of generalized vaginal discomfort and, in particular, pain with penetration

Table 16.1 Genitourinary changes in the older female

Loss of fat and thinning of subcutaneous tissue from the mons pubis
Reduction of pubic hair
Atrophy of labia majora and labia minora
Atrophy of vaginal epithelium
Shortening and decreased elasticity of vagina
Decrease in vaginal secretions

(dyspareunia). In addition, changes in the vaginal epithelium can increase a women's susceptibility to urinary symptoms such as frequency, urgency, dysuria, incontinence, and/or recurrent infections. Reduced estrogen levels may also affect peri-urethral tissues and contribute to pelvic laxity and stress incontinence. In association with lower levels of estrogen, changes in vaginal pH and flora may predispose the peri- and postmenopausal woman to vaginal and urinary tract infections. Atrophy responds well to both local and systemic estrogen administration.[20] However, local hormonal therapy in the form of vaginal creams, tablets, rings, or pessaries is preferred in those who have no other symptoms such as hot flushes, since it avoids systemic side effects.[21] If used in the recommended dose, no added progestogen is required to provide endometrial protection.[21] Many women can also benefit from non-hormonal vaginal lubricants or bioadhesive moisturizers.

A wide array of changes in sexual response can occur in the older woman secondary to both hormonal and non-hormonal changes (see Figure 16.2).

For example, she may experience diminished or delayed arousal to sexual stimulation. Genital blood flow and tissue engorgement may be absent or reduced, affecting sensation and sexual pleasure. Older women are less likely to experience vasocongestion of their breasts and nipple erection. The ability to achieve orgasm usually remains, despite the fact that the overall number and intensity of the orgasm decreases. Older women may occasionally experience painful uterine contrac-

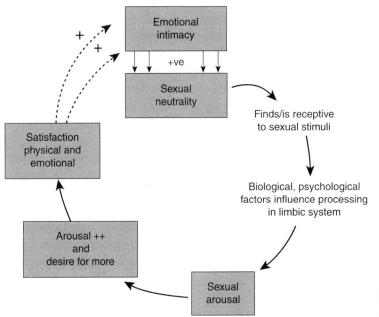

Figure 16.2 The female sexual response. (Adapted from Basson.[60])

tions during orgasm. Such contractions are also present in younger women, albeit usually not painful. Women and their partners need to be aware of these potential changes and educated on various therapeutic approaches (Table 16.2).[22]

CHRONIC ILLNESS, DISABILITY, AND MEDICATIONS

Pain during intercourse afflicts nearly one-third of older women; however, these women are frequently uninformed about possible causes and treatments for their discomfort.[23,24] Other women experience a decline in sexual desire with older age due to diminishing hormone levels as well as disability, chronic illness, or medications, but these etiologies are not always conveyed to them.[25] It is essential that clinicians inform patients of possible sexual changes that can occur over the course of an illness or medical treatment. The remainder of this section explores some common ailments that act as limiting factors of healthy sexual function in older women.

Table 16.2 Age-related changes in sexual response and therapeutic options

Age-related changes
Decreased general muscle tension
Diminished breast size increase and sensation with stimulation
Reduction in vaginal blood flow and genital engorgement
Delayed, diminished or absent vaginal lubrication
Decreased vaginal expansion in width and length
Delayed clitoral reaction time
Fewer orgasms accompanied by diminished vaginal/uterine contractions
Occasional painful contractions with orgasm

Therapeutic options
Hormonal supplements
Genital stimulation devices
Vaginal lubricants
Vary sexual positions
Maximize time for foreplay using non-genital and genital touch
Explore or re-explore self-stimulation
Acknowledge and treat partner's sexual problems
Talk openly with partner about changes in stimulation and response

Arthritis

Approximately 48% of older adults suffer from arthritis.[26] Women are twice as likely to suffer from osteoporosis and arthritis after the age of 70.[27,28] Rheumatoid disorders greatly affect mobility and can significantly limit the variety of sexual positions and masturbation habits of the older female patient. Additionally, certain medications prescribed to reduce the inflammation and pains associated with these disabilities diminish sexual desire.[12] The use of vibrators with and without a partner act as an alternative to intercourse and an effective way to explore one's sexuality. Warm baths may also be incorporated into foreplay to reduce muscle tension and foster intimacy.

Cardiovascular disease

Depending on the severity of the condition, cardiovascular conditions may result in only a temporary delay of sexual activity or long-term absence. Women with heart disease should be stratified into low, intermediate, or high-risk categories based on risk factors for the occurrence of cardiovascular events with sexual activity.[29] Patients in the low-risk category are identified with (1) controlled hypertension; (2) mild, stable angina; (3) successful coronary revascularization; (4) a history of uncomplicated myocardial infarction (MI); (5) mild valvular disease; and (6) no symptoms and <3 cardiovascular risk factors. In low-risk patients, no further work-up is required for the continuation of sexual activity. Intermediate-risk category patients include those with (1) moderate angina; (2) a recent MI (<6 weeks); (3) left ventricular dysfunction and/or class II congestive heart failure; (4) non-sustained low-risk arrhythmias; and (5) ≥3 risk factors for coronary artery disease. Lastly, patients in the high-risk category include those with (1) unstable or refractory angina; (2) uncontrolled hypertension; (3) congestive heart failure (class III or IV); (4) very recent MI (<2 weeks); (5) high-risk arrhythmias; (6) obstructive cardiomyopathies; and (7) moderate-to-severe valvular disease. A consultation with a cardiologist should be obtained for women at intermediate or high risk. Stress testing and/or cardiovascular rehabilitation may be necessary to lower the risk of participating in sexual activity in women at indeterminate or high risk.[29] Individuals with heart disease can be apprehensive about returning to sexual activity and frequently have not had the issue addressed to them by their healthcare practitioner.[30,31] If an individual with heart disease is able to climb two sets of stairs without difficulty, it is a good indication that they can tolerate the cardiovascular demands of sexual activity.[32]

Respiratory disease

Chronic obstructive pulmonary disease or asthma can be debilitating, often leading to muscle weakness, dyspnea, and poor stamina. Older individuals afflicted with respiratory illness usually find themselves too fatigued and short of breath to engage in sexual activity. It is important to periodically reassess the person's respiratory illness and address the issue of intimacy. Maximizing the opportunities for improvement through appropriate medications and/or respiratory rehabilitation can help a person maintain their level of sexual activity.[33,34]

Cancer

Surgery, radiotherapy, and chemotherapy used to treat various cancers can alter women's body image and general physical status. These changes can ultimately affect her sexual health and the level of intimacy she enjoys with her partner. Individuals with a life-threatening diagnosis often experience various psychosocial responses, including anxiety, grief, and depression. Significant challenges in communication with patients induced by the diagnosis of cancer, treatment options, and the fear of recurrence need to be overcome.[35,36] In general, when caring for older individuals, it is imperative to address factors that affect their 'quality of life' before, during, and after they are diagnosed and treated for a significant illness and, in particular, cancer.

Urinary incontinence

Urinary incontinence (UI), most specifically stress urinary incontinence (SUI), is also a common problem in older age, affecting up to half of elderly women; yet, many patients do not volunteer their symptoms to their gynecologists or primary physicians (see Chapter 7).[37,38] Concerns about urine leakage during sex and/or orgasm can result in decreased desire as well as difficulty with sexual response.

Medication

One or more new prescriptions are written in over two-thirds of healthcare office visits in the US.[39] Whereas many prescription medications have been implicated in causing sexual dysfunction, non-prescription medications, homeopathic remedies, illicit drugs, and other substances (e.g. alcohol and tobacco) also have the potential to adversely affect sexual function. The classes of prescription medications most commonly cited to cause sexual dysfunction include the antihypertensives, antidepressants, and antipsychotics.[40] It is important, however, that the healthcare practitioner rules out other possible causes of sexual dysfunction before suggesting a pharmacological etiology. If the prescription or non-prescription medication is thought to cause adverse sexual function, the physician should offer the patient an alternative treatment plan (if the patient desires and treatment is available). Open communication regarding medication side effects and

compliance is vital for every patient's health and safety.

Numerous acute and chronic illnesses can leave the older woman fatigued and reluctant to engage in sexual activity. Alternative forms of intimate physical contact should be encouraged, including hugging, kissing, gentle massage, use of a vibrator, self/mutual masturbation, and intimate verbal communication. A change in sexual positions such as semi-reclining and seated positions may help reduce discomfort and minimize exertion. However, changes in a woman's ability to 'perform sexually' compared to what she did years ago can promote increased anxiety and fear in some individuals. Normalizing the symptoms and sexual side effects of acute and chronic illness as well as educating patients about their options is vital.

PSYCHOLOGICAL CONCERNS

Depression is, unfortunately, a prevalent illness among older women. As many as 10.1% of older women experience a major depressive episode as they age, and nearly 20% of elderly adults report clinical depressive symptoms over the age of 60 (see Chapter 6).[41,42] The deleterious effects of depression on sexual desire and activity have been studied extensively.[43] The litany of sexual side effects caused by antidepressants has also been well-documented.[44,45] It is important to note that many older women manifest their depressive symptoms somatically, as opposed to complaining about feelings of sadness or unhappiness. Thus, a thorough exploration of symptoms is necessary for a proper diagnosis and treatment. Individual therapy is often crucial to the management of depression. Furthermore, couples therapy is also encouraged in order to reduce attributions of blame or guilt and to promote realistic expectations for treatment on the part of the partner.[12]

Older women are often poorly informed of the natural stressors of aging that affect sexual performance and libido, leading them to feel frightened or embarrassed or needing to withdraw from sexual activity. Alone or in combination, changes in a woman's physiology, fear of death and dying, caring for an ill partner, lack of companionship or widowhood, and stress over financial security and retirement contribute to low desire. These concerns are often misinterpreted as evidence that elderly women do not have sexual needs, thereby perpetuating common stereotypes and lack of research in the field.

Changes in a woman's physiology in older age frequently precipitate poor body image. Facial (e.g. wrinkles, age spots), genital (e.g. decreased vaginal lubrication, lessened clitoral sensation), corporal (e.g. poor posture, different fat distribution), and sensory (e.g. hearing, sight, or tooth loss) changes are common sources of anxiety that affect her sexuality. As self-esteem plays a major role in sexual function, normalizing these changes can go a long way toward reversing what may be perceived as a hopeless situation. If the patient is truly struggling with body image or self-esteem issues, it is important to make the appropriate therapy referrals to help her shift her notions of beauty with an eye to increasing her self-esteem.

A large proportion of women (45%) aged 65 or older are widows.[46] Contrary to cultural beliefs, the sexual identities of these women do not die with the death of their spouse. Certainly, sufficient time and energy must be set aside to grieve, but a woman can continue to enjoy a satisfying sexual life after widowhood and into her later years. Unfortunately, many widows experience significant guilt when entering a new relationship, often feeling as if they are cheating on their previous partner. Masturbation, too, also may raise feelings of emptiness and betrayal.[47] Counseling patients about the importance of open communication with a new partner can help to foster greater trust and comfort. It is also helpful to advise older women on alternatives to intercourse, such as erotic kissing and touching, which are often experienced as less frightening and more intimacy enhancing in this population.[48]

Caring for an ill spouse presents an immense emotional burden. Since men die, on average, earlier than women, elderly females are often self- or family-designated as caregivers for their partners (see Chapter 1). Older women who must redefine their role from spouse to caregiver often experience great physical, emotional, and occasional financial distress. Elderly caregivers have a greater risk of mortality due to the impact of these strains.[49] These women experience an array of responses to their new responsibilities, all of which are likely to affect their sexuality: anger and grief over the change in intimacy and spousal roles; guilt over continued sexual desire; and aversion to engaging in sexual contact with their spouse because they feel more like a parent than a lover.[50]

SEXUAL HEALTH ASSESSMENT

Taking a sexual history is an integral part of the overall patient history that should be obtained from women of all ages. Healthcare practitioners should routinely and proactively address sexual health with their patients, as patients prefer that their practitioners initiate these discussions.[51,52] Good communication skills and a sensitive, nonjudgmental approach are essential. A simple question such as, 'Are you sexually active?' suffices to begin. Practitioners should address the needs of both the patient and her partner, being careful to avoid any perception of inappropriateness. Separate time needs to be allotted for both discussions. Practitioners should not assume that their patient is heterosexual. Older lesbian patients may be reluctant to disclose their orientation. Use of gender neutral terms, such as 'partner', may encourage more open communication (Table 16.3).

Offering to undertake a gynecological examination may be helpful. However, it is important to explain why it is being undertaken and what is going to happen. Also, the woman must be told of normality or otherwise as the examination progresses. She must also be reassured that the examination can stop should she find it painful or distressing or wants you to stop.

Until recently, training of health practitioners for assessment of a patient's sexual history and potential problems was relatively limited or absent in many medical and nursing schools. The following represent general recommendations or guidelines that can be followed on behalf of the practitioner in order to ensure a sensitive and comprehensive evaluation. The International Consensus Development Conference on Female Sexual Dysfunction has produced a classification system that divides problems into various categories:[53]

- decreased or absent sexual desire (loss of libido)
- arousal disorders
- lack or loss of orgasm
- painful intercourse
- other, such as gender confusion and paraphilia

Specific questions can also assist in determining if the patient is experiencing signs and symptoms of sexual dysfunction (Table 16.4).

Table 16.3 Tips for taking a sexual history

Initiate and explain the need for discussion
Allow the patient to feel in control
Avoid perception of inappropriateness
Don't be judgmental
Don't assume the patient is heterosexual
Be aware of patient's cultural and religious background
Ensure confidentiality

Table 16.4 Assessing sexual history and problems

Health provider recommendations/guidelines:
- Awareness that sexual assessment takes longer than other gynecological assessments
- Acknowledgment to the patient that sexual matters are private and confidential but that they are important to discuss and can be distressing for some
- Explain to the patient that interviewing partners alone is important because of their different backgrounds and experiences, but it is also helpful to interview them together
- Obtain identifying data:
    - How long the partners have been a couple
    - Occupations; additional household members
    - Medical and psychiatric conditions
    - Medications
    - Concurrent life stressors
    - Personal belief systems

Key questions for assessment of sexual problems (individual and couple):
- What are the sexual problem(s) in their own words? The physician may clarify the details with direct questions, giving options rather than leading questions
- What is the duration of the problem(s)? Are the problem(s) lifelong or acquired; situational or global? Which problem is a priority?
- Determine the context of the sexual problem(s): What are the sexual stimuli? When are sexual attempts made during the day/week? What frequency of sex is expected/attempted? Are their concerns about performance or safety?
- Determine past sexual experiences and their positive and negative aspects

SEXUALLY TRANSMITTED DISEASES

Traditionally, elderly women are not perceived to be at risk of sexually transmitted infections (STIs). As increasing numbers of relationships break down and partners change, such women are at potential risk of acquiring STIs (see Chapter 1). Also, as elderly women no longer need contraception, the use of barrier methods is infrequent, which further increases their risk. In the US, data from the Centers for Disease Control and Prevention (CDC) show a consistently increasing number of older adults who are being infected with STIs, particularly HIV/AIDS. The cumulative number of cases of HIV/AIDS thus reported to the CDC in adults aged ≥50 years old quintupled from 16 288 in 1990 to 90 513 by the end of December 2001.[54] Studies in Washington state (in the US) and in Singapore found an increase of syphilis, gonorrhea, and genital herpes in older persons.[55,56]

Elderly women present with a variety of symptoms that may be attributed to estrogen deficiency or an STI. Often a delay in symptom recognition and healthcare presentation occurs. Thus, older adults are more likely to present with advanced HIV disease, including AIDS, compared with their younger counterparts (36% vs 5%).[57] In older adults, suspicion of HIV is often lacking among patients and doctors, and the pre-AIDS phase is shorter and less symptomatic.[58] Clinical deterioration is more rapid among elderly people infected with HIV than among younger adults. The effect of old age on HIV disease progression is still unclear, but it may be related to the decreased immune function that accompanies advancing age.

CONCLUSION

The most important role for a clinician treating elderly female patients is to create an environment that allows her to explore her sexual feelings and concerns. In order to facilitate an effective dialogue, a practitioner should allocate sufficient time for the patient to discuss her complaints, provide a setting that ensures privacy, exhibit a receptive attitude, use common everyday language, avoid medical jargon, and listen actively to the patient. Beyond any medical treatment, important clinical goals in the treatment of sexual dysfunction among older women include: the encouragement of continued self-exploration through masturbation; promotion of alternative sexual activities; troubleshooting sexual difficulties with practical suggestions (like vibrators and lubricants); and support of open communication with partners to establish trust and comfort with changing sexuality.

It is worth remembering that some women report experiencing greater intimacy with their partners in older age. They attribute this to greater comfort with their bodies, absence of children, and heightened familiarity with their partners.[47] Other women report feeling less lonely in older age than in their younger years.[59] With our continued advancement in the understanding of the physiological and psychological aspects of aging and sexuality, healthcare practitioners have the unique opportunity to help their patients not only add years to their life but also life to those years.

REFERENCES

1. Office for National Statistics (ONS), General Register Office for Scotland and Northern Ireland Statistics and Research Agency. August 25, 2005. Available at www.statistics.gov.uk
2. Masters WH, Johnson VE. Human Sexual Response. Boston: Little, Brown; 1966.
3. Cupach WR, Comstock J. Satisfaction with sexual communication in marriage: links to sexual

satisfaction and dyadic adjustment. J Soc Pers Rel 1990; 7: 179–86.

4. Greeley AM. Faithful Attraction: Discovering Intimacy, Love, and Fidelity in American Marriage. New York: Doherty; 1991.

5. Kurdek LA, Schmitt JP. Relationship quality of partners in heterosexual married, heterosexual cohabitating, and gay and lesbian relationships. J Personality Soc Psychol 1986; 51: 711–20.

6. Haavio-Mannila E, Kontula O. Correlates of increased sexual satisfaction. Arch Sex Behav 1997; 26: 399–419.

7. Lawrance K, Byers ES. Sexual satisfaction in long-term heterosexual relationships: the inter-personal exchange model of sexual satisfaction. Pers Rel 1995; 2: 267–85.

8. Berman LA, Wai S, Demas D, McLean KG, Kolzet J. A survey of vibrator use: prevalence, perceptions and relationship to sexual function and quality of life measures. Draft version under peer review. February 12, 2006.

9. Bretschneider JG, McCoy NL. Sexual interest and behaviour in healthy 80 to 102 year olds. Arch Sex Behav 1998; 17: 109–29.

10. Matthais RE, Lubben JE, Atchison KA, Schweitzer SO. Sexual activity and satisfac-tion among very old adults: results from a community-dwelling Medicare population survey. Gerontologist 1997; 35: 331–3.

11. Janus SS, Janus CL. The Janus Report on Sexual Behavior. New York: John Wiley and Sons; 1993.

12. Hillman J. Clinical Perspectives on Elderly Sexuality. New York: Plenum; 2000.

13. Brogan M. The sexual needs of elderly people: addressing the issue. Nurs Stand 1996; 10: 42–5.

14. Kessel B. Sexuality in the older person. Age Ageing 2001; 30: 121–4.

15. Griffiths E. No sex, please, we're over 60. Nurs Times 1988; 84(1): 34–5.

16. Ehrenfeld M, Tabak M, Bronner G, Bergman R. Ethical dilemmas concerning sexuality of elderly patients suffering from dementia. Int J Nurs Pract 1997; 3: 255–9.

17. Booth B. Does it really matter at that age? Nurs Times 1990; 86: 50–2.

18. Lazarus LW. A program for the elderly at a private psychiatric hospital. Gerontologist 1976; 16(2): 125–31.

19. Hellerstein DJ, Pinsker H, Rosenthal RN, Klee S. Supportive therapy as the treatment model of choice. J Psychother Prac Res 1994; 3(4): 300–6.

20. Castelo-Branco C, Cancelo MJ, Villero J, Nohales F, Julia MD. Management of post-menopausal vaginal atrophy and atrophic vaginitis. Maturitas 2005; 52 (Suppl 1): S46–52.

21. Rees M, Purdie DW. Management of the Menopause: The Handbook, 4th edn. London: Royal Society of Medicine Press; 2006.

22. Walsh KE, Berman JR. Sexual dysfunction in the older woman: an overview of the current understanding and management. Drugs Aging 2004; 21(10): 655–75.

23. Bachmann GA. Influence of menopause on sexuality. Int J Fertil Menopausal Stud 1995; 40: 16–22.

24. Jones J. Embodied meaning: menopause and the change of life. Soc Work Health Care 1994; 19: 43–65.

25. Walker BL, Osgood NJ, Richardson JP, Ephross PH. Staff and elderly knowledge and attitudes toward elderly sexuality. Educational Gerontology 1998; 24: 471–89.

26. Dorgan CA (ed.). Statistical Record of Health and Medicine. New York: Gage Research Inc.; 1995.

27. Sangha O. Epidemiology of rheumatic diseases. Rheumatology 2000; 39(Suppl): 3–12.

28. Wardlaw GM. Putting body weight and osteo-porosis into perspective. Am J Clin Nutr 1996; 63(Suppl): 433–6.

29. DeBusk R, Drory Y, Goldstein I, et al. Management of sexual dysfunction in patients with cardiovascular disease: recommendations of The Princeton Consensus Panel. Am J Cardiol 2000; 86: 175–81.

30. Addis IB, Ireland CC, Vittinghoff E, et al. Sexual activity and function in postmenopausal women with heart disease. Obstet Gynecol 2005; 106(1): 121–7.

31. Thorson AI. Sexual activity and the cardiac patient. Am J Geriatr Cardiol 2003; 12(1): 38–40.

32. Taylor HA Jr. Sexual activity and the cardio-vascular patient: guidelines. Am J Cardiol 1999; 84(5B): 6–10N.

33. Stockdale-Woolley RS. Respiratory disturbances and sexuality. In: Fogel CI, Lauver D, eds. Sexual Health Promotion. Philadelphia: WB Saunders; 1990: 372–83.

34. Walbroehl GS. Sexual concerns of the patient with pulmonary disease. Postgrad Med 1992; 91(5): 455–60.

35. Baker F, Denniston M, Smith T, West MM. Adult cancer survivors: how are they faring? Cancer 2005; 104(11 Suppl): 2565–76.

36. Hendren SK, O'Connor BI, Liu M, et al. Prevalence of male and female sexual dysfunction is high following surgery for rectal cancer. Ann Surg 2005; 242(2): 212–23.

37. Hägglund D, Walker-Engström ML, Larsson G, Leppert J. Reasons why women with long-term urinary incontinence do not seek professional help: a cross-sectional population-based cohort study. Int Urogynecol J Pelvic Floor Dysfunct 2003; 14(5): 296–304.

38. Landi F, Cesari M, Russo A. Potentially reversible risk factors and urinary incontinence in frail older people living in community. Age Ageing 2003; 32(2): 194–9.

39. Copeland C. Prescription drugs: issues of cost, coverage, and quality. EBRI Issue Brief 1999; (208): 1–21.

40. Finger WW, Lund M, Slagle MA. Medications that may contribute to sexual disorders. A guide to assessment and treatment in family practice. J Fam Pract 1997; 44(1): 33–43.

41. Roberts RE, Kaplan GA, Shema SJ. Prevalence and correlates of depression in an aging cohort: the Alameda County Study. J Gerontol B Psychol Sci Soc Sci 1997; S2: S252–8.

42. Ables N, Cooley S, Deitch IM, et al. What practitioners should know about working with older adults. Prof Psychol Res Pract 1998; 29: 413–27.

43. West SL, Vinikoor LC, Zolnoun D. A systematic review of the literature on female sexual dysfunction prevalence and predictors. Annu Rev Sex Res 2004; 15: 40–172.

44. Meston CM. A randomized, placebo-controlled, crossover study of ephedrine for SSRI-induced female sexual dysfunction. J Sex Marital Ther 2004; 30(2): 57–68.

45. Montejo AL, Llorca G, Izquierdo JA, Rico-Villademoros F. Incidence or sexual dysfunction associated with antidepressant agents: a prospective multicenter study of 1022 outpatients. J Clin Psychiatry 2001; 62(3): 10–21.

46. Administration on Aging. A profile of older Americans. Washington, DC: U.S. Department of Health and Human Services; 2000.

47. Foley S, Kope SA, Sugrue DP. Sex Matters for Women. New York: The Guilford Press; 2002.

48. Berman J, Berman L. For Women Only: A Revolutionary Guide to Reclaiming Your Sex Life. New York: Henry Holt & Co; 2001.

49. Christakis NA, Allison PD. Mortality after the hospitalization of a spouse. N Engl J Med 2006; 354: 719–30.

50. Duffy LM. Sexual behaviour and marital intimacy in Alzheimer's couples: a family theory perspective. Sexuality and Disability 1995; 13: 239–54.

51. Sarrel PM. Sexual dysfunction: treat or refer. Obstet Gynecol 2005; 106(4): 834–9.

52. Read S, King M, Watson J. Sexual dysfunction in primary medical care: prevalence, characteristics and detection by the general practitioner. J Public Health Med 1997; 19(4): 387–91.

53. Basson R, Berman J, Burnett A, et al. Report of the international consensus development conference on female sexual dysfunction: definitions and classifications. J Urol 2000; 163: 888–93.

54. Centers for Disease Control and Prevention. AIDS public use data set through year-end 2000. Atlanta, GA: Centers for Disease Control and Prevention; 2000. Database available at: http://www.cdc.gov/.

55. Xu F, Schillinger JA, Aubin MR, St Louis ME, Markowitz LE. Sexually transmitted diseases of older persons in Washington State. Sex Transm Dis 2001; 28(5): 287–91.

56. Tan HH, Chan RK, Goh CL. Sexually transmitted diseases in the older population in Singapore. Ann Acad Med Singapore 2002; 31(4): 493–6.

57. Gott CM, Rogstad KE, Riley V, Ahmed-Jushuf I. Delay in symptom presentation among a sample of older GUM clinic attendees. Int J STD AIDS 1999; 10: 43–6.

58. Mahar F, Sherrard J. Sexually transmitted infections. In: Tomlinson JM, Rees M, Mander A, eds. Sexual Health and the Menopause. London: RSM Press; 2005: 55–62.

59. Friedan B. The Fountain of Age. New York: Simon & Schuster; 1994.

60. Basson R. Rethinking low sexual desire in women. Br J Obstet Gynaecol 2002; 109: 357–63.

Index